Manipal Manual of
MEDICINE for
DENTAL STUDENTS

Other CBS book by the same Author

Manipal Manual of Clinical Medicine

ISBN 81-239-1120-3   Yr 2005   pp. 400 PB

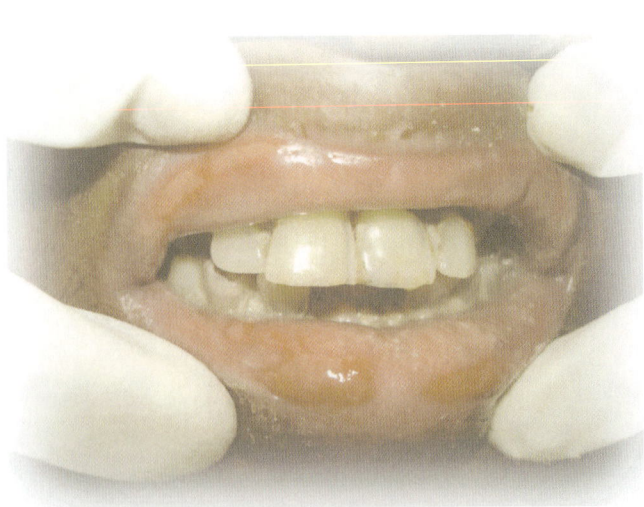

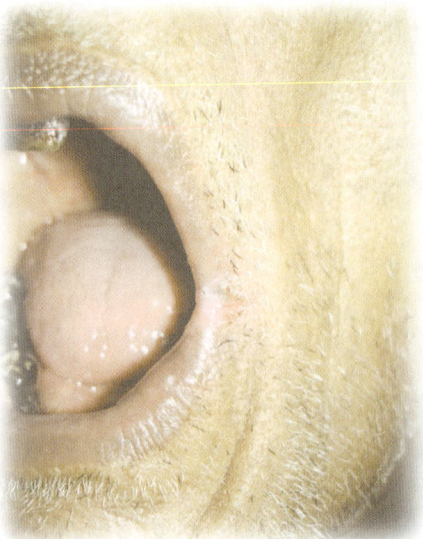

Manipal Manual of
MEDICINE for
DENTAL STUDENTS

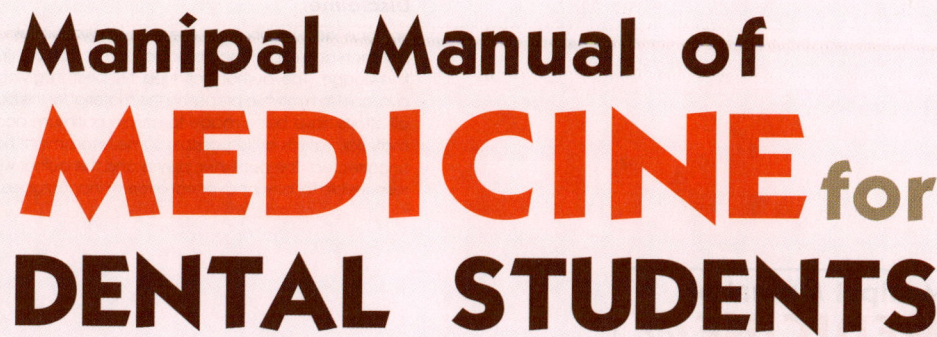

B. A. SHASTRY

Professor of Medicine and Consultant Physician
Kasturba Medical College and Hospital
(A unit of Manipal University)
Manipal 576 104
Karnataka
India

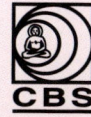

CBS

CBS Publishers & Distributors Pvt Ltd

New Delhi • Bengaluru • Chennai • Kochi • Mumbai • Pune
Hyderabad • Kolkata • Nagpur • Patna • Vijayawada

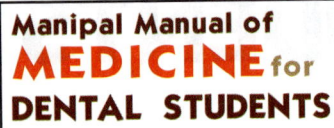

First Edition: 2009

Reprint: 2015

Copyright © Author and Publisher

ISBN: 978-81-239-1742-9

Published by Satish Kumar Jain and produced by Varun Jain for

CBS Publishers & Distributors Pvt Ltd

4819/XI Prahlad Street, 24 Ansari Road, Daryaganj, New Delhi 110 002, India.

Ph: 23289259, 23266861, 23266867   Website: www.cbspd.com

Fax: 011-23243014   e-mail: delhi@cbspd.com; cbspubs@airtelmail.in.

Corporate Office: 204 FIE, Industrial Area, Patparganj, Delhi 110 092

Ph: 4934 4934   Fax: 4934 4935   e-mail: publishing@cbspd.com; publicity@cbspd.com

Branches

- **Bengaluru:** Seema House 2975, 17th Cross, K.R. Road, Banasankari 2nd Stage, Bengaluru 560 070, Karnataka
  Ph: +91-80-26771678/79   Fax: +91-80-26771680   e-mail: bangalore@cbspd.com
- **Chennai:** 7, Subbaraya Street, Shenoy Nagar, Chennai 600 030, Tamil Nadu
  Ph: +91-44-42032115   Fax: +91-44-42032115   e-mail: chennai@cbspd.com
- **Kochi:** 36/14 Kalluvilakam, Lissie Hospital Road, Kochi 682 018, Kerala
  Ph: +91-484-4059061-65   Fax: +91-484-4059065   e-mail: kochi@cbspd.com
- **Mumbai:** 83-C, Dr E Moses Road, Worli, Mumbai-400018, Maharashtra
  Ph: +91-22-24902340/41   Fax: +91-22-24902342   e-mail: mumbai@cbspd.com
- **Pune:** Bhuruk Prestige, Sr. No. 52/12/2+1+3/2 Narhe, Haveli (Near Katraj-Dehu Road Bypass), Pune 411 041, Maharashtra
  Ph: +91-20-64704058/59, 32392277   Fax: +91-20-24300160   e-mail: pune@cbspd.com

Representatives

- **Hyderabad**   0-9885175004
- **Nagpur**   0-9021734563
- **Vijayawada**   0-9000660880
- **Kolkata**   0-9831437309, 0-9051152362
- **Patna**   0-9334159340

Printed at: Paras Offset Pvt. Ltd., C-176, Naraina Industrial Area Phase-I, New Delhi

Foreword

The arrival of Manipal Manual of Medicine for Dental Students marks the culmination of a long-felt need for such a treatise by an Indian author. The author Dr. B. A. Shastry is already popular nationwide through his another masterpiece entitled Manipal Manual of Clinical Medicine for medical students. The neat format of presentation with easy running style and extravagant illustrations make this book a pleasure to read and is bound to capture the imagination of the targeted dental students. That this book encompasses all the essentials of medicine that a dental student needs to know all in just 330 pages, speaks volumes about the author who is a dedicated educationist and an experienced teacher, and it is only natural that all these years of teaching have snowballed into a book of precious pearls. CBS Publishers & Distributors have further added value by the elegant shaping of this all important book — deemed to be a proud possession of every dental student in our country.

Dr. R. Balasubramanian

Professor and Head
Department of Medicine
Kasturba Medical College and Hospital, Manipal

to

my beloved parents
Late Barkur Neelakanta Shastry
and
Indiramma

Preface

Teaching a large number of undergraduate dental students made me realise the need for a book in medicine which is simple and precise for dental students and practitioners. Keeping in view of the vastness of medicine, chapters in the book have been written which are relevant to dentistry. Standard textbooks of medicine and dentistry have been used as reference while preparing the material of this book.

I take this opportunity to express my gratitude to Dr. Kavitha Saravu, Associate Professor, Department of Medicine, and Dr. Keerthilatha Pai, Professor of Oral Medicine, College of Dental Surgery, Manipal, for their help and suggestions.

I would like to thank Mr. Umesh Acharya, Artist, Dental College, for his diagrams and photographs while preparing this book. I am grateful to Mr. Wilfred Lobo of Chetana Printers, Mangalore, for the computer work in preparing this book.

I sincerely thank Mr. S. K. Jain, Managing Director, and Late B. R. Sharma of CBS Publishers & Distributors, New Delhi, for the encouragement and support given to me in preparing the book.

I thank Dr. R. Balasubramanian for his encouragement in the preparation of this book and for having written the Foreword.

I welcome any criticism and suggestions by the students to improve the quality of this book.

B. A. Shastry

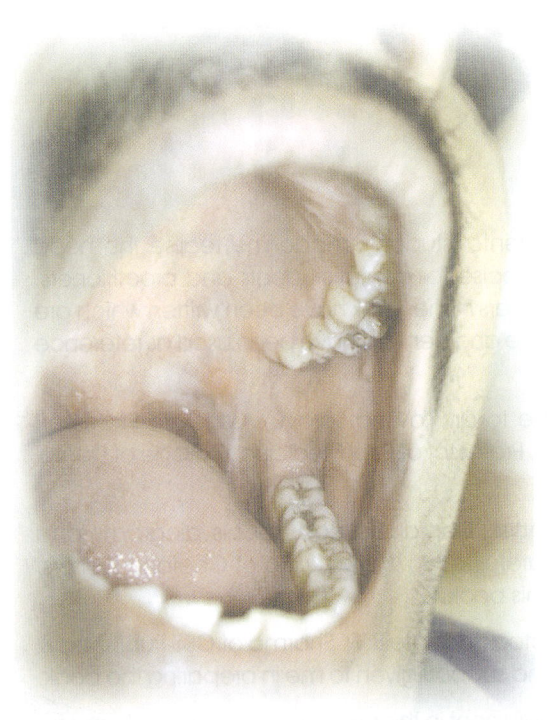
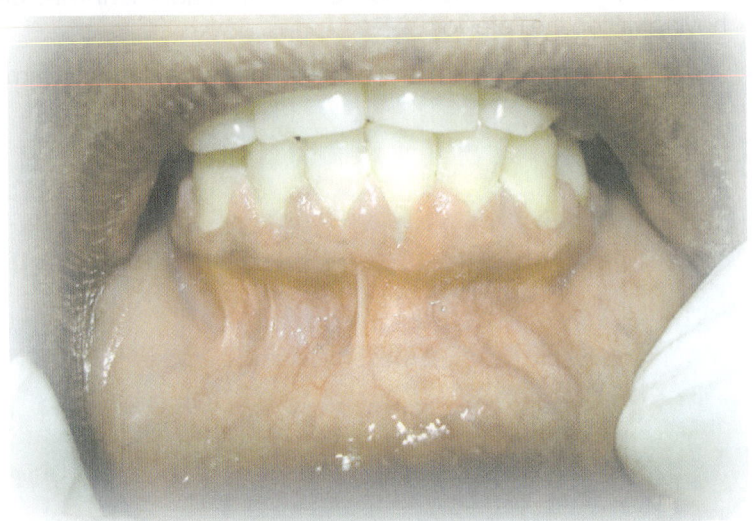

Contents

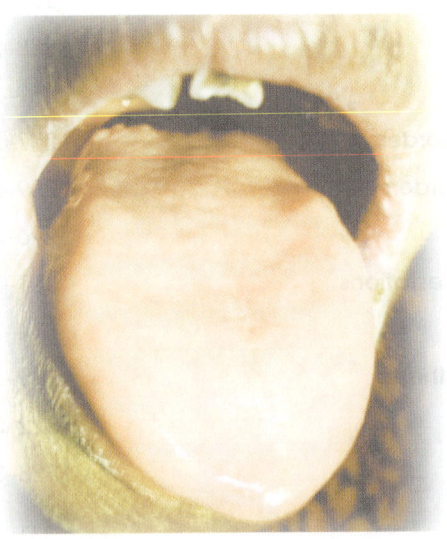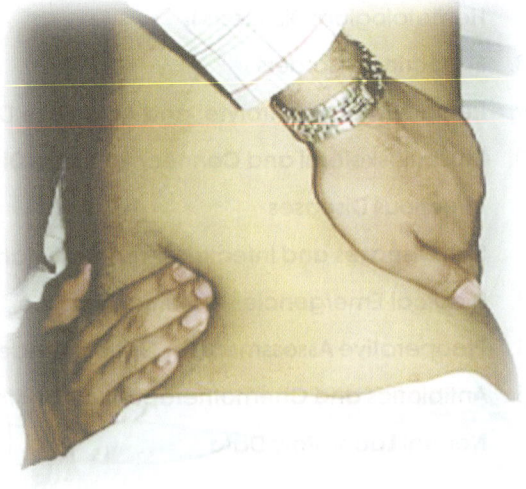

1 Introduction

Persons giving dental care are not only concerned with the treatment of disorders of teeth but also with the patient as a whole for proper patient management. Dental surgeons should be aware of the medical disorders which may interfere with the dental treatment or dental diseases themselves can result in medical illnesses. Detailed knowledge of the drugs prescribed, their interactions, dosage, side effects and contraindications for the use of drugs used in dentistry is of importance while administering dental care.

Approach to a Patient with Medical Disorder

A humanitarian approach is needed while treating a patient of medical disorder and total knowledge of the patient, his illness, mutual understanding and communication between the patient and physician are important for successful patient management.

In the new atmosphere of the hospital, doctor should instill confidence to the patient and make him aware of the laboratory tests and cooperation with the treatment.

History and Physical Examination

A detailed history including patient's presenting symptoms, past illness, previous treatment taken, etc. should be obtained from the patient in his own words in a chronological disorder.

Thorough physical examination and keen observation of the physical findings may reveal the underlying illness. At the end of history elicitation and clinical examination, physician should be able to come to a conclusion regarding the possible diagnosis or differential diagnosis of the underlying illness and plan for further investigation and management. Relevant lab tests, their application and interpretation helps in the diagnosis of the medical disorder. Physician should be aware of the importance of lab tests and should be complementary to the history and clinical examination.

Proper practical guidelines, decision making and assessment of treatment outcome are to be considered while administering medical care. Application of recent advances, practice of evidence based medicine and delivering cost effective medical care are of primary significance in the practice of modern medicine.

Principles of Good Medical Practice

Maintain good doctor-patient relationship with:
- Politeness and honesty
- Respecting the privacy of the patient and confidentiality
- Treating and taking care of each patient as an individual
- Respecting patient's knowledge regarding their illness.

Important Guidelines for Administration of Proper Medical Care
- Taking an informed consent prior to examination and before each procedure.
- Explaining honestly if the things go wrong
- Consideration to patient's carers and partners
- Maintaining proper medical records
- Respecting the colleagues regarding their work, skills and contributions.

1

History Taking
- Informant
- Name of the patient
  - Age
  - Sex
  - Place and address
  - Educational standard
  - Symptoms of present illness in chronological order
- History of present illness
- Past history
- Personal history
- Family history
- Menstrual history and history of previous pregnancies (in a female patient)
- Occupational history
- Treatment history

Examination of the Patient
- General physical examination
- Systemic examination
- Diagnosis/differential diagnosis
- Relevant investigations and treatment
- Name and address of the treating doctor

Name of the patient: Important in identification of the patient.

Age
- Certain diseases are common in particular age group.
- Hereditary/congenital disorders are common in younger age groups.

- Degenerative disorders are common in elderly individuals.

Sex

Coagulation disorders like haemophilia occurs predominantly in males and collagen vascular diseases are common in females.

Place and Address
- Helps in communication with the patient.
- Endemic areas of certain diseases can be identified.

History of Presenting Illness

Detail analysis of presenting symptoms including important negative symptoms.

Past History

Details of previous illness including details of previous treatment received.

Personal History

Personal history includes following details
- Loss of weight/gain in weight
- Appetite loss/appetite increased
- Habits : Details of smoking:
  - Number of cigarettes/beedies and duration of smoking
  - Alcohol intake, amount and duration
  - Pan chewing including tobacco
  - Habits of drug addiction including history of needle sharing
  - Exposure to sexually transmitted diseases

Treatment History

Details of previous treatment helps in identifying the previous diagnosis and planning future treatment.

General Physical Examination

General physical examination includes examination of the patient from head to the toes for the external markers of the disease.

Check list for General Physical Examination

1. Skeletal height
   * Pallor
2. Nourishment (nutritional status)
   * Icterus
   * Cyanosis
   * Clubbing
   * Lymphadenopathy
   * Oedema
3. Vital signs
4. Examination of head, neck and face
5. Examination of hands and feet
6. Examination of genitalia
7. Examination of breasts
8. Examination of skin and hair

SKELETAL HEIGHT

Measurement of Skeletal Height

* Skeletal height is measured from vertex to the sole of the foot.
* Person is standing straight against the wall to which a vertical scale is attached.
* Height is measured from the top of the head (vertex) to the foot.

* *Upper segment:* Measured from the vertex to the upper border of the symphysis pubis (or total height - lower segment).
* *Lower segment:* Measured from the top of the symphysis pubis vertically to the sole of the foot (floor).
* *Arm span:* Stretch the upper limbs horizontally outwards and measure the distance between the tips of the middle fingers of the two out stretched hands.
* *Normal height:* Usually two times the length of pubis to sole of the foot and also equals the arm span.

Note: Measure the skeletal height while:
– The person is standing erect
– Wearing only inner clothes
– Not wearing any foot wear

ABNORMALITIES OF HEIGHT

Increase in the Height

* *Tall stature:* Height more than 97th percentile of the normal population.
* *Causes:* Anterior pituitary hypersecretion before puberty (Gigantism - height > 6 ft 8").
  – Constitutional
  – Marfan's syndrome
  – Homocystinuria
  – Kleinfelter's syndrome
  – Tall thin built with long limbs: Eunuchoidism, Marfan's syndrome.

Clinical Signs Associated with Marfan's Syndrome

1. *Metacarpal index:* Calculate the ratio of total axial length of the 2nd, 3rd, 4th and 5th metacarpals. Total width of the above metacarpals at their mid point. If the ratio is > 8.4, it is suggestive of Marfan's syndrome.
2. *Thumb sign:* Projecting out of thumb beyond the ulnar border when it is completely opposed inside the clenched hand.
3. *Wrist sign:* Overlapping of the distal phalanges of the 1st and 5th digits of one hand when they are wrapped around the opposite wrist.

Decrease in the Height

- *Dwarfism (short stature):* Standing height is below the 3rd percentile for children of similar age and ethnic group (more than 3.5 SD below the mean height).

Causes

1. Endocrine disorders
   - Hypopituitarism
   - Primary hypothyroidism
   - Cushing syndrome
   - Pseudohypoparathyroidism
2. Systemic illness
   - Malabsorption syndrome
   - Chronic systemic disorder (e.g. cardiac/ respiratory)
   - Malnutrition
3. Chromosome abnormalities (e.g. Turner's syndrome)
4. Other causes
   - Intrauterine growth retardation
   - Constitutional dwarfism

Causes of arm span more than the height

1. Marfan's syndrome
2. Homocystinuria
3. Klinefelter's syndrome

Heel Pad Thickness

Calculate the distance at the lower most point (of the X-ray shadows) between the calcaneum and heel pad soft tissue.

Abnormal heel pad thickness for male is > 21 mm and for females is >18 mm.

Causes of increased heel pad thickness

1. Acromegaly
2. Conditions associated with obesity
3. Conditions associated with edema.

NUTRITIONAL STATUS

Assessment of Nutritional Status

Nutritional status is assessed by
- Muscle bulk
- Subcutaneous fat
- Deficiency signs

Note: Presence of edema should be considered while assessing nutrition.

Nutritional Assessment

Measure the muscle bulk and subcutaneous fat while assessing nutrition.

Subcutaneous Fat

Measure the triceps skin fold thickness of the left mid arm. Measurement is ideally done by a calipers (Lange's or Herpenden's).

Average adult measurement of triceps skin fold thickness in males 12.5 mm and in females 16 mm.

Muscle Bulk

Measure the left mid arm circumference. Average measurements in males 25.5 cm and in females 23 cm.

Malnutrition is said to be present when ideal body weight is less than 85%.

Fat Distribution and its Abnormalities

- Localised deposit of fat results in lipomas.
- Localised lipoatrophy may result due to insulin injection.
- Progressive lipodystrophy: Less fat in the upper part of the body with excess fat in the lower part.

Xanthomas

Lipid containing nodules present in the soft tissues and tendons.

Xanthomas may be associated with premature coronary atherosclerosis.

Different Types of Xanthomas and their Clinical Significance

1. Eruptive xanthomas
   * Associated with type I and II hyperlipidemias.
   * Yellow colored nodules distributed all over the body.
2. Tendon xanthomas
   * Associated with type II hyperlipidemias.
   * Swelling in the region of tendons of elbow, tendocalcaneus, etc.
3. Palmar xanthomas
   * Associated with type III hyperlipidemias.
   * Palmar creases will have yellowish discoloration.

Body Weight and Body Mass Index (quatelet's index)

Body mass index (BMI) is measured by weight in kg's/body height sq. ms.

Assessment of Body Weight According to BMI
* Normal weight - BMI 18 to 25
* Overweight - BMI 25 to 30
* Obesity - BMI 30 and above
* Extreme (morbid) obesity - BMI 40 and above
* Underweight—BMI less than 18

BMI less than 18 indicates undernutrition and requires nutritional supplementation.

Waist/Hip Ratio

* Keep the patient erect.
* Measure the waist at the level equidistant between the costal margin and iliac crest.
* Measure hip at the level of greater trochanter.

Significance: Normal waist/hip ratio: < 0.8
* Central abdominal obesity (apple-shaped obesity): waist/hip ratio >0.9

* Gluteofemoral obesity (pear shaped obesity): waist/hip ratio < 0.9
* If waist/hip ratio of > 0.9 in women and >1 in men is abnormal and associated with more incidence of cardiovascular disease, diabetes mellitus, hypertension and insulin resistance.
* Waist measurement of >102 cm in males and >88 cm in females indicates high-risk abdominal obesity.

Cachexia

Severe wasting associated with pallor and wrinkled dry skin, e.g. malignant disorders, infections like tuberculosis and HIV disease, anorexia nervosa.

Pallor

Pallor suggests the pale appearance of skin.

Pale appearance depends on the skin pigmentation and skin thickness.

Anaemia suggests the colour of blood.

Note: Anemia and pallor are not synonymous terms.

Causes of Pallor
* All anaemic disorders
* Hypopituitarism and hypogonadism (due to lack of pigmentation of skin).
* Left heart failure
* Conditions associated with shock (due to decreased blood flow).
* Acute severe blood loss causes constriction of superficial blood vessels with dead white colour of the skin.

Anaemia (see also chapter on hematology)

Definition
Anaemia is defined as the decrease in the hemoglobin level RBCs or decrease in the oxygen carrying capacity of the blood.

Examination of an Anaemic Patient
* Mucous membrane is the ideal site to look for pallor (oral mucosa and tongue).

- *Conjunctival pallor:* Turn down the lower eyelids on both sides simultaneously.
- Conjunctiva becomes pale when Hb% is < 8 gm/dl.
- Palmar crease is lighter in color than the surrounding skin when Hb is < 8 gm/dl.
- Severe pernicious anaemia gives lemon or pale yellow tint to the skin and skin may become ashen grey in acute leukemias.

Sites to look for Pallor

- Oral mucosa
- Tongue
- Conjunctiva
- Nail bed
- Palms and soles

Icterus (Jaundice)

Definition

Yellowish discolouration of skin, sclera and mucous membranes due to excess of circulating bilirubin.

Classification and Causes of Jaundice

1. Unconjugated hyperbilirubinemia
   - Due to increased production, e.g. haemolytic anaemias, ineffective erythropoiesis.
   - Due to defective uptake of bilirubin, e.g. Gilbert's syndrome.

2. Conjugated hyperbilirubinemia
   - Hepatocellular dysfunction
     - Acute and chronic hepatitis
     - Cirrhosis
     - Malignancy of liver
   - Obstruction to outflow of bile from liver to duodenum, e.g.
     - Intrahepatic cholestasis - viral hepatitis
     - Extrahepatic obstruction- gall stones, carcinoma head of pancreas

Classification Depending on the site of Abnormality in a Patient of Jaundice (Table 2.1)

Sites to look for Jaundice
- Sclera
- Sublingual mucosa
- Oral cavity
- Palms and soles
- Skin

Jaundice is best appreciated in day light.
Jaundice becomes clinically detectable when the bilirubin level is >3 mg/dl.

Sclera

- Ask the patient to look downwards and look for the upper sclera for the jaundice (Fig. 2.1).
- Sclera is the first structure to be involved in a patient with jaundice.

Table 2.1 Differences between types of jaundice

	Pre hepatic	Hepatic	Post hepatic
Urine color	Initially normal, but on standing becomes darker due to conversion of urobilinogen to urobilin	Yellow	Deep yellow
Itching	—	– –/+	++
Stool	Normal	pale if cholestasis	Clay colored
Anemia	Severe	+/	+/–
Jaundice	Mild	Moderate/Severe	Moderate/Severe
Hepatomegaly	+/–	+	+/–
Splenomegaly	+	+/–	—
Gall bladder-Enlargement	—	—	+/–
Tests for hemolysis	+	—	—
Abnormal LFT	Only indirect bilirubin h	Direct bilirubin hAST, ALT raise	Direct bilirubin h ALP raise

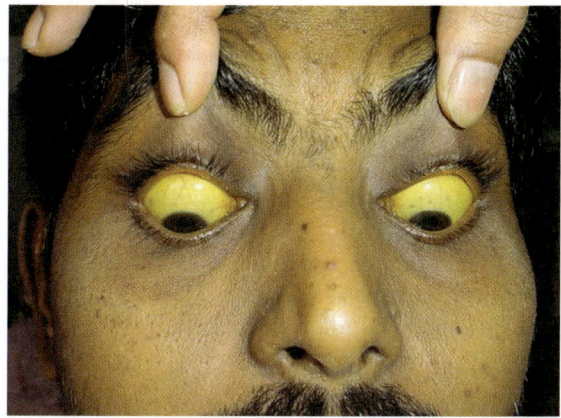

Fig. 2.1 Elicitation of jaundice

- Early involvement of the sclera is due to the high affinity of the elastic tissue to bilirubin.

Latent jaundice: Circulating level of bilirubin is more than normal (but less than 3 mg/dl) but clinically not detectable.

Causes of Yellowish Discolouration Apart from Jaundice

1. Hypercarotenemia
2. Excessive exposure to phenols
3. Quinacrine intake

Hypercarotenemia

- Hypercarotenemia results from consumption of excess carotene containing substances, e.g. carrots.
- Carotene becomes distributed in the subcutaneous fat and stains face, arms and soles yellow.
- Sclera does not become yellow in patients with hypercarotenemia.

KEY POINTS 2.1

- Skin becomes yellowish when the jaundice is severe.
- Sclera becomes lemon yellow in hemolytic jaundice.
- In obstructive jaundice sclera becomes dark yellow or greenish yellow.
- In long-standing jaundice sclera becomes greenish due to oxidation of bilirubin to biliverdin.

Note: Patients with hypothyroidism will have yellowish appearance of face due to impaired metabolism of carotene.

Cyanosis

Definition

Bluish discolouration of mucous membrane and extremities due to decreased oxygenation of blood.

Cyanosis occurs either due to increase in the desaturated haemoglobin or due to abnormal haemoglobins.

Cyanosis appears when the level of desaturated haemoglobin is >5 gm/dl.

Types of Cyanosis (Table 2.2)

- Peripheral cyanosis
- Central cyanosis

a. Peripheral Cyanosis

Mechanism: Peripheral cyanosis occurs due to the decreased capillary blood flow allowing more time for the removal of oxygen by the tissues.

Examples

1. Decreased cardiac output, cardiac failure/shock states.
2. Local vasoconstriction, e.g. cold exposure
3. Arterial and venous obstruction

Sites to Look for Peripheral Cyanosis

- Extremities fingers and toes/tip of nose.

b. Central Cyanosis

Excess of desaturated hemoglobin in the blood leaving the aorta causes central cyanosis.

Table 2.2 Differences between central and peripheral cyanosis

	Central cyanosis	Peripheral cyanosis
Extremities	Warm	Cold
Warming the part	No effect	Cyanosis decreases
Breathing pure O$_2$ 10 litres	May abolish cyanosis	No change occurs

Sites of central cyanosis: Tip of tongue and oral mucosa.

Etiology of Cyanosis

1. Cardiac Causes
- Right to left shunting of blood
  - Reversal of intracardiac shunts
  - Peripheral AV communications
- Defective oxygenation of blood in lungs, e.g. left heart failure.

2. Respiratory Causes
- Ventilation perfusion mismatch with defective oxygenation, e.g. pneumonia/COPD

3. Abnormal haemoglobins
E.g. sulfhemoglobin and methemoglobin

4. Carboxy hemoglobin: Carboxy hemoglobin gives
a cherry red colour to the skin, e.g. CO poisoning.

Clinical Aspects of Cyanosis
- Left heart failure produces both central and peripheral cyanosis.
- Peripheral cyanosis and acutely developed central cyanosis are not associated with clubbing.
- Central cyanosis may appear only on exertion and peripheral cyanosis only on exposure to cold.
- Patient with central cyanosis will also have peripheral cyanosis but warm extremities, except in patients with heart failure (central cyanosis with cold periphery).

Clubbing

Definition
Bulbous enlargement of distal segments of fingers and toes (Fig. 2.2).

Causes
1. *Cardiovascular:* Cyanotic congenital heart disease
   - Reversal of shunts (intracardiac)
   - Infective endocarditis
2. *Respiratory*
   - Suppurative lung disease : Bronchiectasis /lung abscess

- Malignant lung disease: Bronchogenic carcinoma
- Pleural disorders: Empyema thoracis/mesothelioma
- Interstitial lung disease
3. *Gastrointestinal*
   - Ulcerative colitis
   - Crohn's disease
   - Malabsorption syndrome
4. *Hepatic:* Cirrhosis of liver
5. Congenital and idiopathic clubbing

Differential Diagnosis of Clubbing
- Hyperparathyroidism due to resorption of terminal phalanx
- Psoriatic arthritis
- Vinyl chloride exposure
- Pachydermoperiostosis

Grades of Clubbing
Fluctuation: Nail bed becomes soft with redness around and floating of the nail in the nailbed. Minimal fluctuation is normal.

Elicitation of Fluctuation
- Examiner places the terminal phalanx of the patient's finger over the pulp of his two thumbs.
- Gentle pressure is applied with the tips of examiners middle finger over the proximal phalanx of the patient's finger for stabilising the terminal phalanx.

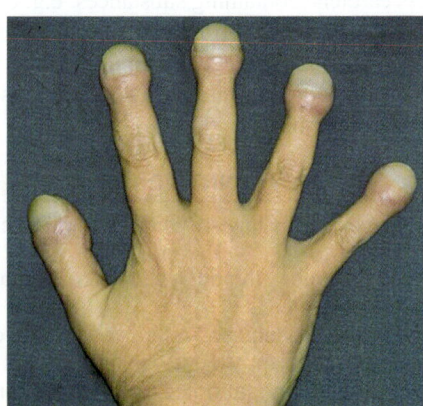

Fig. 2.2 Clubbing of fingers

- Fluctuation is elicited over the patient's nail bed with the tips of examiner's index finger.

Angle Obliteration

Normally there is an angle of about 150 (angle of Lovibond) between the nail and cuticle, in patients with clubbing the angle is lost and may exceed 1800.

Shamroth's Sign

- Ask the patient to keep the two thumbnails opposing each other.
- Observe for the gap in between the nails.
- Reduction or loss of gap between the nails is a manifestation of clubbing.

Change in Curvature of the Nails

- Severe clubbing will be associated with increase in the longitudinal and lateral curvature of the nails.
- In extremely severe cases of clubbing distal phalanx will become bulbous with drumstick appearance.

Hypertrophic Osteoarthropathy

Commonly associated with severe clubbing.
Parts involved: Wrist and ankle with lower ends of long bones like radius, ulna, tibia and fibula.

Features

Wrist and ankle joint will have following features

- Swelling
- Pain
- Stiffness
- Redness
- Rise of temperature
- Joint effusion
- Thickening of periosteum of long bones.

Radiological Changes

- Calcification of the subperiosteal region (separate from bone cortex).

Common Causes of Hypertrophic Osteoarthropathy

- Bronchogenic carcinoma
- Cystic fibrosis
- Bronchiectasis
- Cyanotic congenital heart disease

Pathogenesis of Clubbing

1. *Neurogenic Theory*
   - Reflex vasodilatation of peripheral tissues and nailbed occurs due to brain stem stimulation.
   - Brainstem stimulation may occur as a result of diseased lung and pleura generating impulses reaching the brain stem via the vagi and intercostal nerves.

Note: Features of clubbing and hypertrophic osteoarthropathy may disappear after resection of vagi and intercostal nerves.

2. *Hormonal Theory*
   - Proliferation of distal tissues occur due to hormone like substances released by the diseased tissues.

3. *Shunt Theory*
   - AV shunting allows the substances to bypass the lung (normally these substances are degraded by the lung) which stimulate the distal tissue proliferation.

Proposed Vasoactive Substances in the genesis of Clubbing

- Oestrogen
- Ferritin
- Growth hormone
- Platelet derived growth factor (PDGF)

Growth Factor Theory

- Platelet derived growth factor (PDGF) is released at the distal tissues by the circulating megakaryocytes which bypass the pulmonary circulation.
- PDGF may activate fibroblasts, connective tissues and alter the endothelial permeability resulting in clubbing.

LYMPHADENOPATHY

Lymphatic system includes
- Lymph nodes
- Lymphatic vessels
- Lymphatic tissues

Lymphatic tissue includes tonsils, adenoids, spleen and Peyer's patches in the ileum.

Examination of Lymph Nodes

Check for the following details while examining a lymph node

- Number   -   Mobile/fixed
- Size   -   Tenderness
- Site   -   Fluctuation
- Consistency   -   Surrounding skin
- Discrete/Matted -   Draining area

Characteristics of Different Types of Lymphadenopathy

1. Tuberculous node
   - Soft, non-tender, matted nodes (attached to each other).
   - Discharge, sinus or scar of previous suppuration of untreated cases may be present.
2. Tender node
   - Signifies inflammatory or infective pathology with acute stretching of the capsule.
3. Lymphangitis
   - Superficial lymphatic vessels appear as red streaks running between the nodes and sites of original infection, e.g. filarial lymphangitis.
4. Fixity of lymph node
   - Indicates inflammatory pathology.
   - Deep fixity suggests malignancy.
5. Fluctuation of a lymph node:
   - Suggests abscess forming conditions like sepsis or TB.
6. Lymphoma node
   - Discrete, mobile, non-tender, firm or rubbery (elastic) in consistency.
   - May be symmetrical.
7. Malignant lymph node
   - Hard, non-tender fixed nodes which progressively enlarge.
8. Bubo
   - Inflammatory swelling of one or more lymphnodes in the inguinal region. Masses of lymphnodes may suppurate and drain pus, e.g. chancroid, lymphogranuloma venereum

A. LOCALISED LYMPHADENOPATHY

Enlargement of lymphnodes in a single anatomical area.

Cervical Lymphadenopathy

Causes

- URTI
- Viral illness
- Oral or dental lesions
- Secondaries from primary head, neck, breast, lung and thyroid malignancy.
- Lymphoma and leukemias
- All causes of generalised lymphadenopathy.

Examination of Cervical Lymphnodes

Examine from behind for submental, tonsillar, submandibular, supraclavicular, preauricular and deep cervical nodes.

Scalene Node

Node is present deep to sternomastoid muscle on the scaleneus anticus muscle.

Method of palpation: Finger is dipped through the clavicular head of sternomastoid behind the clavicle.

Significance: Secondary involvement of the lymph node due to bronchial carcinoma.

Jugulo-digastric node

Most commonly enlarged lymphnode, e.g. URTI and tonsillitis.

Palpate just posteriorly to the angle of the mandible.

Examine the posterior triangle of the neck up to the back for posterior auricular and occipital lymphnodes.

Waldeyer's Ring.

Waldeyer's ring constitutes a group of lymphatic structures, which surround the opening of digestive and respiratory tracts.

KEY POINTS 2.2

- Soft, flat lymph nodes of < 1 cm size are usually benign and require follow up. Inguinal lymph nodes of less than 2 cm size are not abnormal.
- Lymph node size > 2 cm or size of 1.5 × 1.5 cm are significant and to be evaluated.

1. Internal ring
   • Adenoids (pharyngeal tonsil)
   • Palatine tonsils
   • Tubal tonsils
   • Lingual tonsil
2. External ring
   • Occipital (posteriorly)
   • Posterior auricular
   • Preauricular
   • Jugular and tonsillar
   • Submandibular
   • Submental (anteriorly)

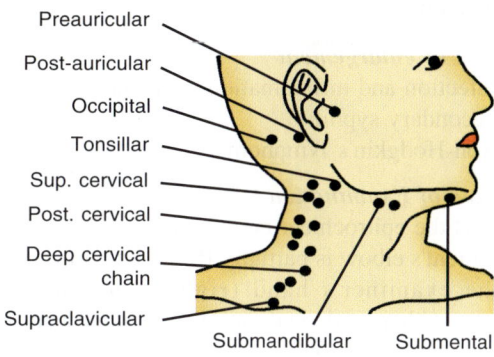

Fig. 2.3 Cervical lymph nodes

Figure 2.3 shows cervical lymph nodes and Figs 2.4a and b methods of their palpation.

Significance
Waldeyer's ring adenopathy occurs with local disease or as a part of generalised lymphadenopathy especially in patients with non-Hodgkin's lymphoma.

Virchow's Node (Troisier's sign)
Enlargement of left supraclavicular node occurs due to metastatic lesion from GIT or testicular malignancy (see also GIT).

Occipital lymphadenopathy: Occurs in scalp infection.

Preauricular lymphnode: Enlargement can occur with conjunctival infection.

Axillary Lymphadenopathy

Causes
1. Infection or injury to the ipsilateral upper limb
2. Breast and chest wall disease
3. Lymphoma

Method of Examination (Figs 2.5a and b)
• Examiner sitting in front of the patient supports the patients upper limb with his own, on the side to be examined.
• Finger tips are inserted into the axillary vault (right finger tips for left axilla and vice versa) and anterior, posterior and medial walls are palpated in turn.

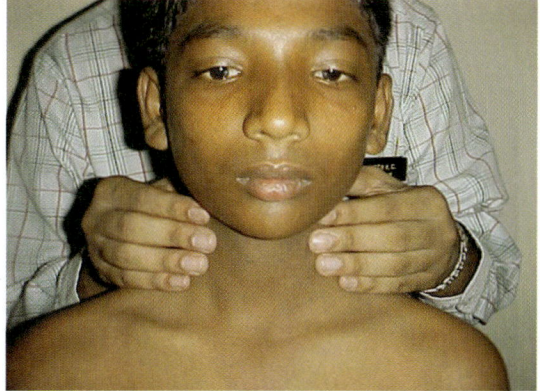

Fig. 2.4a Palpation of the cervical lymph nodes (anterior) from behind

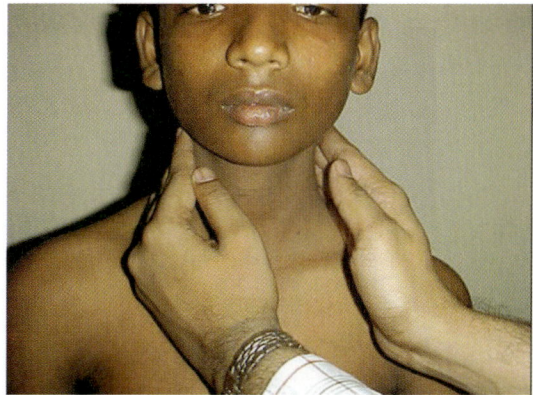

Fig. 2.4b Palpation of the cervical lymph nodes (posterior) from the anterior aspect

Epitrochlear Nodes

Causes of enlargement
- Infection and inflammation of ipsilateral hand
- Secondary syphilis
- Non-Hodgkin's lymphoma

Method of Examination (Fig. 2.6)
- Feel the epitrochlear node with the thumb.
- Patient's elbow is partially flexed and grasped by the examiner's hand (right hand for right epitrochlear node and vice versa) while patient's wrist is supported by the examiner's non examining hand.

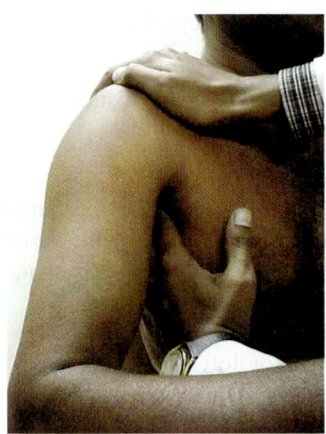

Fig. 2.5a Palpation of axillary lymph nodes (right side)

Inguinal Node (Fig. 2.7)
Palpate horizontal nodes at just below the inguinal ligament and vertical nodes along the saphenous vein.

Causes of Inguinal Lymphadenopathy
- Infection or trauma to the lower extremities
- Sexually transmitted diseases
- Lymphomas
- Metastatic cancer from primary in the rectum, genitalia and lower extremities.

Popliteal Glands
Palpate deeply into the popliteal fossa with both hands with the knee partially flexed.

Causes of Enlargement of Popliteal Glands
- Knee joint disease
- Infection and trauma to the lower limb
- All causes of generalised lymphadenopathy

Intra abdominal Nodes

Para-aortic Nodes
- Palpate deeply in the umbilical region along the aortic pulsation.
- They are felt as round firm, confluent masses and are felt only when significantly enlarged.

Causes of Intra-abdominal Lymphadenopathy
- Tuberculosis
- Lymphomas

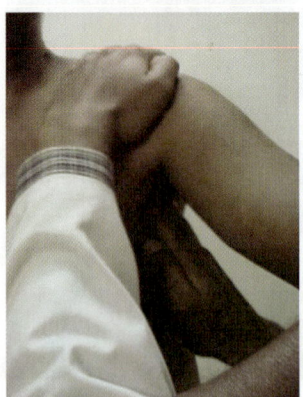

Fig. 2.5b Palpation of axillary lymph nodes (left side)

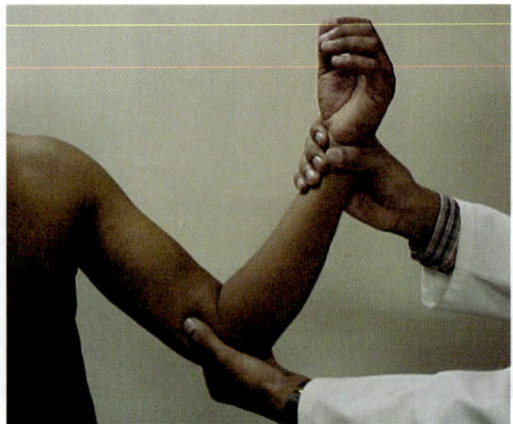

Fig. 2.6 Palpation of epitrochlear lymph node

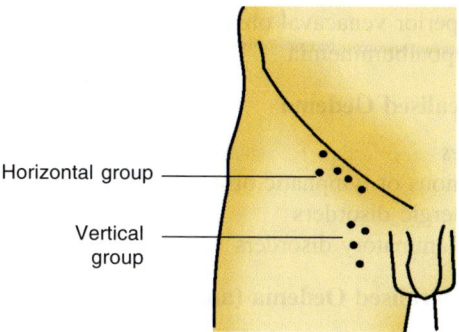

Horizontal group

Vertical group

Fig. 2.7 Inguinal nodes

- Intra abdominal malignant disorders
- Germ cell tumors

Intrathoracic Lymphadenopathy

Mediastinal and Hilar Lymphadenopathy

Causes
- Bronchogenic carcinoma with secondaries
- Lymphomas
- Tuberculosis (usually unilateral)
- Sarcoidosis
- Histoplasmosis

B. GENERALISED LYMPHADENOPATHY

Definition
Enlargement of three or more non contiguous areas of lymph nodes.

Causes
1. Infection
   - Viral infectious mononucleosis
   - HIV infection
   - Disseminated tuberculosis
   - Histoplasmosis, etc.
2. Immunologic
   - Rheumatoid arthritis
   - SLE
   - Sjogren's syndrome
3. Malignancies
   - Hodgkin's and non-Hodgkin's lymphoma
   - CLL
   - ALL

4. Storage diseases
   - Gaucher's and Niemann-Pick's disease
5. Endocrine disorders
   - Grave's disease
6. Drug induced
   - Phenytoin sodium
   - Carbamazepine
   - Allopurinol

Pedal Oedema

Pedal oedema is due to excess collection of fluid in the interstitial tissues causing swelling of the tissues (Fig. 2.8).

Minimal swelling of the feet can normally occur at the end of day due to increased mean capillary pressure on standing.

Sites of oedema
Site of edema collection is predominantly determined by the gravity.

Common sites of oedema
- Legs, thigh, back, face and limbs.
- Sacral oedema is common in bedridden patients.
- Abdominal wall edema can occur in patients with Anasarca (pinch a fold of skin of abdominal wall and look for edema).

Elicitation of oedema
- Apply firm pressure over the lower part of the tibia (above the medial malleolus) or dorsum of feet for about 20–30 sec.
- Observe for pitting nature of oedema.
- Pitting edema appears when the body weight increases by 10–15% due to fluid collection.

Causes
- Acute glomerulonephritis
- Nephrotic syndrome
- Cirrhosis of liver
- Congestive cardiac failure
- Hypoalbuminemia (nutritional)

Facial Oedema

Loose subcutaneous tissue favours the accumulation of the fluid around the eyes.

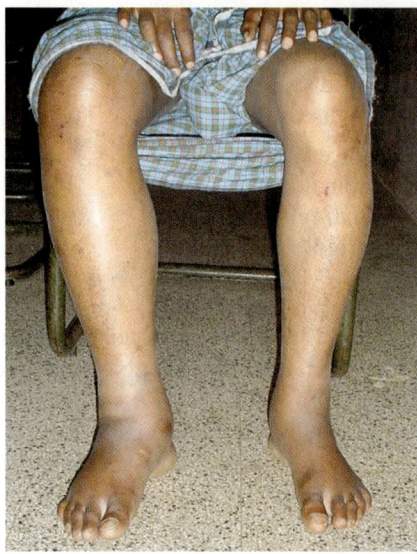

Fig. 2.8 Pedal oedema

Periorbital puffiness occurs predominantly in the morning hours.

Causes of Facial Puffiness
- Acute glomerulonephritis
- Nephrotic syndrome
- Superior venacaval obstruction
- Angioneurotic oedema
- Cushing's syndrome
- Myxoedema

Non-pitting Oedema
Non pitting oedema is characterised by the absence of pitting, on applying pressure but with swollen tissues, e.g. chronic lymphoedema, elephantiasis.

Myxoedema is the collection of firm mucinous material in the subcutaneous tissues.

Different Types and Causes of Oedema
Oedema of upper part of the body can be caused by intra thoracic tumors.

1. Conjunctival Oedema (chemosis)

Causes
- Grave's disease

- Superior venacaval obstruction
- Hypoalbuminemia

2. Localised Oedema

Causes
- Venous or lymphatic obstruction
- Allergic disorders
- Inflammatory disorders

3. Generalised Oedema (anasarca)

Causes
- All causes of hypoalbuminemia
- Cirrhosis of liver
- Nephrotic syndrome
- Nutritional

4. Allergic Oedema
Angioneurotic edema usually involves face and lips, may affect glottis and larynx.

5. Unilateral Oedema

Causes
- Cellulitis
- Lymphatic obstruction
- Deep vein thrombosis
- CNS lesion on one side can affect the vasomotor fibres on that side. Lymphatic and venous drainage is also affected on the affected side causing unilateral oedema.

6. Lymphatic oedema
Normally lymphatics absorb small quantity of albumin filtered from the capillaries.
   Lymphatic oedema due to obstruction to the lymphatic flow.

Causes
- Recurrent filarial lymphangitis–limbs, breast and genitalia.
- After radical mastectomy–upper limb on the affected side
- Radiation for carcinoma breast–upper limb on the affected side
- Lymphatic obstruction due to mass lesion.

Milroy's Disease

Congenital hypoplasia of lymphatic vessels of legs associated with pedal oedema.

VITAL SIGNS

- Pulse (See cardiovascular system)
- Blood pressure (See cardiovascular system)
- Respiratory rate (See respiratory system)

Temperature

Usage of Thermometer (Key points 2.3)

Recording of Temperature
- *Conscious adults:* Record oral or axillary temperature.
- *Unconscious/collapsed/elderly:* Record the rectal temperature.
- *Children:* Record the axillary or rectal temperature.

  Temperature can also be recorded in children in the groin with the thigh flexed over the abdomen.

> *Note:* Rectal temperature is > 0.5°C of oral temperature > 0.5°C of axillary temperature.

Normal body temperature: 36.6°C to 37.2°C or 98–99°F. *Circadian variation* of body temperature is 0.5°C

Normally evening temperature is higher than the normal.
- Lowest level of body temperature is at 6 a.m.
- Highest level of body temperature is at 4 to 6 p.m.

KEY POINTS 2.3

- Thermometer must be accurate.
- Keep the thermometer for at least half a minute for temperature rise to occur.
- While recording the oral temperature, patient should breathe through the nose with lips tightly closed.
- Wash the thermometer with cold water and with antiseptic after usage.
- Shake the thermometer to bring the mercury column below normal before recording the temperature.

Fever

Increase in the body temperature with a rise in the hypothalamic set point.

Morning temperature > 37.2°C (98.9°F) or evening temperature > 37.7°C (99.9°F) is suggestive of fever.

Menstruating women: Temperature becomes 1°F greater (after ovulation) in the morning hours and will remain till the starting of next menstrual cycle.

Hyperthermia
- Increase in body temperature but hypothalamic thermoregulatory set point is not changed.
- Temperature rise exceeds the body capacity for loosing heat, e.g.
  - Heat stroke
  - Thyrotoxicosis
  - Pheochromocytoma
  - Neuroleptic malignant syndrome
  - Malignant hypothermia, e.g. succinyl choline administration.

Hyperpyrexia: Temperature greater than 41.60°C or 107°F

Causes
- Falciparum malaria
- Pontine hemorrhage
- Thyrotoxic crisis
- Neuroleptic malignant syndrome
- Heat stroke

Hypothermia: Temperature less than 35°C or < 95°F.

Causes
- Head injury
- Near drowning
- Alcohol intoxication
- Drug overdose, sedatives and hypnotics
- Severe hypothyroidism

Fever: Different patterns
- *Continuous fever:* Fever does not touch normal within 24 hours but fluctuation is less than 1°C.
- *Remittent fever:* Fever does not touch within 24

hours but fluctuation is more than 2°C., e.g. bacterial infections.

- *Intermittent fever:* Fever is present only in certain parts of a day.
- *Quotidian fever:* Paroxysms of intermittent fever occur daily, e.g. falciparum malaria.
- *Tertian fever:* Fever occurs on alternate days, e.g. vivax malaria.
- *Quartan fever:* Attacks of fever occur with afebrile periods of two days in between, e.g. malariae malaria.
- *Pel-Ebstein fever:* Fever increases and persists for few days (3–10 days) and followed by an afebrile period (3–10 days), e.g. Hodgkin's and other lymphomas.
- *Relapsing fever:* Few days of fever followed by days of afebrile state and then again fever relapses, e.g. Borrelia infection, rat bite fever.
- *Double quotidian fever (double spike):* Two spikes of fever in a day, e.g. visceral leishmaniasis.
  - *Fever with chills and rigors:*
    Examples
    - Malarial paroxysms
    - Pneumonias
    - UTI
    - Septic conditions

Temperature pulse dissociation: For every one-degree increase of temperature pulse rate increases by around ten.

Relative bradycardia: For example typhoid, brucellosis, and leptospirosis

Relative tachycardia: For example myocarditis

State of Hydration

Normal body water constitutes
- 60–65% of total body weight
- Intracellular water–around 30 liters
- Interstitial fluid–around 10 liters
- Blood volume–around 5 liters 7

Assessment of Hydration

Check for the following parameters while assessing the state of hydration
- Skin elasticity
- Intraocular pressure
- Blood pressure recording
- Postural hypotension

Signs of Dehydration

1. Dry tongue (patients with mouth breathing can also have dry tongue).
2. *Skin elasticity:* Pinch a fold of skin, folded skin remains as a ridge which only subsides slowly. Fluid loss of 4–6 litres will result in dry loose and wrinkled skin.
3. *Intraocular pressure:* Intraocular pressure decreases and the eye ball becomes soft in patients with dehydration.
4. Postural hypotension.
5. Supine hypotension (systolic BP less than 90 mmHg).

EXAMINATION OF FACE, HEAD AND NECK

Different Types of Facial Appearances

1. **Endocrine Disorders**
   - *Hypothyroidism:* Dull appearance, facial puffiness
   - *Thyrotoxicosis:* Prominent eyes, startled appearance
   - *Acromegaly:* Prognathism, frontal bossing
   - *Cushing's syndrome:* Moon face
2. **Neuromuscular Disorders**
   - *Facial palsy:* Deviation of angle of mouth to one side.
   - *Third nerve palsy:* Ptosis on the affected side.
   - *Horner's syndrome:* Narrow palpebral fissure on the affected side.
   - *Parkinsonism:* Expressionless, mask like face.
   - *Myotonic dystrophy:* Frontal baldness, ptosis, wrinkling of forehead narrowing of lower half of the face (due to masseter atrophy).
   - *Tetanus:* Risus sardonicus (sustained facial muscle contraction resulting in facial grimace).

Plethoric Appearance of Face
- Polycythemic disorders

- Cushing's syndrome
- Alcoholism

Mitral facies: bluish appearance of face with malar flush

Hemolytic anemia: chipmunk face (frontal bossing, malar prominence, protuberant teeth).

Hippocratic facies: Found in patients with terminal stage of illness.

Characteristics: Sunken eyes, dry skin with flattening of cheek and temporal areas.

Other conditions which can be made out on examination of face
- Butterfly rash of SLE
- Heliotrope rash of dermatomyositis
- Pallor, cyanosis and jaundice
- Wasting of muscles

Table 2.3 Examination of different parts of eye in relation to general medical disorders

	Abnormality	Associated disorder
Conjunc-tiva	Suffused	Polycythemia
	Pallor	Anemic disorder
	Dryness	Sicca syndrome
		Vitamin A deficiency
	Haemorrhage	Leptospirosis
		Bleeding disorder
Sclera	Jaundice	Hepatobiliary disorder
		Hemolytic anaemia
	Scleritis/Episcleritis	Connective tissue disorder
	Blue sclera	Osteogenesis imperfecta
Cornea	Opacity	Keratitis
	K F Ring	Wilson's disease
Iris	Iritis	Inflammatory bowel disease
		Rheumatoid arthritis
		Infectious disorder
	Depigmentation of Iris	Albinism
Lens	Cataract	Diabetes mellitus
		Hypocalcaemia
	Iridodonesis (Tremulousness of iris due to subluxation of lens)	Marfan's syndrome

Examination of Eyes (Table 2.3)

Check for ptosis, squint and pupillary irregularity (for details see nervous system).

Exophthalmos: Prominent eyeball with forward protrusion.

Causes
- *Bilateral* - Hyperthyroidism
- *Unilateral* - Cavernous sinus thrombosis and intra orbital tumors
- *Pulsatile* - Caroticocavernous fistula

Enophthalmos: Inward movement of eyeball

Causes
- Severe wasting
- Extreme dehydration
- Horner's syndrome

Hypertelorism

Characteristics
Increased distance between the two eyes (distance between the two medial canthii is increased).

There will be apparent broadening of the root of the nose.

Defect
Lesser wing of the sphenoid bone is overdeveloped with relatively smaller greater wings.

Significance
Associated with congenital defects/mental deficiency, e.g. Down's syndrome

EXAMINATION OF LIPS, CHEEKS AND GLANDS OF THE FACE

Abnormalities of Lips

- *Cleft lip:* Congenital
- *Chelitis:* Inflammation at the line of closure or mucocutaneous junction of lips. Found in patients with riboflavin deficiency.
- *Angular stomatitis:* Inflamed and painful cracking at the corners of the mouth. Found in patients with iron and riboflavin deficiency.

- *Cold sores:* Vesicles over the lips due to infection with Herpes simplex type I virus. Commonly associated with febrile states.
- *Thick lips:* Acromegaly, myxoedema.

Cheeks

Abnormalities	Associated disorders
Puffiness	Oedema states
Malar flush	Steroid therapy
Butterfly rash	SLE
Mitral facies	Mitral stenosis

Parotid and Lacrimal Glands

Parotid swellings: Present in front of the ear.

Causes
1. Unilateral
   - Acute parotitis (associated with calculus and sepsis)
   - Occasionally mumps
2. Bilateral
   - Mumps
   - Sarcoidosis
   - Sjogren's syndrome
   - Leukemias

Lacrimal Glands

Location: Lacrimal gland lies beneath the lateral part of the upper eyelid visible on everting the eyelid.

Lacrimal sac: Situated between the nose and medial canthus of the eye.

Abnormalities: Damage to the lacrimal gland or lacrimal nerves cause dry eye due to decrease of tears.

Enlargement of Lacrimal Gland

Causes
- Mumps
- Sarcoidosis
- Lymphoma
- Carcinoma

Obstruction to the nasolacrimal duct causes acute dacryocystitis and lacrimal sac abscess.

Note: Different abnormalities of movements of face can occur with nervous system disorders (see nervous system).

EXAMINATION OF HEAD AND NECK

Hydrocephalus

Characteristics
- Increase in the size of the head compared to the body size.
- Protrusion of the forehead.
- Sunken, downward deviated eyes.
- Bulging of the frontanelles due to separation of sutures.
- Increase in the size of the head also occurs in patients with Paget's disease.

Frontal Bossing

Causes
- Chronic hydrocephalus
- Thalassemias
- Rickets

Examination of Neck

Abnormalities
- Thyroid enlargement (goitre)
- Lymphadenopathy
- Neck veins
- Arterial pulsations
- Trachea
- Scar mark

Thyroid Enlargement (Goitre) See also endocrine disorders

Characteristics
- Present in the region of the thyroid (anterior aspect of the neck).
- Swelling moves with deglutition.
- Swelling may be nodular or diffuse.
- Goitre may press over the trachea or may have intra thoracic extension.

- Hyperthyroidism is associated with bruit over the thyroid.
- Thyroid malignancy can involve the recurrent laryngeal nerve.

Palpation of the Thyroid Swelling
Person is comfortably seated and palpation of thyroid is done from standing behind.

Note: Any mass connected with thyroid will move with deglutition.

Minimal thyroid enlargement may be better seen than felt.

Torticollis (wry neck): Causes abnormal positioning of the neck due to spasmodic contraction of muscles supplied by the spinal accessory nerves. Head is drawn to one side with the chin pointing to the other side. For example, congenital, dystonias, stiff and painful neck conditions.

Web neck: Occurs in patients with Turner's syndrome.

Scar mark: Look for the scar of previous lymph node biopsy or thyroid surgery.

Examination of Nose (Table 2.4)

Epistaxis (bleeding from the nose)

Causes
- Local - diseases of nose
- Systemic-bleeding and clotting disorders
- Occasionally in hypertensives

Table 2.4 Examination of nose

Abnormality	Disorder
Enlargement of nose	Occurs in Acromegaly
Reddening of the nose	SLE with butterfly rash
	Alcoholics
Saddle nose (depressed bridge)	Lepromatous leprosy nasal Congenital syphilis
Destruction of nasal structures	Wegener's granulomatosis Tuberculosis (lupus vulgaris)

Examination of Ear

Abnormalities
- Ear discharge–Suggests ear infection
- Vesicles over the ear–Herpes zoster infection
- Tophi–Gouty arthritis
- Prominent crease seen over the ear lobule-Associated with increased incidence of coronary artery disease.
- Bluish appearance–Peripheral cyanosis.

Low Set Ears
Draw a horizontal line from the outer canthus of the eye to the pinna of the ear of the same side. If less than one-third of the pinna is above the line drawn suggests low set ears.

Significance: Low set ears are usually associated with other congenital anomalies.

EXAMINATION OF BREAST

Inspection: Check for

- Symmetry of two breasts
- Presence of ulcers and any swellings
- Inspect also the skin of the breast for:
- Ulceration
- Reddening
- Peau'd orange appearance
- Dimpling of skin

Palpation
- Use the flat of the hand and palpate all the four quadrants of the breast tissue.
- Palpation should also be done with the patient keeping the hand under the head.
- Palpate also with upper limbs above the head and also on leaning forward.
- Examine for any mass lesion. Define the size, shape, surface and fixity of the mass.
- Palpate also the axillary tail, axilla and local lymphnodes for any abnormality.
- Examine the nipple for any discharge (serous, milk or blood).
- Male breast should also be examined for abnormalities like gynaecomastia.

Common Clinical Breast Abnormalities

Skin Changes
- Dimpling of skin-Simple and benign dimpling results in retraction of the skin which is mobile.
- With malignant infiltration of skin-Tumor becomes fixed to skin.
- Peau d'orange appearance - Orange skin like appearance of skin.
- Skin is swollen in between hair follicles.
- Peau d'orange appearance is due to lymphaedema caused by obstruction of the intramammary lymphatics by the tumour.

Lesions of Nipple
1. Nipple inversion
   - Benign - symmetrical slit like appearance due to periductal inflammation.
   - Malignant-distorted asymmetrical inversion.
2. Discharge from nipples
   - Minimal clear fluid - normal on massaging the breast.
   - Blood stained - papilloma, carcinoma
   - Galactorrhea-milky discharge (hyperprolactinemia)
3. Breast abscess
   - Lactational in breast feeding mothers peripheral abscess
   - Non-lactational due to extension of periductal mastitis abscess is at the edge of the nipple.
4. Fibrocystic disease:
   - Common before menstrual periods
   - Irregular nodules of varying sizes found bilaterally.
5. Fibroadenoma
   - Discrete mobile rubbery swellings in the breast.
   - Common cause of lump in the breast in the young (< 35 yrs).

KEY POINTS 2.4

- Explain the purpose of the examination and avoid unnecessary embarrassment to the patient.
- Properly expose the pectoral girdle.
- Ask the patient to keep the hands on the waist for proper examination.

---

6. Carcinoma breast:
   - Firm or hard mass
   - Usually fixed and irregular

HANDS AND FEET

Clinical Abnormalities of Hand

Color
- Nicotine staining of fingers - chronic smokers
- Severe pallor - anaemic disorders
- Palmar erythema - liver disorders, polycythemic disorder
- Bluish discoloration - peripheral cyanosis

Temperature
- Cold hands - Peripheral vasoconstriction
- Warm hands - Hyperthyroidism, CO_2 retention

Size
- Large hands which are thick with spade-like fingers - Acromegaly
- Thick hands - Myxoedema

Importance of Shaking Hands with the Patient
- Delayed relaxation of handgrip - In patients with myotonic dystrophy.
- Cold hands, sweating associates with tremulousness - Anxiety neurosis
- Large hands with increased sweating - Acromegaly
- Warm hands with increased sweating and tremulousness - Thyrotoxicosis.

Shape and Deformities of Hands and Feet

Causes of Deformities and Different Shapes
- Trauma
- Rheumatoid arthritis
- Arachnodactyly - Marfan's syndrome
  Short 4th and 5th metacarpals- Pseudohypoparathyroidism
- Carpal spasm - Tetany

Different Posture of Upper Limb
- Flexed arms and hand on the affected side hemiplegia

- Wrist drop - radial nerve palsy
- Ulnar deviation - rheumatoid arthritis
- Claw hand - ulnar and median nerve palsy

Depuytren's Contracture

Characteristics

Flexion deformities of 4th and 5th fingers due to thickening and shortening of palmar fascia, e.g. alcoholic liver disease, diabetes mellitus

Trophic Ulcers of the Hand

Causes
- Neurologic disease
- Vasculitic syndrome
- Raynaud's disease

Examination of Nails (Table 2.5)

Examination of Feet

Abnormalities of Feet
1. Oedema of feet
   - Renal, cardiac, hepatic disorders
   - Hypoproteinemic states
2. Vascular changes
   - *Chronic venous stasis:* Pigmentation of lower part of legs and feet.

- Eczematous changes and ulceration
- *Arterial ischemia:* Pallor, loss of hair and sensation, ulceration
- *Neuropathic ulcers:* Painless ulcers develop over pressure points.

Bony Abnormalities of Lower Limb

- Knock knees (genu valgum) physiological up to 2 yrs of age.
- Bow legs (genu varum) if persists after 2 yrs, may be due to rickets, renal disease, osteogenesis imperfecta and rarely infection/trauma to growth plate.

Pes Cavus

Characteristics
- Increase in the arch of foot with fixed deformity.
- Foot is usually plantar flexed (equinus).
- Clawing of toes is usually associated.

Causes
- Familial
- Peroneal muscular atrophy
- Friedrich's ataxia
- Syringomyelia

Table 2.5 Examination of nails

Different nail abnormalities	Associated condition
Platynychia (flat nails)	Iron deficiency anaemia
Koilonychia (spoon shaped nails)	Iron deficiency anaemia
Leuconychia (white nails)	Hypoalbuminemia
Nail bed infarct	Vasculitis syndromes
Onycholysis (separation of nail from bed)	Idiopathic, lichen planus, thyrotoxicosis
Missing nail	Nail - patella syndrome
Half and Half nail (red brown distally and white proximally)	CRF
Beau's lines (transverse ridges over the nails)	Indicates stoppage of nail growth temporarily. Affects all nails and appear after few weeks of illness. As the nail grows ridges also move to the distal part.
Nail pitting	Psoriasis
Paronychia (swollen inflamed nail bed)	Repeated trauma, working in wet conditions, diabetes mellitus, poor peripheral circulation
Discolouration of nails	Antimalarials, occupational, Antibiotics, fungal infection, Phenothiazines

Rocker Bottom Feet

- Foot will be associated with protuberance of heel.
- Significance-Edwards syndrome (trisomy 18) with PDA.

Examination of hair (see Chapter endocrine disorders)

Development of hair and different phases of hair growth

- *Lanugo hair:* Acts as a cover to the foetus, fine hairs which are shed a month before birth.
- *Puberty:* Girls- hair development at pubis around the age of 11½ years.
  Boys-pubic hair develops around the age of 13½ years.
  Pubic hairs are coarser in nature and are under the control of adrenal androgens.
- *Axillary hair:* Appears after the pubic hair.
- *Body hair:* Develops and grows through out the period of sexual maturity more in males.

Phases of Hair Growth

- *Anagen phase:* Growing phase of hair. Anagen phase of scalp hair lasts up to 5 years.
- *Telogen phase:* Resting or shedding phase may last up to 3 months.

Scalp Hairs

Total number is around 1 lakh. Check for the presence of nits, lice and dandruff over the scalp.

Nits: Firmly adherent to the hair.

Dandruff: Desquamatory lesions causing hair loss.

Scalp Hair Loss

- Temporal recession of scalp hair occurs in males.
- Predominantly androgen dependant.
- *Alopecia areata:* Patchy scalp hair loss, e.g. local diseases of scalp -fungal infection and secondary syphilis.
- *Alopecia totalis:* Total loss of scalp hair

Causes

- Bacterial infection
- SLE

- Burns
- Radiation
- Fungal infections

Loss of Body Hair

- *Alopecia universals:* Total loss of body hair.

Causes

- Anti malignancy treatment, e.g. cyclophosphamide therapy
- Toxic illness
- Severe starvation
- Hypothyroidism (predominantly - outer one-third eyebrow loss).

Flag Sign

Brownish discolouration of hair interspersed with normal color.

It is a manifestation of protein energy malnutrition.

Loss of Sexual Hair

- Old age
- Hypopituitarism and hypogonadism
- Cirrhosis of liver

Excessive Hair Growth (hypertrichosis)

- *Hirsutism:* Male pattern hair growth over the face, trunk and limbs in a female. It is common after menopause.
- *Virilism:* Development of masculine features in a female. May be a manifestation of androgen secretion.

Causes of Excessive Hair Growth

- Familial
- Sexual precocity
- Adrenal hyperplasia/neoplasia
- Virilising adrenal tumours
- Drug induced - androgens, minoxidil

EXAMINATION OF SKIN

Different Terminologies used when describing Skin Lesions

- *Macule*: Flat and small lesions with altered texture and colour (< 2 cm).

- *Papule:* Solid elevated area of skin (< 0.5–1 cm).
- *Plaque:* Larger (> 1 cm) elevated area of skin.
- *Vesicle:* Small (< 0.5 cm) usually clear fluid containing elevated lesions.
- *Pustule:* Small pus containing lesions in the skin.
- *Bulla:* Large vesicle (> 1 cm).
- *Abscess:* Collection of (> 1 cm in diameter) in the skin with significant depth.
- *Nodule:* Large (1–5 cm) solid lesion in the skin.
- *Wheal:* White compressible raised lesion produced by oedema of dermis.
- *Angioedema:* Oedema involving subcutaneous tissue producing a diffuse swelling.
- *Petechiae:* Bleeding spots (1–2 mm/pin head size) in the skin.
- *Purpur:* Macular or papular collection of blood in the skin (> 3 mm size).
- *Ecchymoses :* Large area of bleeding in the skin.
- *Haematoma:* Collection of blood in the skin with elevation.

Alteration of Skin Color
- Pallor (see under pallor)
- Flushed appearance of skin
  Generalised flushing of skin causes
  - a. Febrile illness
  - b. Hyperthyroidism
  - c. Alcohol consumption
  - d. Corticosteroid therapy
  - e. CO_2 retention

Occasional attacks of flushing
  - a. Menopausal syndrome
  - b. Emotional outbursts

Pigmentation
- *Chloasma:* Mask like pigmentation of face, nipples, areola etc. (e.g. pregnancy).

Localised Pigmentation of Skin
- *Livedoreticularis:* Web-like lesions with reddish blue discoloration, e.g. autoimmune vasculitis
- *Pellagra:* Pigmentation over the exposed parts of the body.
- *Erythema abigne:* Due to long standing siting near the fire-with reticular appearance.

- Café au lait spots (see nervous system)
- Rashes
- Fixed drug eruptions

Characteristics of Different Types of Pigmentation in Medical Disorders
- *Addison's disease*: Bluish or brownish pigmentation
  Sites: Oral cavity, pressure points, bony prominences creases and scars.
- *Haemochromatosis:* Grey/greyish bronze colour of the skin
- *Acanthosis nigricans:* Thick brownish velvety appearance
  Sites: Axilla, sides of neck and groin
  Causes: Internal malignancy, insulin resistance
- Xanthomas and xanthelasma
- Carotenemia and jaundice

Table 2.6 gives different skin lesions associated with general medical disorders. Table 2.7 gives disorders associated with decreased pigmentation of skin.

Systemic Disease
- *Erythema nodosum:* Reddish nodules, tender
  Site: usually on the shin of tibia
  Causes: tuberculosis
- Inflammatory bowel disease
- Sarcoidosis

Table 2.6 Different skin lesions associated with general medical disorders

Disorders	Types of skin lesions
Autoimmune disorders	
SLE	Butterfly rash-see musculoskeletal system
Systemic sclerosis	Scarring and ulceration, acrocyanosis of fingers
Dermatomyositis	Edema of eyelids with heliotrope discolouration (see Locomotor system).
Inherited disorders	
Peutz Jegher's syndrome	Lip and oral cavity pigmentation
Von Reclinghausen's disease	Axillary freckling, Cafe au lait spots
Congenital icthyosis	Scaly skin

Table 2.7 Decreased pigmentation of the skin

Types of pigmentation	Associated disorder
Albinism	Total absence of pigmentation congenital
Piebaldism	Localised absence of pigmentation-congenital
Vitiligo	Patches of depigmentation surrounded by hyper-pigmentation, e.g autoimmune disorders.
Tinea versicolor	Localised hypopigmentation caused by Pityrosporum.
Post inflammatory	E.g. dermatitis/lupus disorders

- Leprosy
- Toxoplasmosis
- Sulfonamides
- *Depigmented macules:* Hansen's disease
- *Purpuric spots:* Bleeding/clotting disorders
- *Pyoderma gangrenosum and skin ulcers:* Ulcerative colitis, rheumatoid arthritis

Systemic causes of Generalised Pruritis
- Diabetes mellitus
- Thyrotoxicosis
- Hepatic failure
- Obstructive jaundice
- Lymphomas
- Drug induced
- Psychogenic

Drug Induced Skin Lesions
- Urticaria - Penicillins
- Morbilliform rash - Ampicillin
- Lichen planus like - Gold and Chloroquine
- Photosensitive - Tetracyclines, Sulphonamides
- Hair loss - Cytotoxic drugs
- Erythema nodosum - Sulphonamides
- Erythema multiformae - Co-trimoxazole

Hyperpigmentation of Skin causes
1. *Localised*
   - Acanthosis nigricans
   - Cafe au lait spots
   - Nevus
   - Fixed drug eruptions (recur in the same areas as circular areas of brown macules, e.g. analgesics, barbiturates, antimalarials).
2. *Generalised*
   - Addison's disease
   - Hemochromatosis
   - Biliary cirrhosis
   - Pellagra
   - Megaloblastic anemia
   - Drugs: Busulphan/cyclophosphomide
   - *Metals:* Arsenic/gold.

Skin Lesions of Leprosy

Tuberculoid Leprosy
- Erythematous maculoanaesthetic patches.
- Lesions are few (single or 2 to 3 in number) and asymmetrical.
- Well defined edges with central flattening.
- Hair growth is decreased with decreased sweating.
- Lesions will have few *Mycobacterium leprae.*
- Person reacts strongly to Lepromin test
- Carries good prognosis

Lepromatous Leprosy
- Multiple lesions, bilateral and usually sym-metrical.
- Erythematous/hypopigmented patches with ill-defined edges.
- Patches may not have loss of sensation or loss of hair growth.
- May have papular, nodular lesions with thick-ening of skin.
- Lesions will have large number of Lepra bacilli.
- Lepromin test is negative and carries bad prognosis.

Cardiovascular System I

Symptoms and History of Present Illness
- Dyspnoea
- Chest pain
- Palpitation
- Syncope
- Cough with expectoration and haemoptysis
- Cyanosis
- Right hypochondrial pain, swelling of feet and decrease in the urine output
- Gastrointestinal symptoms like anorexia, fullness of abdomen and vomiting
- Fatigability
- Fever
- Diabetes mellitus and hypertension

Past History
- Rheumatic fever
- Cyanotic spells
- Recurrent respiratory infections since childhood.
- Detection of murmur/cardiac lesion at school
- Recent dental extraction, genitourinary instrumentation
- Hypertension, diabetes mellitus, ischaemic heart disease or any other significant medical illness.

Family History
- Hypertension
- Ischaemic heart disease
- Congenital heart disease
- Rheumatic heart disease
- Sudden death

Personal History
- Appetite
- Weight loss
- Disturbed sleep
- Bowel and bladder disturbances
- Habits like smoking and alcoholism
- Exposure to syphilis

Menstrual History and History of Previous Pregnancies
Significant in a female patient with cardiovascular disease.

Treatment History
1. Penicillin prophylaxis for rheumatic fever
2. Diuretics
3. Anti hypertensives
4. Salt restriction
5. History of taking sublingual medications
6. History of taking drugs like aspirin, anti-coagulants, beta-blockers, digoxin, etc.

Specific History in a Patient of Suspected Congenital Heart Disease

1. History of heart disease, cyanosis and murmur in family members.
2. History suggestive of maternal rubella (fever with rash) during first 2 months of pregnancy (in patients with PDA, ASD, PS and Tetralogy of Fallot).
3. Syncope, squatting episodes and attacks of cyanosis on straining (in patients with cyanotic heart disease).
4. Detection of murmur in infancy (usual in cases of VSD and PDA) and delayed developmental milestones.
5. Detection of murmur at school (school going age) and restriction from physical activity at school and failure to thrive.

25

6. Recurrent attacks of respiratory infection and pneumonia since childhood (in large left to right shunts).
7. Consanguinity between parents.

APPROACH TO A PATIENT OF CARDIAC DISEASE

Analysis of Presenting Symptoms

Dyspnoea
Definition: Abnormal awareness of breathing with discomfort.

Dyspnoea is a significant manifestation of cardiac failure.

Dyspnoea is more commonly due to left-sided cardiac failure than due to right heart failure.

Mechanism of Dyspnoea in a Patient of Cardiac Failure

Predominant Contributing Factors
1. Decreased lung compliance.
2. Resistance to airflow.
3. Excess respiratory stimulation and drive.
4. Disturbed respiratory muscle function.

Decreased lung compliance is due to
Left heart failure causing pulmonary venous congestion and oedema causing increased stiffness of lungs.

Resistance to air flow is due to
Intra bronchial vessel congestion causing narrow airway caliber.

Excess respiratory stimulation is due to
Stretch of j receptors (juxta capillary) in the pulmonary interstitium, metabolic acidosis and hypoxia.

Disturbed respiratory muscle function is due to
Decreased muscle blood flow, muscle fatigue, altered length and tension relation of the muscle fibres.
Above mechanisms in combination will lead on to increased work of breathing and sensation of dyspnoea in a patient of cardiac failure.

Following details should be enquired with the patient while analysing the symptom of dyspnoea
- Onset
- Duration
- Severity or grade
- Paroxysmal nocturnal dyspnoea.
- Orthopnea
- Wheeze

Onset and Duration
Acute or sudden onset of dyspnoea in a cardiac disease suggests:
Acute left heart failure (acute pulmonary oedema), e.g. in patients with acute myocardial infarction. Patients with mitral stenosis with atrial fibrillation.

Non Cardiac causes of Acute Onset Dyspnoea

1. Respiratory causes
   - Tension pneumothorax
   - Laryngeal oedema
   - Airway obstruction due to foreign body
   - Pulmonary embolism
   - Acute attack of asthma
2. Hysterical hyperventilation (dyspnoea is more at rest than on exertion)

Slowly Progressive Dyspnoea

Causes
1. Left heart disease with chronic left heart failure, e.g. Left sided valvular heart disease, ischaemic heart disease, hypertensive heart disease and cardiomyopathy
2. Non-cardiac disorders like
   - Progressive anaemia
   - Chronic bronchial asthma
   - Chronic obstructive pulmonary disease
   - Interstitial lung disease.
   - Obesity

Severity (Grading)
Functional Grading of Dyspnoea

Grade I: No limitation of any physical activity but dyspnoea occurs on more than ordinary (unaccustomed) exertion.

Grade II: Dyspnoea on ordinary daily activity.

Grade III: Dyspnoea on less than ordinary daily activities.

Grade IV: Limitations of all activities (dyspnoea at rest)

PAROXYSMAL NOCTURNAL DYSPNOEA (PND) - CARDIAC ASTHMA

Significant Symptom of Left Heart Failure (pulmonary venous congestion)

Description of an attack of PND
- Patient goes to sleep without symptoms.
- Sudden awakening of the patient from sleep after about 2–4 hours of sleep.
- Associated with cough, wheezing and sweating with attack of severe suffocation.
- Patient sits up and gasps for breath.
- Symptoms are relieved by sitting or getting out of the bed usually requiring 15 minutes to half an hour (patient may not go back to sleep, as he is afraid of the next attack).

Mechanism of PND
Main factors contributing to pulmonary venous congestion.
After sleeping for 2–3 hours:
- Shifting of fluid from the lower part of the body causing pulmonary venous congestion in patients with pre-existing left heart disease.
- Decrease in the lung expansion due to elevated diaphragm.

- Other mechanisms:
  - Decreased respiratory drive during sleep
  - Loss of sympathetic support to left ventricle during sleep.

All the above mechanisms will lead on to pulmonary congestion and onset of dyspnoea and suffocation resulting in PND.

Sometimes a PND like attack can occur in a patient of chronic airflow obstruction. So it is necessary to differentiate between cardiac asthma (PND with wheezing) and bronchospasm due to airflow obstruction.

Differences between cardiac asthma and bronchospasm of chronic airflow obstruction (Table 3.1).

ORTHOPNOEA

Definition
Dyspnoea that occurs immediately on lying down.

Characteristic Features
- Usually occurs within minutes of assumption of recumbency
- Occurs when the patient is awake
- Indicates the presence of severe left heart failure (Pulmonary oedema) manifests later than PND (in slowly progressive left heart disease).

Non cardiac causes of Orthopnea
Respiratory Causes
- Massive pleural effusion
- Tension pneumothorax
- Severe attack of asthma
- Emphysema
- Bilateral diaphragm paralysis

Table 3.1 Differences between cardiac and respiratory dyspnoea

Cardiac asthma	COPD and bronchial asthma
Dyspnoea precedes cough	Long history of cough, sputum and wheeze. Chronic smoking history may be present.
Symptoms of chest pain, palpitations are usually present.	Usually not present.
Getting up from sleep and sitting relieves dyspnoea	Dyspnoea is relieved by coughing out secretions (or by bronchodilators).
There may be evidence of cardiomegaly and murmurs.	Rhonchi and crepitations may be detectable.

Abdominal Cause

Massive ascites

Mechanism of Orthopnea in Cardiac Failure

Main determining factor of pulmonary venous congestion.

On Assuming Recumbent Position

Pulmonary venous congestion occurs due to shift of fluid from lower part of the body to the lungs, which the failing left heart cannot accept. Raised diaphragm interferes with the lung expansion. Above mechanisms in combination lead on to interstitial pulmonary oedema, decrease in the lung compliance with increased airway resistance resulting in dyspnoea.

Specific other terminologies which are used while describing dyspnoea.

Platypnoea: Dyspnoea occurs on sitting (upright) rather than on lying down position, e.g. left atrial myxoma, left atrial ball valve thrombus and pulmonary A-V fistula.

Trepopnoea

Occurrence of breathlessness only when lying down in lateral position. May be due to ventilation perfusion relationship alteration in certain body position. Trepopnoea is usually associated with heart disease.

Wheeze

Suggests obstructions to the airflow in the medium sized airways, can occur in patients of left sided cardiac failure due to bronchial mucosal congestion

CHEST PAIN

Chest pain of cardiac origin is predominantly due to myocardial ischaemia (ischaemic heart disease) because of coronary atherosclerosis. Chest pain due to ischaemic heart disease is called Angina Pectoris (angina literally means choking).

Description of Angina Pectoris

Site

Usually retrosternal. Sometimes occurs on both sides of the chest.

Type of Pain

Specific character may be difficult to be described. Many patients describe it as a discomfort or an unpleasant sensation in the retrosternal area. [While describing the pain, patient may keep his fist clenched over the precordial area (Levine's sign)]. Sometimes the pain may be described as heaviness, squeezing, burning or constricting band across the chest.

Duration of Pain

- Usually 1–20 minutes
- **Unstable Angina:** Pain typical of angina but lasts for more than 10–15 minutes and also pain may occur at rest.
- **Pain of myocardial infarction:** Prolonged angina like pain persisting for more than few hours.
- If the pain lasts for less than 15 seconds, it is less likely to be angina pectoris.

Aggravating Factors

- Exertion usually precipitates angina.
- Pain of angina occurring at rest may be due to
  – Unstable angina
  – Coronary spasm called Prinzmetal's angina.

Following Factors may also Precipitate an Attack of Angina

- Emotion and fright
- Cigarette smoking
- Exposure to cold
- Heavy meal

Relieving Factors

Taking rest: Pain of angina characteristically subsides by taking rest.

Medication: Taking coronary vasodilators like sublingual nitroglycerine.

Radiation of pain: Usually to the ulnar aspect of the left arm, wrist, epigastrium or left shoulder neck and jaw. Rarely pain of angina can radiate to the right chest.

Associated Symptoms with an Attack of Angina

Nausea, vomiting and sweating: Nausea, vomiting may be more likely associated with acute myocardial infarction.

Cardiac Causes of Precordial Pain apart from Angina Pectoris

- Pulmonary hypertension (due to RV ischaemia or pulmonary artery dilatation).
- Pulmonary embolism
- Aortic dissection
- Mitral valve prolapse
- Pericarditis

Angina Equivalents

Some patients present with symptoms which may not be typical of angina but these symptoms indirectly suggest presence of coronary artery disease. These are called angina equivalents. For example,

- Patient localises the site of origin of dyspnoea at the centre of chest, it is difficult to localise the actual dyspnoea.
- Discomfort felt in the lower jaw, left neck, shoulder and medial aspect of left arm and forearm.
- Dyspeptic symptoms like fullness of epigastrium, nausea and indigestion.

Patient with symptoms of angina equivalents may have other evidence of atherosclerosis like TIA, stroke and pain of vascular claudication.

Nocturnal Angina (Angina decubitus)

Chest pain occurs in recumbent position. Resorption of fluid into the intravascular compartment in recumbent position results in increased myocardial oxygen demand causing chest pain (in patients with coronary artery disease).

Differential Diagnosis of Angina Pectoris

Even though many clinical conditions produce precordial pain following conditions closely resemble angina pectoris and should be differentiated:

1. Costochondritis and myofascial pain
   - Pain is aggravated by movement of the chest and coughing.
   - There may be local costochondral and muscle tenderness over the precordium.
2. Acute pericarditis
   - Acute sharp pain and pain may last for hours.
   - Pain increases on breathing and decreases on sitting up and leaning forward.
3. Reflux oesophagitis
   - Retrosternal/epigastric burning pain.
   - Pain increases on taking food and on assuming recumbent position.
   - Characteristic radiation of pain like angina pectoris.
   - Pain subsides on taking antacids or H2 receptor blockers.

PALPITATION

Palpitation suggests awareness of heartbeat, which may be unpleasant.

Following details should be asked with the patient while analysing the symptom of palpitation

- Onset and duration
- Precipitating factors
- Relieving factors
- Description of palpitation
- Associated symptoms
- Post palpitation diuresis

Onset and Duration

Palpitation which starts and terminates abruptly may be due to:

- Paroxysmal supraventricular tachycardia (PSVT)
- Atrial fibrillation and atrial flutter

Slow onset of palpitation with gradual termination of an attack may be due to:

- Sinus tachycardia
- Anxiety states

Precipitating Factors

- Palpitation on severe exertion is normal.
- Palpitation occurring on minimal exertion may be due to:
  - Anaemia
  - Heart disease and heart failure
  - Atrial fibrillation
  - Thyrotoxicosis

Relieving Factors

- Holding the breath, induction of vomiting decreases the attack of palpitation in patient with PSVT. The

KEY POINTS 3.1

- History of forceful heart beat with throbbing sensation in the neck may be found in patients of aortic regurgitation or conditions associated with wide pulse pressure.
- If the patient feels irregular palpitation, skipped beats it may be suggestive of a rhythm disorder like extra systole or atrial fibrillation.
- Occasionally patient may also give the history of feeling the sensation of the heart as stopped beating. This is due to the compensatory pause of extra systoles.

decrease of palpitation may be due to the increase in vagal tone induced by these manoeuvres.
- Taking rest may relieve palpitation due to cardiac failure and anaemia.

Periodicity and Description of Palpitation
- Recurrent attacks of palpitation with absence of symptoms in between is common with PSVT and intermittent atrial flutter and fibrillation
- History of slow palpitation (due to slow heart rate) is found in patients with complete AV block.

Drug Induced Palpitation
Sympathomimetic amines, caffeine, smoking and vasodilators can cause palpitation. These medications should always be considered while approaching a patient of palpitation.

Associated Symptoms along with Palpitation
Occurrence of syncope following an attack of palpitation may suggest cardiac asystole / Stoke-Adam's attack in a patient with complete heart block.

Stoke-Adam's Attack
Occurs in patients with complete A-V block.

Characteristics
Person looses postural tone.
- Develops pallor and cyanosis
- Becomes flushed on recovery
  Tingling and numbness of hands and feet, feeling of lump in the throat, hyperventilation along with palpitation occurs in patient with anxiety states.

Palpitation may precipitate or aggravate cardiac symptoms like dyspnoea and angina, especially in patient with preexisting heart disease. This may be due to:
1. Increased oxygen demand by the myocardium aggravating the underlying ischaemia causing the chest pain.
2. Increased heart rate causes shortened diastole leading onto decrease filling of the left ventricle and pulmonary congestion leading onto dyspnoea.

Post Palpitation Diuresis
- Occurs usually after an attack of paroxysmal tachycardia.
- Due to the release of atrial natriuretic factor (stored in the atrial myocyte) due to atrial stretch.
- Suppression of ADH secretion may also play a role.
- Causes sodium and water excretion and diuresis.

SYNCOPE

Definition
- Transient loss of consciousness with postural collapse.
- Loss of conciousness lasts for only 30 seconds

Pre-Syncope
A state of dizzy feeling with weakness and tendency to develop loss of postural tone. Consciousness is not lost.

Cardiac Causes of Syncope and Dizziness

Due to abnormal cardiac rhythms
- Bradycardias
  - Carotid sinus syncope
  - Sinus node disease
  - Stoke-Adam's attack
  - Ventricular asystole
- Tachycardias
  - Supraventricular tachycardia
  - Ventricular tachycardias

Due to decreased cardiac output
- Massive myocardial infarction

- Cardiac tamponade
- LV outflow obstruction (severe AS, HOCM)
- RV out flow obstruction (severe PS, massive pulmonary embolism, severe pulmonary hypertension).

Due to decreased venous return to the heart
- Atrial myxoma
- Ball valve thrombus

Differential Diagnosis of Syncope

Syncope which occurs on different body postures
1. On standing for a long time
   - Vasovagal attack (common faint): Note severe pain and emotional stress can also precipitate vasovagal attack.
2. Immediately after getting up from the lying down position:
   - Due to postural hypotension
     Causes: Antihypertensive drugs, autonomic neuropathy, volume depletion
3. Onset of syncope on standing or bending and leaning forward-may also be due to left atrial myxoma and ball valve thrombus.
4. Syncope on movement of the head and neck may indicate
   - Hypersensitive carotid sinus (especially in elderly)
   - Vertebrobasilar insufficiency (may be due to cervical spondylosis).

Syncope occurring at any body position may be due to:
- Complete atrio-ventricular block
- Hypoglycemia
- Hyperventilation disorder.
- Seizure disorder

Syncope on Exertion

Significant symptom of severe aortic stenosis (AS).

Mechanism of Exertional Syncope in Aortic Stenosis

During exertion there will be systemic vasodilatation. In patients with severe aortic stenosis fixed cardiac output causes less blood supply to the brain causing cerebral ischaemia due to peripheral vasodilatation.

Other Related Mechanisms Associated with Syncope in a Patient of Severe Aortic Stenosis
- Transient arrhythmias
- Malfunctioning of baroreceptors

Post Exertional Syncope

Syncope occurs after stopping the exertion.

This is classically found in patients with hypertrophic obstructive cardiomyopathy

Mechanism

After the exertion there will be pooling of blood in the lower limb with decreased venous return to the heart. This leads to decrease LV filling and LV volume causing more severe outflow obstruction in patients with HOCM.

Causes of Syncope Depending on the Onset

Sudden onset of syncope: Stoke-Adam's attack, ventricular tachycardia or may be a seizure disorder.

Gradual Onset of Syncope: *Hyperventilation, Hypoglycemia.*

Following symptoms along with an attack of syncope may suggest the attack may be a seizure disorder rather than syncope
- Clouding of consciousness for a longer time
- Urinary incontinence
- Tongue biting and body injury
- Preceding aura

Significance of Associated Symptoms along with an Attack of Syncope
- Intake of insulin–Hypoglycemia
- Intake of antihypertensives–Postural hypotension
- Occurrence of chest pain–Acute myocardial infarction, pulmonary embolism.
- Occurrence of neurological deficit–Cerebrovascular disturbance
- Sudden getting up after micturition in elderly–Micturition syncope.

Cough with Expectoration

Cough with sputum can occur in patients with cardiac disease under following circumstances
- Dry, irritating nocturnal cough may be present in

patients with pulmonary venous congestion secondary to left heart failure.

- Left heart failure results in pulmonary venous congestion and pulmonary oedema in which patient may bring out pink frothy sputum.
- Attacks of recurrent bronchitis are common with left heart disease (oedematous bronchial mucosa predisposes to recurrent infection).
- Patients with congenital shunt lesions like VSD, PDA, etc. can develop recurrent respiratory infection.

Following Cardiac Conditions may also Present with Cough with Hoarseness of Voice without Upper Respiratory Infection

- Aortic arch aneurysm.
- Enlarged left atrium (severe mitral valve disease-Ortner's syndrome)
- Enlarged pulmonary artery (severe pulmonary HT)

Hoarseness of voice in above conditions is due to the pressure effect on the left recurrent laryngeal nerve.

Haemoptysis

It is the expectoration of blood with or without sputum which can occur in a patient of cardiac disease.

Mechanism of Hemoptysis in a Cardiac Disease

- Pink frothy sputum production in acute pulmonary oedema.
- Rupture of collaterals between bronchial venous and pulmonary system can occur in patients with mitral stenosis causing haemoptysis.
- Oedematous bronchial mucosa in patients with mitral stenosis may predispose to the development of chronic bronchitis with recurrent haemoptysis (winter bronchitis).
- *Pulmonary infarction:* Due to congestive cardiac failure with mitral stenosis (late stages).

Pulmonary Apoplexy

This is the term used for the sudden severe haemoptysis which may be life threatening.

Occurs in patients with early mitral stenosis. Due to the rupture of this walled bronchial veins as a result of sudden rise of left atrial pressure.

CYANOSIS

History of cyanosis is relevant and may be present in the following cardiac conditions

a. Cyanosis beginning in infancy indicates the presence of congenital cardiac malformations with right to left shunt (E.g. Fallot's tetralogy).
b. Cyanosis beginning to appear after 6 weeks of age may be an indication of VSD with slowly progressive right ventricular outflow obstruction.
c. History of cyanosis in a suspected patient of congenital heart disease between the age of 5–20 years indicates reversal of left to right shunt (Eisenmenger's reaction).

Cyanosis predominantly occurring in the tongue suggests central cyanosis and can be due to

a. Cyanotic congenital heart disease
b. Reversal of left to right shunt
c. Left heart failure

Note: Cyanosis may not be present at rest and may appear only on exercise.

Bluish discolouration without cardiac disease can occur in patients with congenital methaemoglobulinaemia.

Arterial or venous obstruction, Raynaud's phenomenon can cause peripheral cyanosis.

Pedal Oedema, Right Hypochondrial Pain and Decreased Urine Output

Presence of swelling of feet along with right hypochondrial pain suggests right ventricular failure (always associated with dyspnoea) in a patient of cardiac disease.

Swelling of Feet (pedal oedema)

Right heart failure causes systemic venous congestion with increased hydrostatic pressure in the lower limb veins. This results in the transudation of fluid causing oedema.

Ankle oedema is more common in ambulatory patients. Bed ridden patients develop sacral edema.

Right Hypochondrial Pain

This is due to the enlarged and congested liver and stretching of its capsule.

Decreased Urine Output

In the presence of cardiac failure due to decreased cardiac output, renal blood flow decreases with decrease in the glomerular filtration rate. This causes decrease of urine output in patients with cardiac failure.

Oedema of Cardiac Cause but not Associated with Cardiac Failure (dyspnoea and orthopnoea are absent)

- Tricuspid regurgitation
- Tricuspid stenosis
- Constrictive pericarditis

Patient with advanced heart failure can also develop generalised oedema of the body (anasarca).

Nocturia (more urine produced during night)

Due to increase of renal blood flow during recumbency and redistribution of intravascular blood volume. May be an early manifestation of heart failure.

Gastrointestinal Symptoms

Patient with right heart failure can have symptoms of anorexia, abdominal fullness and right hypo-chondrial pain. This may be due to abdominal visceral congestion secondary to heart failure.

Occasionally patients of acute myocardial infarction and digitalis effect may also present with nausea and vomiting.

Easy Fatigability

Many patients with chronic heart disease complain of easy fatigability.

It signifies impaired cardiac function and low cardiac output with impaired skeletal muscle blood flow.

Excessive use of diuretics in patients with CCF, severe reduction in the blood pressure and use of beta blockers can also cause severe fatigue in patient with cardiac disease.

Fever

Fever may be the presenting symptom in patients with infective endocarditis, rheumatic fever or other systemic infections with cardiac disease.

Rheumatic Fever

Following history suggests an attack of rheumatic fever

- Usual age group involved 5–15 years.
- Symptoms of sore throat (pharyngitis) 2–3 weeks prior to the onset of joint pain.
- Joint pain, i.e. migrating joint pain that involves major joints.
- Joints will be swollen, red and extremely painful.
- Joint pain will subside within 2–3 weeks (occasionally even without treatment) without residual deformities.

Symptoms of Rheumatic Carditis

Chest pain, dyspnoea and palpitation suggest the presence of carditis.

Occasionally patient may present with symptoms of chorea (Sydenham's chorea) like involuntary movements and higher mental function abnormalities. Chorea may occur as alone manifestation after about 3 months after the initial attack of rheumatic fever.

Symptoms and signs of rheumatic fever respond effectively to acetyl salicylic acid (aspirin).

Infective Endocarditis

Suspect infective endocarditis in any patient who has fever with cardiac murmur especially with recent history of undergoing dental extraction or geni-tourinary instrumentation.

Miscellaneous History

History of diabetes mellitus, hypertension and bronchial asthma should be enquired in all patients with heart disease.

Diabetes mellitus: Predisposes to coronary artery disease and cardiac muscle abnormality.

Hypertension: Can cause LVH, cardiac failure, coronary artery disease and aortic valve disease.

Bronchial asthma: Beta blockers should be

cautiously administered in a patient of bronchial asthma with hypertension. It may precipitate bronchospasm.

Past History

1. *Rheumatic fever:* Enquire about the previous illness suggestive of rheumatic fever or rheumatic chorea. 50% of patients with rheumatic valvular disease may not give the history of rheumatic fever, as it would have been subclinical.
2. Recurrent attacks of lower respiratory infections since childhood is common in adults with left to right intracardiac shunts.
3. Detection of murmur at school going age may be an indication of presence of cardiac lesion since childhood. (example: congenital shunt lesions-VSD, PDA)
4. Enquire about the recent dental extraction or genitourinary instrumentation in patients with cardiac lesion and fever to rule out the possibility of infective endocarditis.
5. Previous history of angina should be elicited in patients presenting with myocardial infarction or CCF.
6. Previous history of diabetes mellitus and Hypertension should be enquired because of their importance in causing coronary artery disease and heart failure.
7. Enquire attacks of cyanotic spells and squatting after exertion which are common in patients with Fallot's Tetralogy.

Squatting After Exertion

Child assumes squatting position after exertion. Squatting results in increased peripheral vascular resistance and decreased venous return and decreased right to left shunt and decrease of dyspnoea.

Cyanotic Spells

Child becomes bluish, hyperventilates and may develop syncope and convulsion usually after feeding or crying. Due to decreased pulmonary blood flow and increased right to left shunt.

Family History

Following cardiac diseases can affect more than one family member. Enquire the patient about these cardiac diseases in other family members.

- Essential hypertension and hypertensive heart disease.
- Coronary artery disease
- Congenital heart disease
- Rheumatic fever
- Rheumatic fever can manifest in more than one members of a family because of transmission of streptococci due to over crowding or close contact.
- Sudden death of a first degree relative in a family-one should search for causes like hypertrophic obstructive cardiomyopathy, prolonged QT interval and coronary artery disease in other close family members.
- Marfan's syndrome can cause aortic regurgitation and dissecting aneurysm of aorta and can run in the family.
- Enquire also about the history of murmurs, cyanosis in other family members in a suspected patient of congenital heart disease.

Personal History

Appetite loss and fullness of the epigastrium are common in patients with CCF and on digitalis therapy.

Weight loss: Severe weight loss is common in patients with chronic heart failure.

Sleep: Sleep may be disturbed due to PND and Orthopnea in patients with cardiac failure.

Smoking: Enquire the duration and amount of cigarette smoking. Smoking is a significant risk factor for coronary artery disease.

Alcoholism: Enquire the duration and the amount of alcohol consumption. Alcohol in large amounts can cause Cardiomyopathy, CCF and cardiac arrhythmias.

Urine output: Amount of urine passed should be enquired in all patients with cardiac disease (as discussed earlier).

Menstrual History and Previous Pregnancies

Menstrual flow may be decreased in female patients with chronic CCF.

Pregnancy and Heart Disease

Detailed history of previous pregnancies should be elicited in a female patient with cardiac disease.

Altered Hemodynamics during Pregnancy and its effect on Cardiac Function

- Blood volume increases rapidly during pregnancy starting from 6th week of gestation up to mid-pregnancy. Thereafter increase of blood volume occurs in a steady manner.
- Stress, labour pain and contractions of uterus alter haemodynamics during labour and delivery.
- Immediately after delivery excess venous blood will be shifted to systemic circulation. Contraction of empty uterus and release of inferior venacaval compression (compressed by foetus) will also add to the blood volume.
- Patients with significant cardiac disease may not tolerate the pregnancy because of the increase blood volume and altered haemodynamics and can develop cardiac failure.

Treatment History

- Patient with previous attack of rheumatic fever may be taking long acting penicillin (benzathine penicillin) once in 3 weeks suggesting the prophylaxis against rheumatic fever.
2. Taking sublingual nitrates may indirectly indicate the presence of ischaemic heart disease.
3. Detailed enquiry should be made about anti-hypertensive medications. These drugs may produce postural hypotension, fatigability and palpitation (due to tachycardia).
4. Drugs like sympathomimetics and digoxin can induce cardiac arrhythmias and beta-blockers may precipitate an attack of cardiac failure in susceptible patients.
5. Antineoplastic drugs like doxorubicin, cyclophosphamide can also induce LV dysfunction.

EXAMINATION OF CARDIOVASCULAR SYSTEM

Scheme of Examination

General Examination
- Build
- Nourishment
- Pallor
- Cyanosis
- Clubbing
- Jaundice
- Pedal edema
- Lymphadenopathy

External Markers of Cardiac Disease
- Examination of face
- Eyes
- Skin and mucosa
- Extremities

Vital Signs
- Pulse
- Blood pressure
- Respiratory rate
- Temperature

Examination of the Peripheral Cardiovascular System
Radial pulse:
- Rate
- Rhythm
- Volume
- Character
- Condition of vessel wall

Examination of
- The carotids
- Other peripheral pulses
- Jugular venous pulse and pressure
- Peripheral signs of wide pulse pressure (in relevant situations)
- Peripheral signs of infective endocarditis
- Peripheral signs of rheumatic fever

Examination of the Precordium

Inspection
- Precordial bulge
- Position of the apical impulse
- Pulsation's in the left parasternal region, 2nd left intercostal space, 2nd right intercostal space, epigastric pulsation, suprasternal pulsation.
- Engorged veins over the chest
- Spine (kyphoscoliosis)

Palpation
- Apical impulse-Position and character
- Left parasternal heave
- Palpation of epigastric pulsation
- Thrills
- Palpable sounds

Percussion
- Right cardiac border
- Left cardiac border
- Left and right 2nd intercostal space

Auscultation
Mitral, tricuspid, aortic, pulmonary and other additional areas for
- 1st and 2nd heart sounds
- Additional sounds
- Murmurs

Examination of Other Systems
- Respiratory system
- Gastrointestinal tract
- Central nervous system
- Musculoskeletal, endocrine, etc. (if necessary)

Examination of Cardiovascular System

Build
Short stature and growth retardation can occur in children with severe congenital heart disease.

Tall Stature

Marfan's habitus - Associated with aortic regurgitation, dissecting aneurysm of aorta and MVP

Features of Marfan's Syndrome
- Long extremities
- Arm span more than the total height
- Longer lower segment than the upper segment
- Arachnodactyly (long, spider leg like fingers)
- High arched palate
- Iridodonesis (due to subluxation of lens)
- Abnormal metacarpal index (see general physical examination)

Nourishment

Severe emaciation can occur in severe chronic heart failure due to
1. Excess metabolic demand
2. Intestinal congestion causing decreased nutrient absorption.
3. Loss of appetite, nausea and vomiting occurs due to hepatic congestion or digoxin therapy.
4. Protein losing enteropathy associated with severe right heart failure.
5. Excess concentration of tumor necrosis factor.

Obesity (Predominantly abdominal) can be associated with coronary artery disease (see general physical examination).

Examination of Face
Following features may be indicative of underlying cardiac abnormality while examining the face. Abnormalities

Elfin facies: Receding jaw, flarred nostrils, pointed ears

Condition associated: Supravalvular aortic stenosis.
Mitral facies: Malar flush and pinkish purple

Mitral stenosis with decreased cardiac patches over the cheek output and systemic vasoconstriction.

High Arched Palate: Marfan's syndrome.

Ear
Presence of crease in the pinna of the ear is associated with increased incidence of coronary artery disease.

Eyes
Exophthalmos associated with thyroid heart disease.

Blue Sclera
Osteogenesis imperfecta with aortic regurgitation.

Ophthalmic Fundus
Look for
* Arterosclerotic changes
* Hypertensive retinopathy
* Roth's spots (of infective endocarditis)
* Arterial pulsations in AR
* Cork screw arteries — Coarctation of aorta.

Skin and Mucus Membranes
Look for
* Cyanosis, jaundice
* Bronze pigmentation (haemochromatosis with cardiomyopathy)
* *Xanthomas:* Fat filled nodules found in the skin, tendon or soft tissues, associated with early coronary Atherosclerosis (see general physical examination).
* *Xanthelasma:* Deposition of lipid in the skin of eye lids (upper and lower eye lids) (may be associated with hyperlipidemia).

Extremities
Marfan's syndrome: Arachnodactyly with long extremities
Turner's syndrome:
* Short stature, cubitus valgus, medial deviation of extended forearm.
* Associated cardiac condition–Coarctation of aorta
Holt Oram's syndrome
* Thumb with an extra phalanx
* Thumb lies in the same plane as other fingers
* Radius and ulna may be deformed
* Associated cardiac condition-ASD

General examination also includes the following signs:

Clubbing
Cardiac Causes
* Cyanotic congenital heart disease
* Reversal of left to right shunt
* Infective endocarditis

Pallor
Severe anaemia may be associated with
* Chronic CCF
* Infective endocarditis

Severe anemia can itself cause cardiac failure or aggravates the underlying heart disease.

Patient with cyanotic congenital heart disease may have polycythemia with suffused conjunctiva.

Cyanosis
Central cyanosis occurs in the following cardiac conditions
* Cyanotic congenital heart disease
* Reversal of left to right shunt
* Intra pulmonary right to left shunt
* Pulmonary edema (left heart failure)
Peripheral cyanosis occurs in
* Congestive cardiac failure
* Peripheral vascular disease

Differential Cyanosis
Feet and toes are blue but hands and fingers are not cyanosed, e.g. PDA with pulmonary hypertension with reversal of shunt.

Reverse Differential Cyanosis
Fingers are more cyanosed than toes, e.g. transposition of great vessels with pulmonary hypertension with preductal coarctation with reversed flow through PDA.

Cyanotic congenital heart disease may be associated with hypertrophic pulmonary osteoarthropathy.

Jaundice
Following cardiac conditions may be associated with jaundice.
* Congestive cardiac failure with congestive hepatomegaly
* Cardiac cirrhosis
* Pulmonary infarction

Pedal Oedema
Pitting oedema of the feet can occur in
* Congestive cardiac failure
* Constrictive pericarditis
* Tricuspid valve disease

Lymphadenopathy
Conditions associated with generalised lymphadenopathy may involve the cardiovascular system, e.g. lymphoma, SLE, etc.

Vital signs
- Pulse rate, rhythm, volume, character and condition of the vessel wall
- Blood pressure
- Respiratory rate
- Temperature

SYSTEMIC EXAMINATION OF CARDIOVASCULAR SYSTEM

Peripheral Vascular System

Pulse
Definition: Waveform felt regularly over an artery due to expansion and elongation of the arterial walls passively produced by pressure changes during ventricular systole and diastole.

Radial Pulse (Fig. 3.1)
Compress the vessel against the lower end of the radius and feel the vessel with tips of fingers just lateral to the tendon of flexor carpi radialis.

Felt 80 milliseconds after cardiac systole.

Brachial Artery
Feel the vessel immediately medial to the tendon of Biceps by compressing the vessel against the humerus.

Felt 60 milliseconds after the cardiac systole.

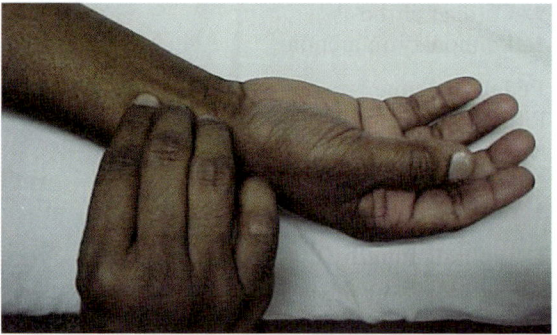

Fig. 3.1 Palpation of radial pulse at wrist

Carotid Artery
Press the thumb against the transverse process of cervical vertebra gently backwards. Feel the vessel at the medial border of the sternomastoid at the level of larynx.

Left thumb is used for right carotid and vice versa.

Both carotids should not be palpated simultaneously.

Careful palpation is required in patients with carotid atheroma or hypersensitive carotid sinus.

Carotid pulse is felt 30 miliseconds after the cardiac systole.

Importance of Carotid Examination in Cardiac Disease
Carotid pulse should be examined for
- Presence of thrill–associated with valvular aortic stenosis
- Character–slow upstroke with severe aortic stenosis
- Dancing carotids–severe aortic regurgitation
- Jerky carotids–obstructive cardiomyopathy.

Femoral Artery
Feel the artery against the femur at a point midway between the iliac crest and the pubic ramus. Felt 75 milliseconds after the cardiac systole.

Popliteal Artery
Feel the artery deep in the popliteal fossa with the fingertips pressed when the patient's knee is slightly flexed.

Posterior Tibial
Feel the artery behind the medial malleolus when the patient's foot is partially dorsiflexed.

Dorsalis Pedis (Fig. 3.2)

Palpate on the dorsum of the foot lateral to the tendon of extensor hallusis by compressing against the tarsal bones.

Following parameters should be recorded while feeling for the pulse
- Rate
- Rhythm
- Volume

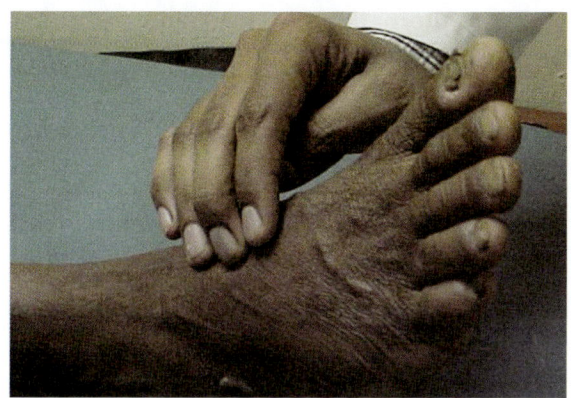

Fig. 3.2 Palpation for dorsalis pedis artery pulsation

Table 3.2 Difference between multiple ectopics and atrial fibrillation

Ectopics	Atrial fibrillation
Occasionally irregular	Irregularly irregular.
Pulse apex deficit minimum	Pulse deficit large.
Exercise abolishes ectopics	Exercise will not abolish irregularity.
'a' wave is present in the JVP	'a' wave is absent in the JVP.

- Character
- Condition of the vessel wall

Rate: Normal rate–60 to 100 /minutes. Count at least for 30 seconds

Abnormalities of the pulse rate

a. Bradycardia: Rate < 60/min
Causes
1. Physiological–Athletes
2. Pathological–Complete AV block, Beta-Blocker therapy, hypothyroidism.

b. Tachycardia : Rate > 100/min
Causes
1. Physiological–Exercise, anxiety
2. Pathological–Supraventricular tachycardia, tachyarrythmias, thyrotoxicosis, sympathomimetic drug therapy, etc.

Rhythm

Normal: regular sinus rhythm.
Abnormal: irregular rhythm

Sinus Arrhythmia
Physiological acceleration of heart rate during inspiration and slowing at the beginning of expiration. Common in young adults with increased vagal tone.

Sinus arrhythmia is not seen in patients with CCF and autonomic neuropathy.

Abnormal Rhythms (Table 3.2)

Irregularly irregular
- In atrial fibrillation
- Extrasystoles (occasionally irregular)
- Paroxysmal atrial tachycardia and atrial flutter with varying block.

Regularly irregular pulse
- Pulsus bigeminus
- Pulsus trigeminus
- Paroxysmal atrial tachycardia and atrial flutter with fixed block.

Apex Pulse Deficit in Atrial Fibrillation

Count the pulse rate and heart rate for full one minute simultaneously. Note the difference between the heart rate and the pulse rate. In patients with atrial fibrillation heart rate will be significantly more than the pulse rate.

Mechanism of Pulse Deficit
- There will be varying length of the LV diastole in patients with atrial fibrillation, if there is shorter diastole (less of LV filling producing decreased stroke volume). Aortic pulse will be weak and may not be felt in the peripheral pulse.
- Longer diastole will lead onto increased LV filling with increased stroke volume resulting in stronger ventricular contraction causing peripheral pulse to be felt. This causes difference in the heart rate and the pulse rate causing pulse deficit.
- Varying length of the diastole is due to the varying refractory period of the AV node.

Tracing of a Normal Pulse Wave (Fig. 3.3)

p- percussion wave

n- dicrotic notch

d- dicrotic wave

p- Percussion wave due to rapid rise of ventricular pressure and increased velocity of blood ejected from the ventricle.

n- A sharp downward deflection related to the fall of aortic pressure due to backward flow of blood

D- Dicrotic wave, i.e. small rise of pulse wave due to return of blood column due to closure of semilunar valves and also due to reflected waves from the periphery.

Special Characters of Pulse

1. Volume alteration in the pulse, i.e.
   a. Anacrotic pulse, alternans pulse
   b. Bisferien's
   c. Collapsing
   d. Dicroticus
   e. Paradoxus
   f. Parvus et tardus
2. Rhythm alteration in the pulse, i.e. irregularly irregular pulse, pulsus bigeminus, pulsus trigeminus.

Pulse Volume

Represents the degree of amplitude (expansion) of the pulse: rough guide to indicate the stroke volume.

Volume Alternations in the Pulse

High volume pulse (bounding), e.g. fever, anemia, AR, MR (Fig. 3.4).

Low volume pulse: State of shock, CCF and severe aortic stenosis (Fig. 3.5).

Pulsus parvus et tardus: Low volume pulse with slow peaking, e.g. aortic stenosis. Signifies fixed severe obstruction to the aortic outflow. Best appreciated in the carotids.

Collapsing pulse (Corrigan's or water hammer pulse): Rapid upstroke followed by precipitous fall (Down stroke) of the pulse and made prominent by raising the patient's arm (Fig. 3.6).

Water hammer effect: Extremely rapid and forceful upstroke of pulse, e.g. of collapsing pulse are severe AR, PDA, and large arteriovenous communication.

Mechanism of Rapid Upstroke

It is due to
- Greatly increased systolic pressure.
- Large LV stroke volume ejected into the empty arterial system.

Rapid Down Stroke

- Due to diastolic leak back in to the left ventricle with sudden fall of aortic pressure.
- Peripheral vasodilatation and decreased peripheral resistance with rapid peripheral run off of blood.

Note
- Peripheral resistance may also decrease due to stretch of carotid and aortic sinus due to increased stroke volume.

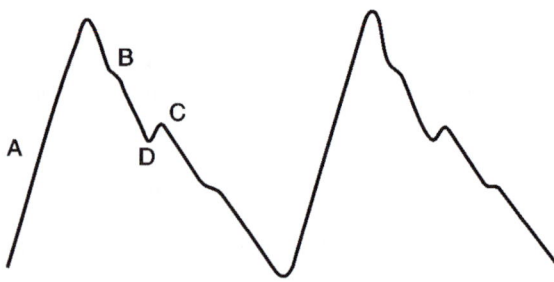

A = Primary wave B = Pre-dicrotic wave
C = Dicrotic wave D= Dicrotic notch

Fig. 3.3 Radial pulse tracing

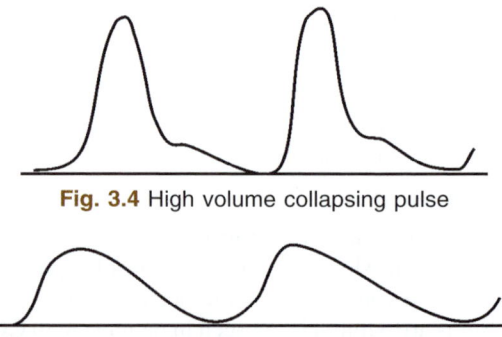

Fig. 3.4 High volume collapsing pulse

Fig. 3.5 Low volume slow rising pulse

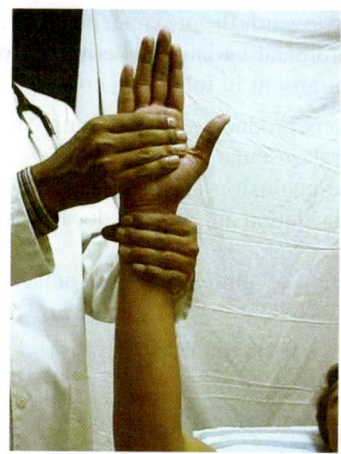

Fig. 3.6 Palpation of collapsing pulse

Note: Patients of AR with CCF will have high diastolic pressure due to increased peripheral resistance.

Importance of raising the arm while detecting the collapsing pulse:

On raising the arm, peripheral run off is better appreciated may be due to the effect of gravity.

Bisfereins Pulse (Fig. 3.7)

Pulse with 2 peaks (in systolic upstroke) separated by a dip (mid systolic)

For example, in moderate AS with severe AR and in severe aortic regurgitation

Best appreciated in the carotids.

Anacrotic Pulse

Slow raising pulse, peaking late in systole and will have a notch on the upstroke of carotid pulse 'Anacrotic notch'. For example, patient with severe aortic out flow obstruction-severe AS.

Dicrotic Pulse

- Pulse with two peaks, one in systole and other one in diastole.
- Peak occurring in diastole is due to increased and palpable dicrotic wave occurring after the 2nd heart sound .
- Best felt in the carotids.
- Occurs in conditions with low cardiac output, soft elastic aorta and a high peripheral vascular resistance.

For example, dilated cardiomyopathy and severe CCF, cardiac tamponade, young febrile patient without any other abnormality, hypovolemic shock.

Pulsus Alternans (Fig. 3.8)

Alternating large and small beats due to alternating strong and weak cardiac contractions.

Occurs with regular rhythm and better appreciated with sphygmomanometer.

Better felt in peripheral vessels (brachial/ radial) it is ideal to hold the breath while checking for pulsus alternans.

E.g. Severe left ventricular failure.

PULSUS PARADOXUS

Felt as decrease in the pulse volume during normal inspiration due to accentuated fall in inspiratory systolic pressure.

For example, cardiac tamponade, constrictive pericarditis, severe air flow obstruction.

Normally there is inspiratory decrease of systolic pressure of around 10 mm Hg.

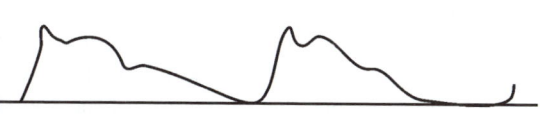

Fig. 3.7 Bisferiens pulse

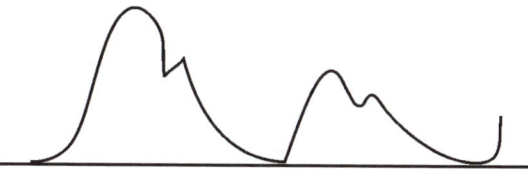

Fig. 3.8 Pulses alternans

In conditions like cardiac tamponade, severe air flow obstruction there is accentuated fall of systolic arterial pressure during inspiration.

This causes decrease of pulse volume or disappearance of pulse during inspiration.

Alterations in the Rhythm of Pulse

Pulsus Bigeminus (Fig. 3.9)
Premature ventricular contraction occurring after each normal beat.

Premature beat is always followed by a short interval (pause), e.g. digitalis toxicity.

Delay in the Femoral Pulse (radiofemoral delay)
Delayed femoral pulse when compared to the appearance of right radial pulse occurs in a patient of coarctation of aorta.

Delay of radial pulse: Thoracic outlet obstruction, aorto arteritis (involving the aortic arch).

Condition of Vessel Wall
- Estimated by applying pressure with the fingertips over the artery or to roll the artery.
- Normal artery is not palpable (vessel wall merges with the surrounding tissues).
- In atherosclerosis the artery can be palpated and rolled with the fingers.

Locomotor Brachii
- Dancing movement of thickened and tortuous brachial artery (arm is flexed at the elbow around 110° to make it easily visible).
- Indicates thickened vessel wall (e.g. atherosclerosis)

Importance of Examination of Peripheral Pulses in a Cardiac Disease
All peripheral pulses should be palpated. Start the palpation from peripheral pulse like dorsalis pedis

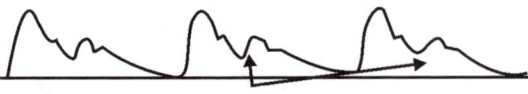

Fig. 3.9 Pulses bigeminus

and proceed towards the proximal pulses. Apart from certain anatomical variations. Peripheral pulse may be feeble or absent in following conditions.

1. Conditions producing hypovolemic shock
2. Peripheral vascular disease
3. Embolic occlusion arising from the heart, e.g. Atrial fibrillation, infective endocarditis, left atrial myxoma
4. Coarctation of aorta-lower limb pulses are feeble

BLOOD PRESSURE

Definition
Lateral pressure exerted by the blood on the vessel walls while flowing through it.
Measurement of blood pressure by cuff method

BP Cuff Measurement

For the Upper Limb
In adults, width 12 cms (should cover the 2/3 of the arm). Length of the cuff is 25 cms. Cuff width in obese is 8 inches. Cuff width for the lower limb on adults is 18 cms.

Recording of Blood Pressure by Cuff Method
- Sphygmomanometer and observer's eye should be at the same level of the cuff on the patient's arm.
- Apply the cuff with its lower border 1 inch above the cubital fossa.
- Inflate the cuff to a pressure of 20–30 mm Hg above the level at which the radial pulse disappears. Place the stethoscope over the brachial artery.
- Reduce the cuff pressure 3 mm of Hg every second until the Ist sound is heard over the stethoscope (Korotkoff sound). Radial pulse becomes palpable. This indicates systolic pressure.
- Deflate the cuff until the sounds become faint (muffled) (4th phase of Korotkoff sound).
  Continue to reduce the pressure until the sound disappears (5th phase of Korotkoff sounds).

Diastolic Blood Pressure

The level of the pressure at which the Korotkoff's sound disappear is taken as diastolic BP.

- If the Korotkoff sounds do not disappear even at zero mm of Hg, then muffling of sounds (4th phase of Korotkoff) can be taken as diastolic BP. This is possible in conditions with extremely low diastolic BP such as severe AR.
- It is advisable to take 3 recordings (in basal conditions) a week apart to avoid anxiety associated hypertension (white coat hypertension) before defining the person as having hypertension.

If the diastolic BP increases on standing it is suggestive of essential hypertension.

If the systolic BP decreases on standing it may be suggestive of secondary hypertension (not on anti hypertensive medication).

Postural hypotension can occur in patients with Autonomic neuropathy or in patients on anti-hypertensive drugs.

BP Recording in Patients with Atrial Fibrillation (AF)

Multiple recordings of BP and average of that are advisable in patients with atrial fibrillation.

Systolic pressure in a patient of AF: Level of blood pressure at which majority of Korotkoff sounds appear.

Diastolic pressure in a patient of AF: Level of blood pressure at which most of Korotkoff sounds disappear.

Normal Blood Pressure

Systolic blood pressure: 100–140 mm of Hg
Diastolic: 60–90 mm of Hg
Mean blood pressure: Diastolic BP+1/3 of pulse pressure. Represents tissue perfusion pressure.

Indications for Recording Lower Limb BP

1. If the pulse pressure is wide.
2. If the lower limb pulses are feeble

Recording of Lower Limb Blood Pressure

- Patient is lying on his abdomsen, BP cuff is applied above the knee around the thigh (cuff size 18 cm width).
- Auscultate over the popliteal artery in the same way as for recording of upper limb blood pressure.
- Normally lower limb systolic BP is 10–20 mm of Hg higher than the upper limb (diastolic is identical).

Importance of recording lower limb blood pressure

Lower limb blood pressure is decreased in patients with

1. Coarctation of aorta
2. Aortoarteritis of the abdominal aorta
3. Aortic dissection

Lower limb systolic BP will be more than upper limb by 20 mm of Hg or more in patients with severe AR (Hill's sign).

Difference in the Blood Pressure in the Upper Limb

1. Supravalvular aortic stenosis-BP is higher on the right upper limb.
2. Subclavian steal syndrome-BP is reduced on the affected side.

White coat hypertension: Clinical or hospital recording of BP is higher than home recording.

Border line hypertension: Initial diastolic blood pressure exceeds 90 mm of Hg, but repeated recordings will be below this level. Annual checking of blood pressure is required.

Systolic hypertension: Usually defined as systolic blood pressure more than 140 mm of Hg.

Causes
- Aortic regurgitation
- AV fistula
- Thyrotoxicosis
- Hyperkinetic circulation
- Beri beri
- Arteriosclerosis of aorta
- Patent ductus arteriosus

Accelerated Hypertension

Sudden rise of blood pressure above the previous recordings with fundal haemorrhages but without papilloedema.

Malignant Hypertension

Recording of diastolic blood pressure above 140 mm Hg associated with papilloedema.

Pseudo Hypertension
- Condition characterised by high systolic and diastolic or mean BP measured indirectly by cuff method.
- Direct intra-arterial recording of blood pressure is normal.
- There is no evidence of hypertension induced target organ involvement (like retina, heart or kidney).
- It is due to sclerosis of arteries, e.g. in elderly person, conditions like Monckeberg's arteriosclerosis.

Demonstration of Pseudohypertension

Inflate the BP cuff above the systolic pressure until the radial pulse has disappeared.

In patients with thickened arteries, radial/brachial artery will be felt even after the disappearance of pulse.

JUGULAR VENOUS PULSE AND PRESSURE (JVP)

Jugularvenous pulse and pressure represents the pressure changes within the right atrium

Clinical Aspects of JVP

Internal jugular vein on the right side is preferred for examination of JVP as it is straighter than the left.

External jugular vein can also show the pulsations but less reliable than the internal jugular vein because of the following reasons.
1. It passes through fascial planes and extrinsic compression can alter with the blood flow.
2. Because of the presence of venous valves, transmission of pressure can be interfered in the external jugular vein.

Note: Internal jugular pulse should not be confused with the carotid pulsation.

Differentiating Features Between JVP and Carotid Pulse (Table 3.3)

Normal Wave Pattern of Jugular Venous Pulse (Fig. 3.10)

Three positive waves (due to increase of pressure in the atrium)

a wave due to atrial systole

c wave due to movement of tricuspid valve into the right atrium during ventricular systole. Carotid pulsation impact on the jugular vein may also contribute)

v wave due to venous filling of right atrium when the tricuspid valve is closed (phase of ventricular systole)

Two negative waves (due to decrease of pressure in the atrium)

X descent due to atrial relaxation and due to downward movement of the tricuspid valve during early right ventricular systole.

Y descent due to tricuspid valve opening with right atrial pressure decrease. 'A' wave usually precedes the carotid up stroke and 'v' wave follows it. So waves of the JVP are timed with carotid upstroke.

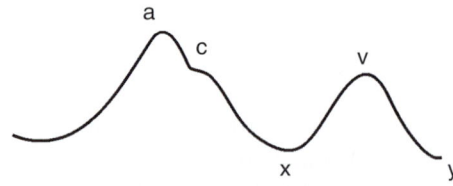

Fig. 3.10 Normal JVP

Table 3.3 Differentiating features between JVP and carotid pulse

	JVP pulse	Carotid pulse
Effect of posture	Varies with posture	Does not change
Effect of respiration	Changes with respiration	Does not change
Wave form	Present and better visible	Single up stroke better felt
Form of pulsation	Predominantly inwards	Predominantly outwards
Effect of finger pressure at the root of the neck	Abolishes the pulsation	No change and cannot be obliterated.

Significance of Waves in the JVP

Prominent (giant) 'a' wave represents forceful contraction of right atrium.

Causes
a. Against stiff right ventricle
  • RVH secondary to any cause
  • Pulmonary hypertension
  • Pulmonary stenosis
b. Tricuspid stenosis

Prominent V wave due to venous filling of right atrium, e.g. tricuspid regurgitation.

Prominent X descent due to ASD, RV volume overload, constrictive pericarditis

Rapid Y descent due to constrictive pericarditis, tricuspid regurgitation.

Absence of a wave due to atrial fibrillation

Cannon 'a' wave produced when the right atrium contracts against a closed tricuspid valve, e.g. regular cannon wave due to atrial flutter with fixed block, junctional rhythm.

Irregular cannon wave due to complete heart block, premature ventricular beats.

Method of Examination of JVP
Patient should be comfortably lying in the bed at 45° position (for more effective examination 45° position is ideal. Keep the patient at 90° straight if venous pressure is very high).
• Neck can be slightly turned to the left side.
• Shine the torch tangentially across the neck
• Observe the lower part of the neck (at the medial border of the sternomastoid).
• Simultaneous palpation of the left carotid artery helps to differentiate between venous and arterial pulsations.
• Look for the wave forms

Measurement of Jugular Venous Pressure
(Fig. 3.11)

Patient is at 45° position

1. Sternal angle is used as the reference point because the right atrium lies approximately 5 cms below the sternal angle at whatever body position.

2. Venous pressure (indirectly reflecting JVP) is measured from the center of right atrium. Measure the vertical distance between the top of venous column and the level of the sternal angle. Normal distance is around 3–4 cm (cms of blood) which represents the normal jugular venous pressure.

Normal central venous pressure is equal to 4 cm + 5 cm (depth of center of right atrium from the sternal angle) = around 9 cm.

JVP is said to be raised, if it is above 4 cm from the sternal angle.

Commonest cause of JVP raise is right sided cardiac failure.

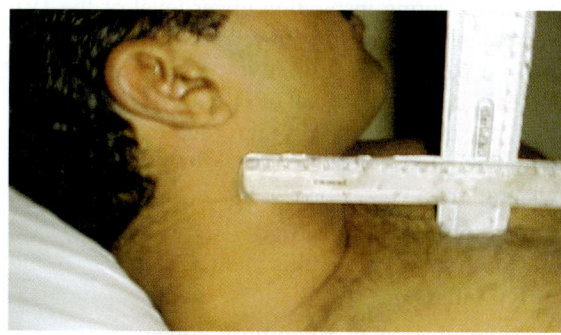

Fig. 3.11 Measurement of JVP

Abdominal jugular reflux (can be conventionally called hepatojugular reflux)

Helpful in detecting early right ventricular failure in patients who have normal JVP (at rest).

Technique of Elicitation

Apply firm pressure with the palm to the right upper quadrant of the abdomen for 10–30 seconds while patient is breathing normally.

Observe the jugular vein for any change in the level of pulsation.

Normally there is no significant change in the JVP.
Positive test: In early right ventricular failure, there will be sustained increase in the upper level of venous pulsation (more than 4 cm). Can also be positive in a patient of tricuspid regurgitation. This test is negative in patients with Hepatic outflow obstruction.

Causes of JVP Raise

1. Cardiac causes: Right ventricular failure. pericardial diseases, pericardial effusion. Constrictive pericarditis.
2. Congested states (no cardiac failure) volume overload conditions.
3. Non cardiac cause: Superior vena caval obstruction (waveforms are absent into the JVP).

Note: Unilateral raise of JVP can occur in innominate vein occlusion.

Massive ascites and pleural effusion can also raise JVP.

Kussmaul's Sign

Normally during inspiration upper level of the JVP decreases with negative intrathoracic pressure.

In a patient of constrictive pericarditis, there is increase in the upper level of JVP during inspiration. This is called Kussmaul's sign (due to interference with the blood flow to the right atrium during inspiration).

Causes of Kussmaul's Sign

- Constrictive pericarditis and CCF
- RV infarction

Peripheral signs of Rheumatic Fever

1. *Arthritis:* Major joints, swollen, warm, tender.
2. *Erythema marginatum:* Red macular lesions with central pallor, non itching and round margins found on trunk and proximal extremities.
3. *Subcutaneous nodules:* Nodule size is 0.5–2 cms, non tender and firm. Found over the extensor surfaces of knee, elbow and occiput.

Jaccoud's Arthritis

This occurs due to repeated attacks of rheumatic fever. Patient may develop marked ulnar deviation of the metacarpophalangeal joints due to subluxation.

In patients with collapsing pulse and wide pulse pressure, it is essential to look for other peripheral signs, e.g. in a patient of severe chronic AR.

Peripheral Signs of Chronic Severe AR

1. Collapsing pulse (water hammer or Corrigan's pulse) already discussed.
2. *Corrigan's sign:* Dancing carotids (prominent carotid pulsation in the neck).
3. *Demusset's sign:* Nodding of head with each systolic pulsation.
4. *Quincke's sign:* Apply firm pressure to the nail tip.
   - Observe for alternate flushing and blanching of the nail bed.
5. *Pistol shot sounds (Traube's sign):* Systolic sound is heard over the femorals when the stethoscope is placed on it.
6. *Duroziez's sign:* Systolic and diastolic murmur is heard over the femoral artery.
   Proximal compression of the artery - systolic murmur is heard.
   Distal compression of the artery - diastolic murmur is heard.
7. *Hill's sign:* Systolic pressure in the lower limb is more than the upper limb by more than 20 mm of Hg. (Higher the pressure difference - more severe the AR).
8. *Other less prominent signs*
   - Pulsation of uvula - Müller's sign
   - Pulsation of the retinal artery -Becker's sign
   - Alternate blanching and flushing of face- light house sign

- Pulsation of liver - Rosenbach's sign
- Pulsation of spleen - Gerhardt's sign

Peripheral Signs of Endocarditis

In all patients with fever and underlying cardiac lesion check for the peripheral signs of infective endocarditis. These signs may not be present in all cases of endocarditis.

Signs of Endocarditis

1. Fever
2. Pallor
3. Clubbing
4. Petechael haemorrhages
   Evidence of septic embolisation
5. Splinter haemorrhage
   - At the nail bed of fingers and toes
   - Flame shaped or dark linear streaks
6. *Osler's nodes:* Tender subcutaneous nodules at pulp of fingers. May be purplish red.
7. *Janeway lesion:* Haemorrhagic or reddish macular lesions. Non tender lesions, over palms and soles.
8. *Roth spots:* Pale centered oval haemorrhagic spots in the retina.
   Evidence of systemic embolisation and spleno-megaly are other features of endocarditis.

EXAMINATION OF PRECORDIUM

Precordium: Area or part of the anterior chest wall which overlies the cardia (heart).

Important Anatomical Landmarks

1. Mid-clavicular line: Draw a line vertically downwards from the mid point which is in between the suprasternal notch and tip of acromion.
2. Anterior, mid and posterior axillary lines: Draw vertical lines downwards along the anterior, mid and posterior axillary borders respectively.
   Inspection and palpation can be suitably combined while examining the precordium.
   It is considered separately here, in order to maintain the schematic presentation.

INSPECTION

Examiner can stand at the side of the bed or at the foot end for inspecting the precordium.

Precordial Shape

a. *Bulge (prominence):* Suggests cardiac enlargement before the occurrence of puberty.
b. *Pectus excavatum (sternal depression):* Pectus excavatum may be associated with ejection systolic murmur without any organic cardiac abnormality.
c. *Shield chest:* Present in patients with Turner's and Noonan's syndromes.

Characteristics of shield chest: Nipples are widely placed. Angle between the manubrium and body of the sternum is more than normal.

Note: Well-built muscular chest with less developed lower extremities can be present in patients with coarctation of aorta.

APICAL IMPULSE

Definition

Outermost and lowermost definite cardiac impulse seen or felt.

Normal Apical Impulse

Seen when the patient lies supine or with the upper part of the body inclined to 30°. If not localized in supine position then patient can be made to sit and stoop forward (or patient laterally rotated to left).

Normal position: Left 5th intercostal space, 1cm medial to the left mid clavicular line or 9 cm lateral to the mid sternal line on the left side.

Pulsations Over the Precordium

Look for the following pulsations over the precordium.

1. Left parasternal
2. Left 2nd space
3. Right 2nd space
4. Epigastric
5. Suprasternal pulsation
   Details of these pulsations will be discussed under palpation.

Whole of Precordium may Pulsate Under the Following Conditions
- Severe aortic or mitral regurgitation
- ASD, VSD, PDA
- Hyperkinetic states (e.g. thyrotoxicosis)

Note: Conditions like Fallot's tetralogy is associated with relatively quiet precordium.

SCAR MARK

Observe for midline scar over the sternum
- Indicative of previous open cardiac surgery like coronary bypass graft or valve replacement.
- Left inframammary scar indicative of closed mitral valvotomy done for mitral stenosis.

Spine: Look for kyphoscoliosis
- Severe kyphoscoliosis may lead to hypoxia and pulmonary hypertension.

PALPATION OF THE PRECORDIUM

Apical impulse (Figs 3.12a and b)

Palpation of Apical Impulse
- Patient is in the supine or sitting up position.
- Place the right hand over the left chest wall with the middle finger in the 5th intercostal space with its tip to locate the apex.
- Ideally patient should not be turned to the left lateral side for locating the apex, as cardia moves to a variable extent (around 0.5 to 1 cm) on turning to the left.

Normal Apex

- Palpating the cardiac apex for the character (patient is in the left lateral position).
Normal apex is in the 5th intercostal space 1 cm medial to left MCL felt as a gentle tap and it is about 1cm in diameter (may be up to 2.5 cm) and persists only up to 1/3 of systole.
- Apical impulse which is outside 10 cm to the left from the mid sternal line is suggestive of cardiomegaly.

KEY POINTS 3.4
- Use fingertips for palpating sounds, distal palm or heads of metacarpals for palpating thrills and proximal palm for palpating heaves or lifts.
- Time the palpatory events whenever necessary with simultaneous palpation of cardiac apex or carotid upstroke.
- 2nd costal cartilage corresponds to the sternal angle from which the inter costal spaces can be counted for localisation of different cardiac areas.
- Look for precordial tenderness (due to costo-chondritis) for the differential diagnosis of precordial pain.

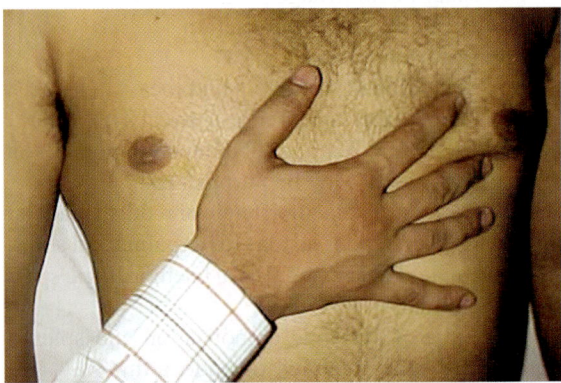

Fig. 3.12a Localising the cardiac apex with the finger (patient is supine)

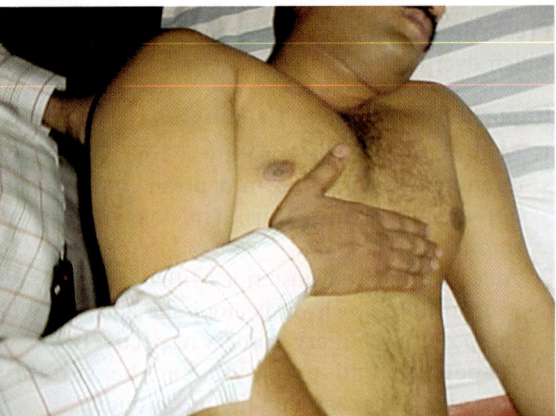

Fig. 3.12b Palpating the cardiac apex for the character (patient is in the left lateral position)

- In patients with hypertrophic cardiomyopathy apical impulse will have two outward systolic movements (better seen than felt).

Dyskinetic Segment

This appears as a systolic bulge in patients with left ventricular aneurysm.

It is present in the left mid precordium about 1 or 2 intercostal spaces above and 1–2 cm medial to the apex.

Shifting of the Cardiac Apex Occurs in Following Conditions

Cardiac cause: Cardiomegaly

Non cardiac causes

- Pleural or pulmonary disease
- Scoliosis
- Pectus excavatum
- Conditions associated with elevated diaphragm (pregnancy, massive ascites)

Conditions where in the Cardiac Apex may not be Detectable

- Obesity
- Pleural or pericardial effusion
- Dextrocardia
- Emphysema

Different Positions and Characters of Apical Impulse

For detection of character of the apex, patient may be turned to the left (lateral side).

Tapping Apex

- Felt as a hard knock (like the knock on the other side of the closed door).
- Found in patient with mitral stenosis
- It is the palpable loud 1st heart sound (closing snap)

Hyperdynamic Apex (Forceful)

- Apex is shifted outwards and downwards.
- With less sustained lift (more than 1/3 of systole but not throughout systole).
- Signifies left ventricular enlargement (volume over load).

- Apex is diffuse and may be more than 3 cm in diameter, e.g. AR, MR

Heaving Apex

- Sustained outward lift of the apex (duration more than 2/3 of systole).
- Position of the apex may not shift if it is concentric hypertrophy.
- Heaving apex suggests pressure overload of left ventricle (LV hypertrophy), e.g. AS, systemic hypertension

Different Terminologies used While Describing Cardiomegaly

Cardiac enlargement: Suggests dilatation or increase in the chamber volume.

Cardiac hypertrophy: Increase in the thickness of musculature and chamber volume is not increased.

Concentric Hypertrophy

- Uniform increase in the musculature with decrease in the cavity size
- Dilatation may occur later
- Occurs in conditions with LV pressure overload, e.g. systemic hypertension, aortic stenosis (severe).

Eccentric Hypertrophy

Dilatation of the cardiac chamber with later hypertrophy. Hypertrophy is not proportionate to dilatation. Occurs in conditions with LV volume overload, e.g. mitral regurgitation, aortic regurgitation.

Significance of Other Pulsations over the Precordium

Left parasternal pulsations and heave

Significance: Usually produced by the right ventricular enlargement or hypertrophy.

Method of Palpation

Patient is made supine and palpate during expiration. Best felt by the proximal part of the palm or finger tips kept over the left lower parasternal area. Appreciate the lift or heave.

Left parasternal lift (less sustained pulsation) signifies right ventricular volume overload conditions without hypertrophy, e.g. atrial septal defect, tricuspid regurgitation.

Left parasternal heave (sustained outer lift)
- Suggests right ventricular hypertrophy
- Occurs in conditions with RV pressure over load, e.g. pulmonary hypertension, pulmonary stenosis.
  In patient with emphysema, hyper-inflated lungs intervene between the heart and chest wall, making it difficult to feel the left parasternal right ventricular pulsation. In such situations, it is ideal to appreciate the RV pulsation in the epigastrium.

Conditions Presenting with Left Parasternal Pulsation apart from RVH

Left 2nd intercostal space pulsation

Occurs in conditions producing dilatation of pulmonary artery e.g. severe pulmonary hypertension. Idiopathic dilatation of pulmonary artery. Post-stenotic dilatation of pulmonary artery.

Technique of Palpation for Pulmonary Artery Pulsation
- Patient is sitting and leaning forward. Press firmly with the finger over the left 2nd intercostal space. Prominent systolic pulsation can be felt in the left 2nd intercostal space just to the left of sternum.
- Suggests enlarged pulmonary artery pulsation. Sometimes only a palpable shock (sound) or tapping sensation felt which is due to loud pulmonary component of 2nd heart sound (P2).
- This is found in patients with pulmonary artery hypertension.

Pulsation due to Massively Enlarged Left Atrium
- Pulsation appears and ends later than the apex felt at left of the sternum.
- Pulsation is due to regurgitation of large volume of blood into left atrium.

Note: Pulsation due to RVH appears and disappears along with the apex.

Right Parasternal Pulsation

- Occurs due to ascending aorta aneurysm
- Massively enlarged right atrium

Rocking Movement of Ventricles
- LV hypertrophy produces lateral outward movement with left parasternal retraction.
- RV hypertrophy produces left parasternal outward movement with lateral retraction.
- Bi-ventricular hypertrophy produces left parasternal and apical outward movement with an area of retraction in between.

Subxiphoid (Epigastric) Pulsation

Causes: Right ventricular pulsation, prominent aortic pulsation.
Method of palpation: Tip of the index finger or the thumb is inserted upwards and obliquely beneath (towards left) the xiphoid process with breath held in inspiration.
RV pulsation: Pulsation is felt by the tip of the finger.
Aortic pulsation: Felt by the pulp or beneath the pulp of the trigger.

Suprasternal Pulsation

Causes
- Unfolding of aorta or aneurysm of arch of aorta.
- Hyperkinetic states.

Pulsatile Liver

Palpate the liver bimanually. Hold one palm over the anterior surface of liver and the other palm over its posterior lateral surface. Feel for the pulsation of the liver (see also gastrointestinal tract).

Causes
Systolic pulsation: Tricuspid regurgitation, aortic regurgitation.
Pre-systolic pulsation: Tricuspid stenosis.

Thrills and Palpable Sounds

Thrills: Vibratory sensations (described as purring of cat) which are palpable manifestations of a murmur.

Method of Palpation of Thrill
Best appreciated with the head of metacarpal bones (distal palm).

Significance of Thrill

- Suggests presence of a murmur
- It localises the site origin of a diffuse murmur
- Favours (usually) presence of an organic valvular lesion
- Thrills are more common with obstructive lesions with narrow orifice, thin chest wall and in conditions with rapid blood flow.
- In patients with valvular aortic stenosis thrill can be appreciated over the carotids.
- Diastolic thrill of mitral stenosis is better appreciated on turning the patient to left lateral side.
- Diastolic thrill in a patient of aortic regurgitation suggests severe AR.
- Continuous thrill is present in patients with PDA.

Sudden Appearance of Thrill

May occur in the following situations

- Development of infective endocarditis causing valvular damage.
- Failure of prosthetic valve.

Palpable Sounds

Loud Ist sound of mitral stenosis: Felt as tapping apical impulse (closing snap)

Palpable 2nd Heart Sound

Palpable P2

- Palpable pulmonary component of 2nd heart sound.
- Felt as knocking sensation in the left 2nd intercostal space (patient is upright and leaning forward).
- Due to forceful closure of pulmonary valve under abnormally high pressure.
- Found in patient with significant pulmonary arterial hypertension.

KEY POINTS 3.5

- Always identify the area from where the thrill is felt.
- If the thrill coincides with the carotid, it is systolic and if it does not it is a diastolic thrill.

Palpable A2 (Aortic component of the 2nd heart sound)

- Felt as a tapping sensation in the right 2nd intercostal space.
- Due to forceful closure of aortic valve - under an abnormally high pressure.
- Found in patients with systemic hypertension

Prominent 3rd and 4th Heart Sounds

Palpable as diastolic movement at the cardiac apex (left sided 3rd and 4th heart sounds). Further details will be discussed under auscultation.

PERCUSSION

- Percussion gives less information in patients with cardiac disease.
- It is discussed here for completing the schematic presentation.

Percussion of Cardiac Borders

Right Cardiac Border

Define the upper border of the liver by percussing downwards in the mid-clavicular line from the right second intercostal space (normally upper border of the liver is in the right 5th intercostal space).

Percuss the intercostal spaces above the liver dullness in the mid-clavicular line moving towards the right sternal border.

Observe for the change of percussion note (from the normal lung resonance to dull note).

Normally the right cardiac border corresponds to the right sternal border.

Cardiac Causes of Dull Note Outside the Right Sternal Border

- Cardiomegaly
- Pericardial effusion

Percussion of the Right 2nd Intercostal Space

- Normally resonant
- In aneurysmal dilatation of the root of the aorta, right second intercostal space becomes dull on percussion.

Percussion of the Left Cardiac Border

1. Find the apical impulse.

2. Start percussion from outside the apex in the 5th intercostal space (or from the mid-axillary line, if the apex is not felt) moving medially towards the left sternal border.
3. Percuss parallel to the left sternal border.
4. Observe for the changing percussion note from the normal lung resonance.
5. Percussion note changes to dullness when one reaches the left cardiac border (apex).
6. Repeat the percussion in the same way in the upper intercostal spaces above the apex till the change of note to delineate the left cardiac border (3rd and 4th spaces).

Normally in the adult male, left cardiac border is within 10 cms from the mid-sternal line in the left 5th intercostal space.

In the 3rd intercostal space if the left cardiac border is > 4 cm from the mid sternal line signifies cardiomegaly.

Conditions with Displacement of the Left Cardiac Border Outside the Normal Position

1. *Cardiomegaly:* Left cardiac border will be corresponding to the apex.
2. *Pericardial effusion:* Left cardiac border will be outside the apex (cardiac dullness outside the apex).

Percussion of the left 2nd Intercostal Space
Normally resonant

Cardiac Conditions Producing Dullness in the Left 2nd Space

1. Enlarged pulmonary artery
2. Pericardial effusion

Important Clinical Aspects of Cardiac Percussion
Cardiac percussion is helpful in delineating the left border of the heart if the apex is not felt. In patients with emphysema cardiac dullness is reduced or absent due to hyper inflated lungs.

Greatly enlarged right atrium can produce dull note in the right lower parasternal area.

Cardiac malpositions can be detected by percussion (position of the heart can be compared with the position of the stomach).

Auscultation
Important guidelines for proper cardiac auscultation
- Identify the different areas of auscultation correctly for detection of auscultatory events.
- Simultaneous palpation of the carotid artery is essential to time the event as systolic or diastolic.
- A good stethoscope and a quiet room are required for efficient auscultation.

Parts and Requirements of a Good Stethoscope

Shallow Bell
- Useful in detecting low frequency sounds (3rd and 4th heart sounds) and low pitched murmurs.
- Should be applied lightly against the skin.

Smooth Thin Diaphragm
- For high frequency sounds and murmurs (first heart sound, second heart sound, opening snap and high pitched murmurs).
- Diaphragm should be applied firmly against the skin.

Tubing
- Ideally should be 12 inches long, internally smooth and 4–6 mm in circumferential diameter.
- It is better to have stethoscopes with double tubings for efficient auscultation.

Ear Tips
Larger ear tips, which are slightly soft and made of rubbery material are ideal for use.

Auscultatory Areas (Fig. 3.13)

Mitral area-corresponds to the apex.

Tricuspid area-left of the lower part of the sternum (4th and 5th intercostal space).

Aortic area-right of the sternum in the 2nd intercostal space).

Pulmonary area-left of the sternum (2nd intercostal space).

Additional Areas of Auscultation
- Left axilla-for pan systolic murmur of mitral regurgitation (MR).

- Interscapular area for pan systolic murmur of MR.
- Anterior chest-3rd intercostal space on the left side for the murmur of AR (Erb's area).
- Left infra clavicular area for-MR murmur, PDA murmur
- Left 3rd and 4th intercostal space (sternal border) for murmur of VSD.

Sequence of Cardiac Auscultation
- Start from the apex
- Proceed along the left sternal border below (tricuspid area) and pulmonary (above).
- Then auscultate the right 2nd space (aortic area).
- Auscultate additional areas whenever necessary.
- For auscultating aortic and pulmonary area, ask the patient to sit and stoop forward.
- Perform different auscultatory maneuvers if required.

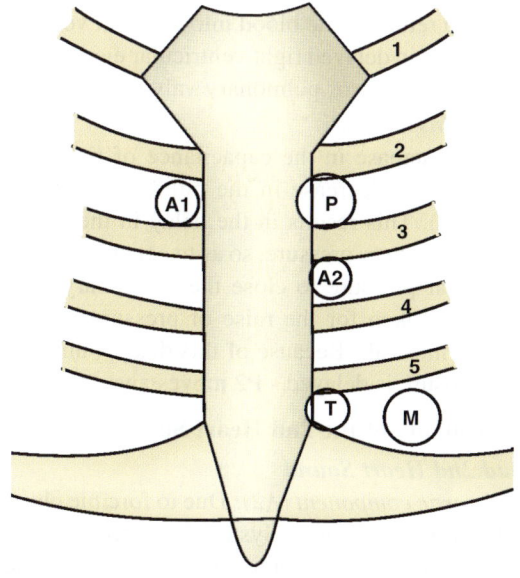

Fig. 3.13 Areas over the pericordium over which different auscultatory areas of the heart are represented: A1 - aortic area 1; A2 - Erb's area, M- Mitral area; T- Trcuspid area

HEART SOUNDS

KEY POINTS FOR AUSCULTATING HEART SOUNDS
- Sound intensity may be increased or decreased.
- Sounds may be abnormally split
- Low frequency extra sounds may appear, i.e. 3rd and 4th heart sounds.
- Additional sounds: Originating from the abnormal valves may be heard, e.g. clicks, snaps, etc.
- Decrease in the intensity of the heart sounds may be due to non cardiac causes like obesity, emphysema and pericardial effusion.

1st Heart Sound (Loud)

Produced by the closure of mitral (M1) and tricuspid valve (T1) simultaneously, so heard as a single sound.

1st heart sound indicates the onset of ventricular systole.

Method of Identification
- Heard as a lub in (lub-dub), while auscultating for heart sounds.
- Immediately precedes/coincides with the apex or carotid pulse.
- Loudest at the apex

Abnormality of 1st Heart Sound (S1)

Causes of loud 1st Heart Sound
- Tachycardia
- Mitral stenosis
- Tricuspid stenosis
- Hyperkinetic states
- Indicates pliable anterior leaflet of the mitral valve.

1st heart sound can also be loud in ASD (due to loud tricuspid component)

Mechanism of loud 1st Heart Sound in Mitral Stenosis

In patients with Mitral stenosis mitral valve moves over a greater distance with higher velocity causing loud 1st heart sound due to

1. High left atrial pressure causing the valve leaflets to be kept in a doomed position in LV cavity.
2. Valve closure occurs at a time when the LV pressure is very high.

Soft (muffled) 1st Heart Sound

Causes
- Cardiac failure
- Bradycardia
- Mitral regurgitation
  Soft first heart sound may also indicate calcified anterior mitral leaflet.

Varying Intensity of First Heart Sound
Beat to beat variation of the 1st heart sound occurs in atrial fibrillation.

Cannon sound is intermittently loud 1st heart sound in patients with complete heart block.

Splitting of the 1st heart sound occurs in complete RBBB due to delayed tricuspid component.

2nd Heart Sound

Genesis of 2nd Heart Sound
- Produced by the closure of aortic valve (A2) and pulmonary (P2) valves.
- Pulmonary valve closes later (due to lower pressure in the pulmonary artery) and aortic valve closes earlier due to early raise of left ventricular pressure and early activation of the LV.
- As a result 2nd heart sound is heard as 2 components, A2 (aortic component) and P2 (pulmonary component).

Method of Identification
- Heard as dub (in lub-dub) while auscultating for the heart sounds.
- Follows the apical impulse and carotid pulse.
- Better heard at the pulmonary and aortic areas.

Splitting of the 2nd Heart Sound

Normal (physiological) Splitting (Fig. 3.14)
- 2nd heart sound is heard as A2 (aortic) and P2 (pulmonary) component as a split.
- Split increases during inspiration (normal split - 0.06 seconds) with P2 moving away from A2.
- Split decreases during expiration (0.02 seconds).
- Physiological split is common in children and young adults.
- Split is best appreciated in the pulmonary area.

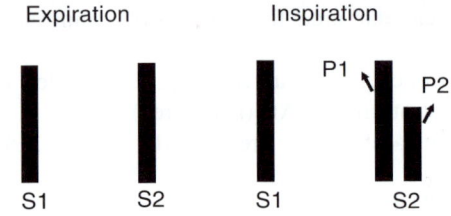

Fig. 3.14 Physiologic splitting of 2nd heart sound

- A2 - Aortic component can be heard in all areas.
- P2 - Pulmonary component is best appreciated in the pulmonary area.
- P2 - Heard loud at the apex may be suggestive of pulmonary hypertension.

Mechanism of Physiological Split of 2nd Heart Sound

During Inspiration
Due to negative intrathoracic pressure, there is increased return of the blood into the right ventricle. This results in delayed right ventricular ejection time with later closure of pulmonary valve - P2 delayed.

During Inspiration
There is increase in the capacitance of pulmonary vascular bed (decrease in the pulmonary vascular resistance). This results in the delay in the raise of Pulmonary artery pressure, so as to equalize the right ventricular pressure to close the pulmonary valve. This time taken for the raise of pressure is called hangout interval. Because of this delay, pulmonary valve closure is delayed - P2 moves away from A2.

Abnormality of the 2nd Heart Sound

Loud 2nd Heart Sound
Loud aortic component (A2): Due to forcible closure of the aortic valve, e.g. Systemic hypertension. Aortic root dilatation (aorta is closer to the chest wall).
Loud pulmonary component (P2): Due to forcible closure of the pulmonary valve, e.g. pulmonary artery hypertension.

Causes of Loud P2 without Pulmonary Hypertension

- ASD
- Straight back syndrome
- Idiopathic dilatation of pulmonary artery

Muffled (soft) 2nd Heart Sound

Due to muffled Aortic component (A2): Severe AS or Aortic atresia (only pulmonary component is heard as a single sound).

Due to muffled P2 (pulmonary component): Severe PS or pulmonary atresia (only aortic component is heard) and Fallot's Tetralogy.

Abnormal Splitting of 2nd Heart Sound

- Persistent (wide) split Fixed and not fixed
- Paradoxically split
- Narrow split

Persistent (wide) Split (Fig. 3.15)

- Not a fixed split. Split is audible in both inspiration and expiration but duration is not fixed, e.g. due to delay in the pulmonary component - RBBB, LV ectopic beat.
- Due to early timing of aortic component; severe MR
- Due to prolonged right ventricular contraction- Pulmonary embolism.

Wide and Fixed Split of 2nd Heart Sound

A2 and P2 are audible in both the phases of respiration and the duration of the split is fixed, e.g. uncomplicated osteum secondum ASD.

Mechanism of Wide Splitting in ASD

- Right heart receives additional volume of blood due to inter atrial shunt.

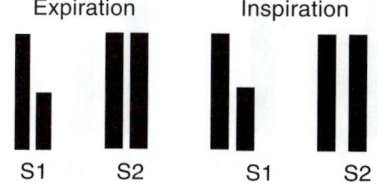

Fig. 3.15 Pathologic splitting (wide spitting)

- RV ejection time is prolonged due to additional volume of blood in the right RV due to inter atrial shunting causing delayed P2 (pulmonary valve closure).
- Increased pulmonary capacitance in ASD causes increased pulmonary hang out interval with delaying of P2.
- Above 2 mechanisms result in widening of the split.

Fixed Splitting of the 2nd Heart Sound in ASD (Fig. 3.16)

Free communication between right atrium and left atrium causes equal amount of blood flowing to RV and LV both during inspiration and expiration causing fixed time for valve closure.

Paradoxically Split (Reverse split) (Fig. 3.17)

- Pulmonary component occurs before the aortic component.
- On inspiration-A2 and P2 gap narrows.
- On expiration - split audible with separation of A2, and P2, e.g. LBBB

Severe AS: LBBB causes early right ventricular septal repolarisation with early P2 and delayed A2.

Severe AS: Causes prolonged LV ejection delaying A2.

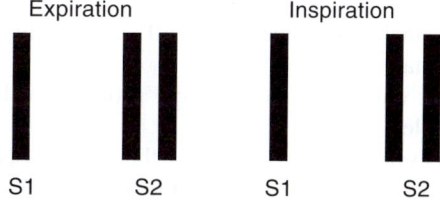

Fig. 3.16 Fixed spitting

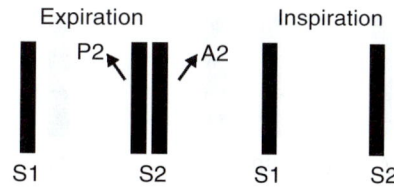

Fig. 3.17 Paradoxical (reverse) spitting

Narrow Splitting of the 2nd Heart Sound

In patients with severe pulmonary hypertension increased pulmonary artery pressure causes decrease of hangout interval with early closure of the pulmonary valve (P2 occurs early).

Single 2nd Heart Sound

- Due to absent of A2 - Severe AS
- Due to absent of P2 - Severe PS and Fallot's Tetralogy.

3rd Heart Sound (S3) (Fig. 3.18)

Genesis of 3rd Heart Sound

Sound is produced due to the rapid filling of the ventricle during early diastole leading to sudden limitation of expansion of the ventricle causing vibrations. 3rd heart sound can be physiological under following circumstances, e.g. healthy young adults, athletes, pregnancy and fever.

Characteristics of 3rd Heart Sound

Low frequency sound, heard better with the bell of the Stethoscope.

Heard in diastole (early part of diastole) - protodiastolic, during maximum (rapid) filling phase of ventricular filling (0.15 seconds after 2nd heart sound).

Abnormal (Pathological) S3

- S3 occurring after the age of 40 years is always abnormal.
- Occurs due to altered physical property of left ventricle.

3rd heart sound occurs whenever there is increased rate and volume of flow across the atrioventricular valve and raised end diastolic pressure of the ventricle.

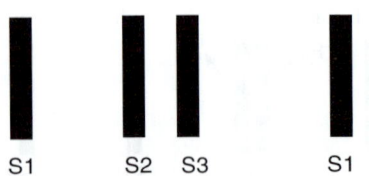

S1   S2   S3   S1

Fig. 3.18 Third heart sound (S3)

Causes of Abnormal S3

Cardiac failure, mitral regurgitation, dilated cardiomyopathy.

Fourth (4th) Heart Sound (Presystolic Gallop) (Fig. 3.19)

Characteristics

- Low frequency sound
- Heard in the later part of the diastole (pre-systolic) in patients with sinus rhythm.
- Better felt than auscultated
- Disappears in patients with atrial fibrillation

Genesis of 4th Heart Sound

- In conditions with decreased ventricular compliance there will be increased atrial contraction producing ventricular distention causing the sound during the presystolic phase.
- 4th heart sound occurs during the atrial filling phase of the ventricular diastole.

Characteristics of 4th Heart Sound

- They can be produced either from the right or left side of the heart.
- Better felt than auscultated
- Low frequency sounds are better heard with the bell of the stethoscope.
- Occurs in conditions with freely communicating atrioventricular orifices.

Left sided 3rd and 4th heart sounds are better heard
- At the apex
- Left lateral position
- During expiration

Right sided 3rd and 4th heart sounds are better heard: At the lower left sternal border (tricuspid area) during inspiration.

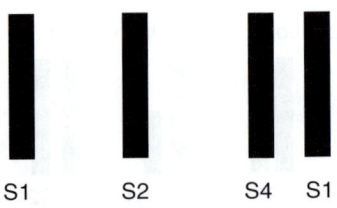

S1   S2   S4   S1

Fig. 3.19 Fourth heart sound (S4)

Causes of 4th heart sound: Conditions associated with LVH and RVH.

Triple rhythm - Combination of first heart sound, second heart sound and third or fourth heart sound.

Gallop rhythm - In patients with tachycardia, diastole becomes shortened. This causes 3rd and 4th heart sounds to coincide. This results increase in the amplitude of the heart sounds making it easily detectable.

This type of summation of sounds result in summation gallop. Presence of S1, S2 and S3 or S4 together with tachycardia produces a gallop rhythm.

Additional Sounds

Ejection clicks: Occurs due to sudden opening of semi lunar valves with their forward movement (Fig. 3.20).

Aortic Ejection Click

Occurs after the 1st heart sound.

- Indicates abnormality of the aortic valves, e.g. valvular aortic stenosis.
- Absent in supra or sub-valvular aortic stenosis.
- In patients with bicuspid aortic valve, there can be only click without murmur.
- In calcified aortic valve ejection click will be absent.

Pulmonary Ejection Click

Present in patients with valvular pulmonary stenosis (e.g. congenital pulmonary stenosis). Only auscultating event occurring in the right side of the heart which is better heard on expiration, becomes soft on inspiration.

Respiratory Variation of Pulmonary Ejection Click

Mechanism

On Inspiration

Forward movement of the pulmonary valve occurs due to the transmission of high force of right atrial contraction to right ventricle and pulmonary valve. This leads to minimal forward movement of the valve on systole causing decreased intensity of ejection click on inspiration.

Non Ejection Mid Systolic Click (Fig. 3.21)

- Occurs in patients with Mitral Valve Prolapse.
- May be associated with late systolic murmur.

Genesis of Mid Systolic Click

Occurs due to the vibrations produced by the sudden tensing of redundant leaflet of the valve when they prolapse into the atrium.

Ejection Sound of Dilated Arteries

- Occurs in patients with dilated aorta or pulmonary arteries.
- Aortic ejection sound occurs in patients with dilated aorta and systemic hypertension.
- Pulmonary ejection sound occurs in patients with dilated pulmonary artery with severe PAH.

Ejection sounds are due to

- Semi lunar valve opening producing resonation in the dilated artery.
- Sounds produced by wall of the dilated arteries.

Differentiation Between Split 2nd Heart Sound and 2nd Heart Sound with Opening Snap

- Sometimes opening snap may be heard over the pulmonary area and one may mistake the opening snap for the split 2nd heart sound.

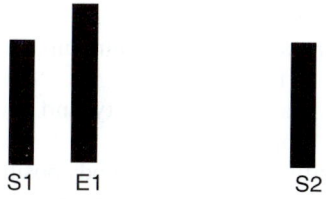

Fig. 3.20 Ejection click

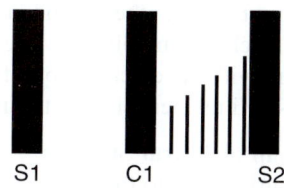

Fig. 3.21 Mid systolic click

- In such situations. It is better to make the patient stand and auscultate.
- On standing 2nd heart sound OS interval increases due to decrease venous return and decrease left atrial pressure
- On standing split 2nd heart sound (A2- P2) gap decreases due to decrease venous return to right heart

Tumour Plop Sound

Occurs in cases of atrial myxoma. Myxomas are usually mobile with attachment to the atrial septum by a long stalk. Sound occurs when the leaflet prolapses in to the atrium.

Prosthetic Valve Sounds

- Both opening and closing sounds are produced by mechanical prosthetic valves.
- Closing sounds are louder compared to the opening sound.
- Metallic type first heart sound produced by mechanical mitral valve.
- Metallic type of second heart sound produced by mechanical aortic valve.
- Bioprosthetic valve sounds sounds are similar to normal heart sound.
- Diminished intensity of prosthetic valve sound indicate LV dysfunction, arrhythmias, malfunctioning of valves.

Opening Snap (Fig. 3.22)

Produced due to sudden opening of mitral or tricuspid valve.

Characteristics
- High pitched sound
- ccurs in diastole after the 2nd heart sound
- Indicates thickened mobile valve leaflets
- Disappears with the calcification of valves
  Examples: Mitral stenosis and tricuspid stenosis

Opening Snap of Mitral Stenosis
- Better heard medial to the apex
- It may radiate to the base of the heart

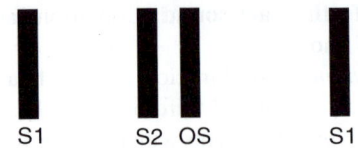

Fig. 3.22 Opening snap

- Interval between the 2nd heart sound and the opening snap (0.04 to 0.12 seconds) varies inversely with severity of mitral stenosis.

Genesis of Mitral Opening Snap
In patients with mitral stenosis LA pressure is increased. This leads to abrupt opening of mitral valve. But because of the commissural fusion the valve cannot open fully and the valve stops opening suddenly. This abrupt stoppage of opening causes vibrations producing a snapping sound.

MURMURS

Genesis of Murmurs
Murmurs are due to the vibrations produced by the turbulent flow at:
1. The region of the valve
2. Near the valve
3. Abnormal communication within the heart
   Mechanisms such as formation of sound currents due to sudden decrease of pressure may also play a role in the genesis of murmurs.
Following points should be noted while auscultating for a murmur
1. Timing with the cardiac cycle - systolic/diastolic.
2. Behaviour with respiration - Better heard on inspiration or expiration.
3. Low pitched or high pitched.
4. Character - soft, blowing, rumbling, etc.
5. Presence of thrill
6. Point of maximum intensity and direction of selective propagation.
7. Any specific manoeuvres or body positions which make the murmur more prominent.
   Murmur may be systolic, diastolic or continuous.

Systolic murmurs coincide with the carotid upstroke. Diastolic murmurs follow the carotid upstroke.

SYSTOLIC MURMURS

Mechanism of Production of Systolic Murmurs

1. Increased flow through a normal valve, e.g. flow murmurs.
2. Normal or decreased flow through the stenotic valve, e.g. aortic/pulmonary stenosis.
3. Systolic leak from high to low pressure chambers, e.g. MR, TR, VSD, etc.

Different types of Systolic Murmurs are as follows

- Early systolic
- Ejection systolic
- Late systolic
- Pan systolic or hollow systolic

Early Systolic Murmur

Murmur begins with the 1st heart sound and diminishes in intensity and stops well before the 2nd heart sound (before mid systole), e.g. acute MR, acute TR, small VSD, VSD with severe pulmonary hypertension.

Ejection (Mid Systolic) Murmur (Fig. 3.23)

Characteristics

- Commences after the 1st heart sound.
- Peaks in mid systole
- Stops before the 2nd heart sound.

- There will be a definite gap in between the murmur and the 1st and 2nd heart sound.
- Phonocardiogram depicts the murmur as diamond shaped.

Following circumstances produce ejection systolic (mid systolic) murmur

a. Obstruction to the ventricular outflow, e.g. aortic stenosis, pulmonary stenosis.
b. Due to ejection of blood into the dilated aorta or pulmonary arteries, e.g. ejection systolic murmur in patients with AR and PR.
c. Accelerated systolic flow into the aorta and pulmonary arteries, e.g. ejection systolic murmur which occurs in patients with systemic and pulmonary hypertension.

> *Note:* Ejection systolic murmurs depend on the forward flow of blood. So in patients with irregular rhythm they vary from beat to beat in contrast to pan systolic murmurs

Late Systolic Murmur (Fig. 3.24)

Murmur begins well after the 1st heart sound (clear gap between the murmur and the Ist heart sound) and continues up to the 2nd heart sound, e.g. mitral valve prolapse, papillary muscle dysfunction.

Pan (Holo Systolic) Murmurs (Fig. 3.25)

- Murmur begins with the Ist heart sound and ends with the 2nd heart sound or its component (A2 or P2).

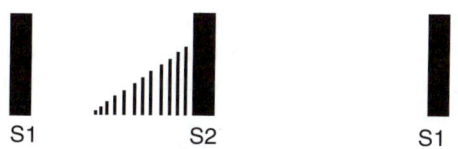

Fig. 3.24 Late systolic murmer

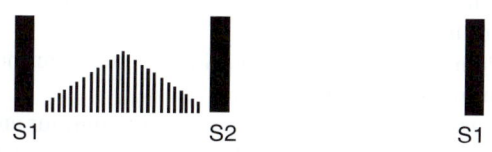

Fig. 3.23 Ejection systolic (mid systolic murmer)

Fig. 3.25 Pan systolic murmer

- 1st heart sound is usually muffled, intensity of the murmur is uniform throughout the systole, e.g. MR, TR, and VSD

Genesis of pan systolic murmur: Generated whenever pressure between the two chambers or vascular bed is high throughout the systole and blood flow becomes turbulent.

Grading of Murmurs

Systolic Murmurs are Graded as Follows
Grades
  I. Heard with great difficulty under ideal conditions.
  II. Easily detectable
  III. Loud without a thrill
  IV. Murmur is associated with thrill
  V. Very loud, heard over wide area or can be heard with the edge of the chest piece of the stethoscope applied to the chest wall.
  VI. Extremely loud, heard without the stethoscope or with the chest piece of the stethoscope just held away from the chest wall.

Innocent Murmurs

These murmurs are present in persons with normal cardiovascular system and normal carotid, brachial and femoral arteries.

There is no physiological or structural abnormality in the cardiovascular system.

They are ejection systolic in nature, less than grade 3 in intensity.

Murmur varies in relation to change in body position, level of activity, examination to examination.

They are not associated with thrill, not conducted to axilla or carotids.

They arise from flow across a normal LV or RV outflow tract, e.g. young children (3–8 years). Vibratory systolic murmur - Still's murmur. Adult > 50 years, ejection systolic murmur.

Flow Murmurs

These murmurs are produced due to the altered physiological state and they are flow related and are usually associated with increased stroke volume.

Characteristics
- Usually mid systolic (ejection systolic) in pattern.
- Predominantly heard at the pulmonary area.
- Intensity of the murmur increases by the manoeuvres that increase cardiac output.

Genesis of Flow Murmurs
- Due to abnormally rapid flow of blood through a normal valve or ejection of blood into a dilated vessel, e.g. anemia, thyrotoxicosis, hypertension.
- Due to increased transmission of the sound across a thin chest wall, e.g. systolic murmur heard in patient with straight back syndrome.

Note: Systolic flow murmurs can also be heard in children and in pregnancy.

To and Fro Murmurs

In this situation both systolic and diastolic murmurs are heard but the 2nd heart sound is well heard (murmur does not envelope the 2nd heart sound).

In contrast to continuous murmur (where the blood flow is in one direction throughout systole and diastole), in cases of to and fro murmurs, blood flow in systole and diastole will be in opposite direction, e.g. ejection systolic murmur due to AS and early diastolic murmur of AR.

Diastolic Murmurs

Diastolic murmurs are heard after the 2nd heart sound and before the subsequent Ist heart sound.

Types of Diastolic Murmurs

Early Diastolic Murmur (Fig. 3.26)
Murmur starts just after the 2nd heart sound and gradually decreases in intensity (persists up to the opening of mitral and tricuspid valves), e.g. aortic regurgitation.

Pulmonary regurgitation (Graham steel murmur of pulmonary hypertension).

Auscultation for aortic regurgitation murmur and for cardiac apex (especially for the murmur of mitral stenosis are shown in Figs 3.27a and b.

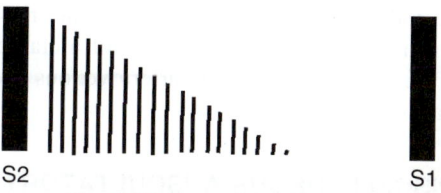

Fig. 3.26 Early diastolic murmer

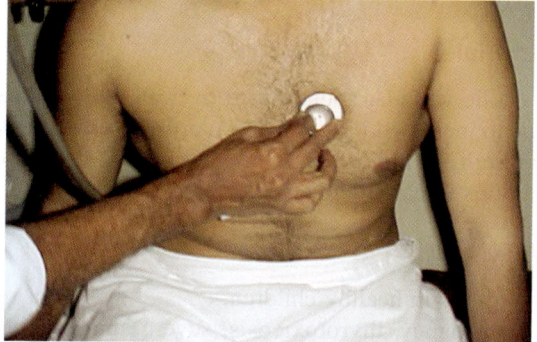

Fig. 3.27a Auscultation for aortic regurgitation murmur (patient is sitting and leaning forward)

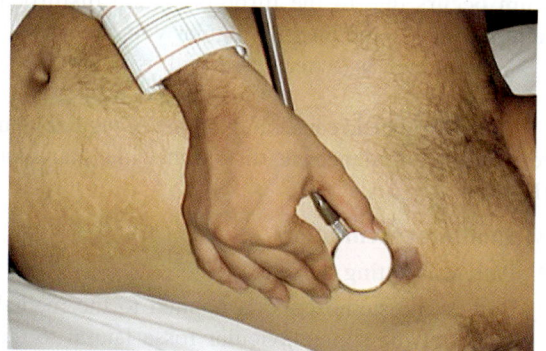

Fig. 3.27b Auscultation for cardiac apex patient is in left lateral position (especially for the murmur of mitral stenosis)

Mid Diastolic Murmur (Fig. 3.28)

Murmur begins well after the 2nd heart sound and may persist up to the next 1st heart sound (during passive ventricular filling), e.g. mitral stenosis, tricuspid stenosis, Austin Flint murmur, Carey-Coombs murmur.

Austin Flint Murmur

Soft mid diastolic murmur heard at the apex, in patients with severe AR.

Genesis of Austin Flint Murmur

In patient with severe AR, left ventricle fills from the regurgitant flow of blood from the aorta and also from the left atrium during diastole.

Blood leaking from the Aorta will be jetting over the anterior mitral leaflet.

Both of the above events together will result in relative approximation of mitral leaflets causing turbulence and vibrations producing a mid diastolic murmur.

Carey-Coombs' Murmur

Mid-diastolic murmur which is heard in patients with acute rheumatic fever.

Murmur occurs due to inflammation of the mitral valve cusps in acute rheumatic valvulitis with turbulence of flow.

Mid Diastolic Flow Murmurs

These are due to increased volume and velocity of blood flow across a normal atrioventricular valve during diastole, e.g. MDM across the mitral valve. In patients with mitral regurgitation and VSD, PDA. MDM across the tricuspid valve. Tricuspid regurgitation, ASD.

Mid diastolic flow murmurs may be associated with left sided 3rd heart sound in contrast to organic mitral stenosis.

Conduction and Radiation of Murmurs

It is the murmur, which is heard with the same intensity or with decreased in intensity at the different

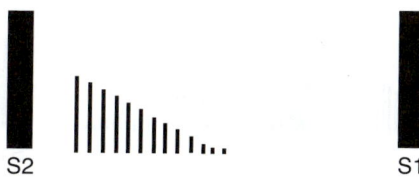

Fig. 3.28 Mid diastolic murmur

area of the chest or precordium. It is due to the selective propagation of murmur from its original site of production.

Examples of Murmur Conduction

Murmurs	Areas of conduction
• Aortic stenosis	Right sternal edge, neck (carotids), apex
• Aortic regurgitation	Left sternal border, right sternal border
• Mitral regurgitation	Axilla, interscapular area, left and 2nd inter costal space
• Mitral stenosis	Localised to the apex (conduction unusual)

Continuous Murmurs

Characteristics
Murmur begins in the systole (after the 1st heart sound) and continues without interruption through the 2nd heart sound (2nd heart sound is not heard) into all or part of the diastole (Figs 3.29, 3.30).

Genesis of Continuous Murmurs
Blood flows without interruption from a vascular bed of higher resistance into a vascular bed of lower pressure or resistance without interruption between

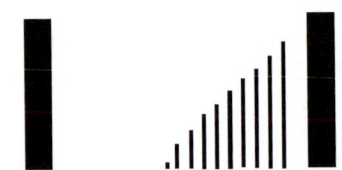

Fig. 3.29 Presystolic (late diastolic) murmur

S1   S2   S1

Fig. 3.30 Continuous murmur

systole and diastole, e.g. patent ductus arteriosus - Gibson's murmur (heard in the left infra clavicular and left 2nd intercostal space), arteriovenous fistula, Coronary AV fistula.

MISCELLANEOUS AUSCULTATORY CARDIOVASCULAR EVENTS

Arterial Bruit
Systolic vascular sound heard over an artery either due to increased flow across a narrow artery or flow through an abnormal artery, e.g. Bruit over the carotids in carotid atherosclerosis.

Venous Hum in the Neck
- Occurs in healthy children.
- Pregnancy, thyrotoxicosis, severe anaemia etc. Hum is heard due to increased venous flow.

Genesis of Venous Hum in the Neck
Hum occurs due to the turbulence and disturbed laminar flow in the internal jugular vein.

Venous hum is better heard with rotation of the head.

Rotation of head causes angulation of jugular vein resulting in turbulence and disturbance in it's laminar flow.

Method of Auscultation
- Patient is sitting upright.
- Bell of the stethoscope is applied to the medial aspect of the supraclavicular fossa lateral to the sternomastoid.
- Turn the patient's neck to the opposite side.
- Hum may be continuous, but louder during diastole.
- Hum is better heard on the right side and on deep inspiration (right internal jugular is larger than the left).
- Venous hum disappears by proximal compression of the ipsilateral internal jugular vein by fingers.

Mammary Souffle (Continuous Arterial Murmur)
- Heard at second to sixth intercostal space during pregnancy
- Lactation

PERICARDIAL DISORDERS

Pericardial Rub

Superficial coarse scratchy sound

Characteristics
- Due to abnormal pericardial layers rubbing against each other.
- It has got 3 components due to atrial systole, ventricular systole and rapid early diastolic filling of the ventricle.
- Pericardial rub may not disappear by the appearance of massive effusion (some portion of 2 layers of the pericardium will be still in contact).
- It is a high pitched leathery and scratchy sound.

Technique of Auscultation
- Patient is upright and leaning forward.
- Firm pressure of the stethoscope diaphragm to be applied over the precordium towards lower left of the sternum.
- Better heard on expiration.

Pericardial Knock

Occurs in patient with constrictive pericarditis. It is a low frequency diastolic sound.

Genesis of Pericardial Knock
Constrictive pericarditis results in sudden stoppage of ventricular filling during early diastolic phase causing vibration.

Dynamic Auscultation
By altering the circulatory dynamics auscultatory events in the cardiovascular system can be made more prominent or less prominent. Circulatory dynamics can be altered by certain body maneuvers and vasoactive substances.

Manoeuvres or vasoactive substances used for dynamic auscultation
Manoeuvres
- Respiration
- Postural change
- Isometric exercise
- Valsalva manoeuvre

Vasoactive amines : Amylnitrate, phenylephrine

Exercise: Patient lying on a couch—sit up and lie down quickly (about 10 times).

Valsalva maneuver: Patient is asked to take relatively deep inspiration followed by forced expiration (for about 10 to 12 seconds) against a closed glottis.

Variations of Murmurs During Dynamic Auscultation

Systolic Murmurs
1. *Valvular AS:* Increases with passive leg raising, sudden squatting, with valsalva release or amylnitrate decreases with hand grip, valsalva stain
2. *HOCM:* Louder with valsalva strain, standing and amylnitrate, decreases with squatting and hand grip.
3. *PS:* Increases on inspiration, amylnitrate.
4. *Rheumatic MR:* Increases with squatting, hand grip and phenylephrine, decreases with amylnitrate.
5. *MVP*
   Early click and early murmur - standing valsalva strain, amylnitrate.
   Late click and murmur - squatting, recumbency.
6. *TR:* Increases with inspiration and amylnitrate

Diastolic Murmurs

AR - Increases with squatting and hand grip or phenylephrine and increases with amylnitrate
PR - Increases on inspiration and amylnitrate
MS - Increases with exercise, left lateral position, hand grip or amylnitrate.
TS - Increases with inspiration and amyl nitrate.

Mitral Stenosis

Causes

1. Rheumatic heart disease
2. Calcified mitral valve
3. Congenital mitral stenosis
4. Mucopolysaccharidoses
5. Collagen disease

Clinical Findings

- Tapping apical impulse
- Diastolic thrill at the apex
- Loud first heart sound
- Presence of an opening snap
- Mid diastolic murmur at the apex

Murmur of Mitral Stenosis - Mid Diastolic Murmur at the Apex

- Low pitched rough and rumbling
- Heard with the bell of the stethoscope and in the left lateral position - associated with presystolic accentuation. Breath held in expiration.

Pre Systolic Accentuation

Occurs due to

1. At the last part of the diastole contraction of the left atrium causes increased flow across the mitral valve.
2. Due to the effect of onset of the ventricular contraction mitral valve starts to close causing turbulence.

   (The 2nd mechanism contributes for the presence of presystolic murmur even in patients with atrial fibrillation).

Following Features Suggest Severe Mitral Stenosis

1. Longer duration of mid diastolic murmur
2. Decreased interval between the 2nd heart sound and opening snap
3. Severe pulmonary hypertension

Mitral Stenosis with Soft First Heart Sound

Causes

- Calcified mitral leaflets (opening snap also disappears)
- Associated significant mitral regurgitation.
- Severe mitral stenosis with extreme clockwise rotation of the heart (RV occupies the apex).

Silent Mitral Stenosis

- Severe form of mitral stenosis.
- Marked pulmonary hypertension, RVH with decreased cardiac output.
- MDM murmur is not heard (or only heard in the axilla).

Causes of Mid Diastolic Murmur at the Apex Apart from Organic Mitral Stenosis

- *Conditions which mimic - Mitral stenosis:* Left atrial myxoma and left atrial ball valve thrombosis
- *Organic disease of the heart but mitral valve is not damaged:* Austin - Flint and Carey-Coombs murmur
- Mid diastolic flow murmurs at the apex: VSD and PDA.

Juvenile Mitral Stenosis

- Mitral stenosis can occur at early ages as a consequence of rheumatic fever (as early as 3–8 years).
- In South East Asian region rheumatic fever assumes aggressive course due to lack of immunity, overcrowding and improper prophylaxis. This results in early valvular damage.

Differences Between Organic Mitral Stenosis and other Causes of MDM at the Apex (Table 3.5)

Mitral Regurgitation

Causes

1. Rheumatic
2. Mitral valve prolapse
3. Ischaemic damage to papillary muscle
4. Rupture of chordae tendinae (trauma, ischaemia, infective endocarditis)
5. LV dilatation with enlargement of mitral annulus

Table 3.5 Differences between organic mitral stenosis and other causes of MDM at the apex

Organic mitral stenosis		Other causes of MDM at the apex
Diastolic thril	- present	absent
Ist heart sound	- very loud	normal or soft
Opening snap	- present	absent
Murmur	- rough and rumbling	soft and short and of longer duration.
Pre systolic accentuation	- present	absent

Clinical Features

- High volume pulse
- Hyper dynamic apical impulse
- Systolic thrill at the apex
- Soft Ist heart sound
- Presence of left sided 3rd heart sound
- Pansystolic murmur at the apex

Murmur of MR

Pan systolic-soft blowing high pitched, heard better with diaphragm of the stethoscope and on expiration.

- Conducted to axilla if the anterior leaflet is involved (rheumatic).
- Conducted to the base of the heart (2nd left intercostal space) if the posterior leaflet is involved.

MR with Loud First Heart Sound: consider associated dominant mitral stenosis.

MR with Normal First Heart Sound: consider MVP, papillary muscle dysfunction.

Soft First heart sound in MR: *Due to*
1. Defective closure of deformed valve leaflets.
2. Murmur starting with the first heart sound.

Mitral Regurgitation with Late Systolic Murmur

Causes

1. MVP
2. Ischaemic- papillary muscle dysfunction.

Differences Between Acute and Chronic MR
(Table 3.6)

Severe MR: Presence of loud S3, pan-systolic murmur and mid diastolic flow murmur across the mitral valve suggests severe MR.

Aortic Stenosis

Causes
1. Rheumatic
2. Congenital
3. Calcified aortic valve

Clinical Findings
1. Low volume and slow raising pulse (pulsus parvus et tardus) and apicocarotid delay-severe aortic stenosis.
2. Heaving apical impulse
3. Systolic thrill over the aortic area and over the carotids (in valvular stenosis)
4. Ejection click (in valvular stenosis)
5. 2nd heart sound - soft or single or paradoxically split.
6. Ejection systolic murmur at the aortic area.

Table 3.6 Differences between acute and chronic MR

	Acute MR	Chronic MR
Apex	not displaced	displaced
Murmur	soft, low pitched and short	harsh and pansystolic
Thrill	absent	present
Location of murmur	base	apex
Severe LVF	usually present	±

Murmur - Ejection systolic murmur with late peaking conducted to the carotids (in valvular stenosis).

Better heard on expiration with patient sitting up and stooping forward.

Sometimes the ejection systolic murmur of aortic stenosis can be heard at the apex with a different quality. This is called Gallaverdin phenomenon.

Gallaverdin Phenomenon

Harsh ejection systolic murmur of aortic stenosis is heard as musical quality murmur at the apex, occurs in elderly with aortic valve calcification and sclerosis.

Mechanism

Harsh aortic area murmur is due to high velocity of blood flow causing turbulence at the aortic root.

Musical component at the apex is due to high frequency vibration produced by the valve conducted to the apex.

Aortic Regurgitation

Causes

AS with AR
- Rheumatic fever
- Bicuspid aortic valve

Only AR
- AR due to syphilitic aortitis
- Marfan's syndrome

Acute AR
- Infective endocarditis
- Dissecting aneurysm of aorta.
- Trauma to the chest

Signs of AR

1. Peripheral signs of AR
2. Hyper dynamic or heaving apex (later stages)
3. Diastolic thrill at the aortic area (severe AR)
4. 2nd heart sound loud or musical
5. Murmur
   - Early diastolic murmur of longer duration.
   - Decrescendo and high pitched on expiration heard with diaphragm of the stethoscope and on sitting up and stooping forward (Fig. 3.31).

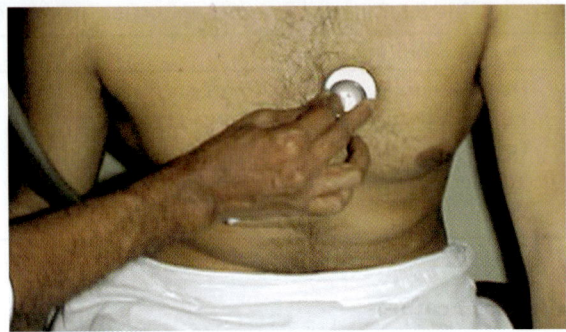

Fig. 3.31 Auscultation for aortic regurgitation murmur patient is sitting and leaning forward

If the murmur of AR is better on right sternal border signifies dilatation of the aortic root, e.g. syphilis.

Marfan's Syndrome

If the murmur of AR is better heard on the left sternal border signifies AR of valvular origin, e.g. rheumatic heart disease.

Musical murmur of AR (Cooving dove): Due to either eversion or perforation of aortic cusps

Severe AR
- Dominant peripheral signs of AR
- Diastolic thrill at the apex
- Long duration of early diastolic murmur

AR associated with AS
- Bisferien's pulse (if AR is dominant)
- Systolic blood pressure decreases (systolic decapitation - if AS is dominant).

Differences between acute and chronic AR
(Table 3.7)

Table 3.7 Differences between acute and chronic AR

	Acute AR	*Chronic AR*
Peripheral signs	Absent	Present
Apex	Not Hyper dynamic and not displaced	Hyper dynamic and displaced
AR murmur	Shorter	Longer

Cole Cecil Murmur

Murmur of AR radiates to axilla and apex.

Differences between syphilitic AR and rheumatic AR (Table 3.8).

Aortic Aneurysm

Signs of Aneurysm of Ascending Aorta
- Right parasternal pulsation and bulge
- Aortic regurgitation
- Loud A2
- Compression of right main bronchus, phrenic nerve and cervical sympathetic chain.
- Signs of aneurysm of Arch of aorta: Supra sternal pulsation.
- Tracheal tug
- Pressure effect on left recurrent laryngeal nerve, cervical sympathetic and phrenic nerve.

Tricuspid Stenosis

Causes
- Rheumatic
- Tricuspid atresia
- Carcinoid syndrome

Signs
1. Opening snap
2. Mid diastolic murmur at the tricuspid area better heard on inspiration.

Tricuspid Regurgitation

Causes
Usually secondary to right ventricular dilatation causing stretching of the tricuspid annulus in patients with severe pulmonary hypertension.

Table 3.8 Differences between syphilitic and rheumatic AR

Syphilitic AR	Rheumatic AR
H/o exposure to syphilis	H/o Rheumatic fever
Not associated mitral valve disease	Usually associated with mitral valve disease
Peripheral signs predominant	Peripheral signs less dominant
No associated AS	May be associated with AS

Other Causes
- Rheumatic and carcinoid syndrome
- Right sided infective endocarditis
- Ebstein's anomaly

Signs
- Prominent 'V' wave in the JVP
- Pulsatile liver

Murmur

- Pan systolic murmur high pitched
- De Carvallo's sign – TR murmur is better heard on inspiration. This sign is absent in severe RV failure and hepatic outflow obstruction.
- Heard at the tricuspid area
- Right sided S3 may be present

Myxoma

- Tumour of the atrium raising from the inter atrial septum
- Commonly found in the left atrium.
- Can cause embolisation.
- Left atrial myxoma may obstruct the mitral valve and can produce mid-diastolic murmur at the apex.

Mid-Diastolic Murmur of Left Atrial Myxoma

Characteristically appears on standing and may disappear on lying down. MDM may be associated with tumor plop sound rather than an opening snap.

Pulmonary Stenosis (Usually Congenital)

Signs
- Right ventricular hypertrophy is usually present.
- Ejection click is heard in the pulmonary area which is better heard on expiration (valvular stenosis).
- 2nd heart sound- pulmonary component may be soft and may be delayed.
- Ejection systolic murmur which is heard over the pulmonary area and better heard on inspiration.

Atrial Septal Defect (ASD)

Signs
- Left parasternal lift (due to right ventricular volume overload).

- Fixed and wide splitting of the 2nd heart sound.
- Ejection systolic murmur at pulmonary area (due to increased flow across the pulmonary valve).
- Mid diastolic murmur at the tricuspid area due to increased flow across the tricuspid valve.

ASD without fixed split: Sinus venosus type of ASD.

ASD with thrill in the pulmonary area: Large ASD/ASD associated with valvular PS.

Ventricular Septal Defect (VSD)

Signs

1. Hyper dynamic apex
2. Systolic thrill at the lower end of the left sternal border.
3. Pan systolic murmur at the left lower part of the sternum.
4. Murmur does not radiate to axilla

Roger's Melady: Small VSD with high velocity prominent pan systolic murmur.

Patent Ductus Arteriosus (PDA)

1. Continuous murmur and thrill at the pulmonary area-machinery murmur (accentuation of the murmur at the 2nd heart sound).
2. Functional mid diastolic murmur at the mitral area.
3. Peripheral signs of wide pulse pressure
4. With the onset of pulmonary hypertension, diastolic component of the murmur will be shortened.

Pulmonary Hypertension

Causes

1. All causes of left heart disease, e.g. mitral valve disease, ischaemic heart disease.
2. *Reversal of left to right shunt:* Eisenmenger's syndrome.
3. *Respiratory causes:* Cor pulmonale, COPD, pulmonary embolism.
4. Primary pulmonary hypertension

Signs

- Prominent a wave in the JVP (due to stiff right ventricle)

- Left parasternal heave (due to RVH)
- P2 palpable and loud.
- Ejection systolic murmur at the pulmonary area.
- Early diastolic murmur (Graham steel murmur) heard at the pulmonary area, better heard on inspiration due to dilatation of the pulmonary valve and pulmonary regurgitation.

Coarctation of Aorta

Signs

- Radiofemoral delay
- Left ventricular hypertrophy
- High blood pressure recorded in the upper limbs compared to lower limbs.
- Ejection click at the aortic area
- ESM at the aortic area due to bicuspid aortic valve.
- Collaterals around the scapulae.

Ebstein's Anomaly

Signs

- Central cyanosis
- Systolic thrill and murmur of TR
- Wide split of 1st and 2nd heart sounds with 3rd and 4th heart sounds

Fallot's Tetralogy

Components

- Pulmonary stenosis (usually infundibular)
- Ventricular septal defect
- Right ventricular hypertrophy

Table 3.9 Differences between aortic (AR) and pulmonary regurgitation

AR	PR
Associated with peripheral signs of AR	Signs of severe Pulmonary hypertension.
A2 loud	P2 loud.
Murmur better heard in expiration.	Murmur better heard on inspiration.
Associated with LVH	Presence of RVH

- Overriding of the aorta (aorta arises from either ventricle)

Signs
- Central cyanosis
- Clubbing
- Relatively quiet precordium
- Ejection systolic murmur at the pulmonary area.
- Single second heart sound (P2 is absent)

Acyanotic fallot (pink fallot): Interventricular shunt with mild RV outflow obstruction.

Triology of fallot: Pulmonary stenosis with reversed inter atrial shunt.

Pentalogy of fallot: Tetralogy with ASD.

Hypertrophic Obstructive Cardiomyopathy (HOCM)

Characterized by inappropriate hypertrophy of the left ventricle and septum.

Signs
- Jerky or sharp carotid pulse (due to abnormal pattern of blood flow from left ventricle).
- Double apical impulse
- Stiff left ventricle produces loud S4 at the apex
- Obstruction to the LV outflow produces ejection systolic murmur at the left sternal border, murmur not conducted to the carotids.
- Papillary muscle abnormality in HOCM causes mitral regurgitant murmur at the apex.

Congestive Cardiac Failure

Signs
- Patient may be orthopnoeic (severe left heart failure)
- Pulse rate > 120/min
- Cheyne - Stokes breathing (due to prolonged circulation time to the medullary respiratory centre).

Left Sided Heart Failure
- Low volume pulse
- Pulsus alternans

- Bilateral basal crepitations
- Left side 3rd heart sound
- Central cyanosis

Right Sided Heart Failure
- JVP increased
- Congestive hepatomegaly (some times congestive splenomegaly)
- Ascites and pleural effusion may be present.
- Pedal oedema

Chronic Congestive Cardiac Failure
Severe weight loss (cardiac cachexia), jaundice and ascites

Atrial Fibrillation

Signs
- Irregularly irregular pulse
- Pulse apex deficit (large)
- A wave absent in the JVP
- Varying intensity of the Ist heart sound

Causes
Causes of atrial fibrillation can be remembered with the pneumonic THRIL

T - Thyrotoxicosis
H - Hypertensive heart disease
R - Rheumatic heart disease
I - Ischaemic heart disease
L - Lone atrial fibrillation

Pericardial Effusion

Signs
- Apex not felt
- Cardiac dullness increased out side the apex
- Heart sounds muffled
- Pericardial rub may be audible

Ewart's sign - Dullness/bronchial breathing below angle of left scapula due to compression of the left lung base by the pericardial effusion.

Pericardial Tamponade
- Pulsus paradoxus may be present
- Signs of pericardial effusion present

Constrictive Pericarditis

- Kussmaul's sign present
- Pericardial knock present

Acute Rheumatic Fever

Signs of Carditis
- Tachycardia (disproportionate to fever)
- Cardiomegaly
- Cardiac failure
- Carey-Coombs' murmur
- MR murmur
- Pericardial rub

Examples of Congenital Heart Diseases and their Associated Malformations (Table 3.10)

EXAMINATION OF PERIPHERAL VASCULAR SYSTEM

Venous System

Deep Vein Thrombosis
Features
- Sudden onset of pain in the limb with swelling
- Associated with mild degree of fever
Signs
- Oedema of limbs
- Tenderness in the muscles (calf tenderness in the DVT of leg)

Homan's sign: Person feels pain in the calf when he dorsiflexes the foot.

Table 3.10 Examples of congenital diseases and their associated malformations	
Malformations	*Associated Cardiac Anomalies*
1. **Holt Oram's syndrome**	
Thumb with an extra phalanx	ASD
Thumb lies in the same plane as other fingers	
Radius and ulna may be deformed	
2. **William's syndrome**	
Microcephaly, Elfin facies	Supra valvular AS
Hypercalcemia, mental retardation	
3. **Down's syndrome**	
Mongoloid facies, hypertelorism and mental retardation	Endocardial cushion defect
	ASD, VSD, tetralogy of fallot
4. **Turner's syndrome**	
Short statured female, broad chest	Coarctation of aorta
Webbed neck, lymphoedema, cubitus valgus	Bicuspid aortic valve, Aortic dilatation
5. **Noonan's syndrome**	
Webbed neck, pectus excavatum and cryptorchidism	Pulmonary valve dysplasia, Cardiomyopathy
6. **Rubella syndrome**	
Deafness, cataract	PDA, ASD
Microcephaly	Valvular pulmonary stenosis
7. **Marfan's syndrome**	
Arachnodactyly, iridodonesis	AR
High arched palate, Ht < arm span	Aortic dissection
Upper segment < lower segment	
8. **Foetal alchohol syndrome**	
Cataract, deafness	VSD

Moses sign: Person feels pain on squeezing the calf muscles.

Risk factors for DVT
- Long term immobilisation
- Post operative states
- Polycythemic states
- Protein C and S deficiency
- Oral contraceptive intake

Thrombophlebitis
- Reddish discouloration of the part affected
- Tenderness
- Cord like feeling of veins

Varicose Veins
- Due to incompetence of venous valves veins become tortuous and dilated

Complications
- Venous stasis and ulcers
- Oedema of limbs and Thrombophlebitis

Predisposing factors for varicose veins
- Occupations associated with long term standing
- Congestive cardiac failure
- Extreme obesity
- Pregnancy
- Venous obstruction due to pelvic tumors

Effect of chronic venous stasis
- Varicose ulcers
- Varicose pigmentation
- Oedema of limbs
- Usual sites of chronic venous stasis
- Lower part of the lower limb on its medial aspect usually above the ankle.

Anatomy and Physiology of Cardiovascular System

Heart is a muscular pump consisting of 4 main chambers and 4 valves with right heart pumping blood into the lungs and left heart pumping blood into the systemic circulation supplying the entire body system.

Different Chambers of Heart (Fig. 3.32)

Right side of the heart consists of right atrium (RA) and right ventricle (RV).

Left side of the heart consists of left atrium (LA) and left ventricle (LV).

Right atrium receives unoxygenated blood from upper part of the body through superior vena cava (SVC) and from lower part of the body through inferior vena cava (IVC) (Fig. 3.34)

Right ventricle receives unoxygenated blood from right atrium and pumps it to the lungs through pulmonary artery where it gets oxygenated.

Left atrium receives oxygenated blood from the lungs through 4 pulmonary veins. Left ventricle receives oxygenated blood from left atrium and pumps it into various parts of the body through the aorta.

Different Valves of The Heart

Mitral Valve

Mitral valve lies in between the left atrium and the left ventricle. During left atrial contraction mitral

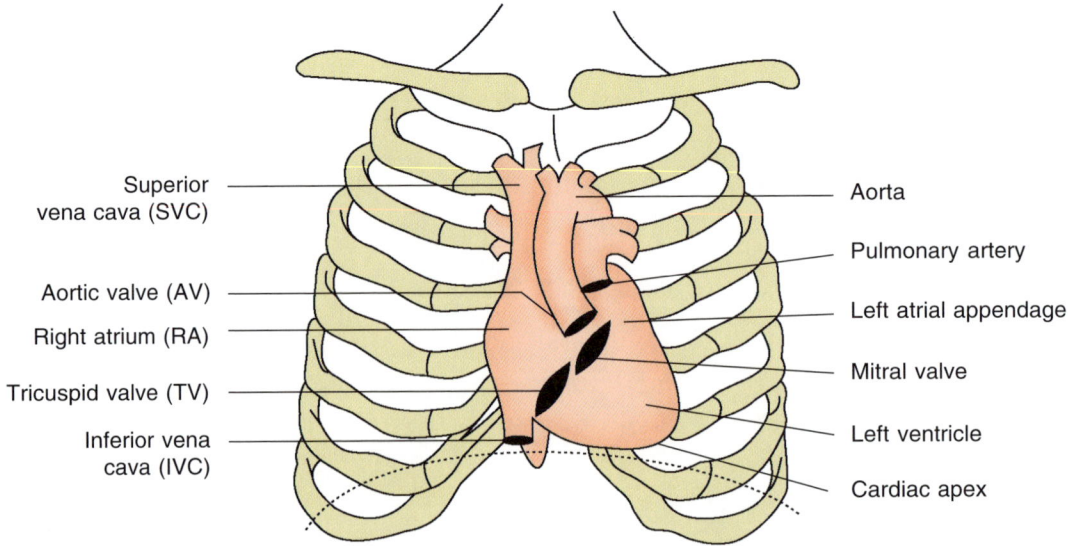

Fig. 3.32 Position of the heart in the thoracic cavity with cardiac chambers, valves and great vessels

valve opens and blood enters into the left ventricle. During left ventricular contraction mitral valve closes so as to prevent the blood from flowing backwards into the left atrium.

Aortic Valve

Aortic valve lies in between the aorta and the left ventricle. During left ventricular contraction aortic valve opens and allows the blood entering into the aorta and then closes (during ventricular dilatation) to prevent the blood from getting back into the left ventricle.

Tricuspid Valve

Tricuspid valve lies in between the right atrium and the right ventricle. During right atrial contraction tricuspid valve opens and blood enters into the right ventricle. During right ventricular contraction tricuspid valve closes so as to prevent the blood getting back from right ventricle to right atrium.

Pulmonary Valve

Pulmonary valve lies in between the right ventricle and pulmonary artery. During right ventricular contraction pulmonary valve opens allowing the blood entering into the lungs and then it closes (during RV dilatation) to prevent the blood from getting back into the right ventricle.

Blood Supply and Nerve Supply of the Heart

Cardiac muscle is supplied by 2 arteries called coronary arteries (Fig. 3.33).

Left Coronary Artery

Arises from aorta and gives rise to left anterior descending and circumflex arteries which give rise to different branches supplying different parts of left heart.

Right Coronary Artery

Arises from aorta and supplies various parts of right ventricle.

Venous system of the heart follows arterial system and then drains into the coronary sinus and then to the right atrium.

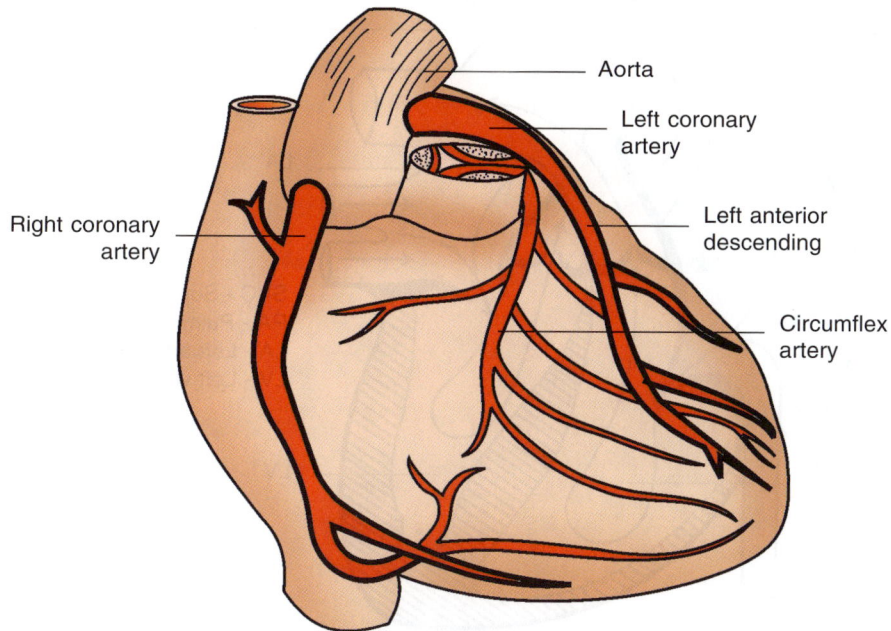

Fig. 3.33 Blood supply of the heart

Nerve Supply

Heart is supplied by both adrenergic and cholinergic system (parasympathetic). Sympathetic stimulation causes increase in the heart rate and parasympathetic (via vagus) stimulation causes decrease in the heart rate.

Physiology of the Heart

Heart muscle (myocardium) acts as a pump by mechanism of contraction (systole) and dilatation (diastole). During atrial contraction ventricle dilates and during ventricular contraction atria dilate (Fig. 3.34).

Myocardial Contraction

Contraction of the cardiac muscle cell (myocyte) is carried out by sarcomere which is the basic unit of contraction. Cardiac muscle contraction is regulated by the inward movement of calcium ions through calcium channels.

Cardiac Output

It is the amount of blood pumped from each ventricle/minute during cardiac contraction.

Stroke Volume

It is the amount of blood pumped from each ventricle/minute. Normal value=70 ml\ minute.

Blood Pressure

Definition

Blood pressure is the lateral pressure exerted by the contained column of blood on the wall of arteries.

Systolic Blood Pressure

* Maximum pressure exerted in the arteries during cardiac systole.

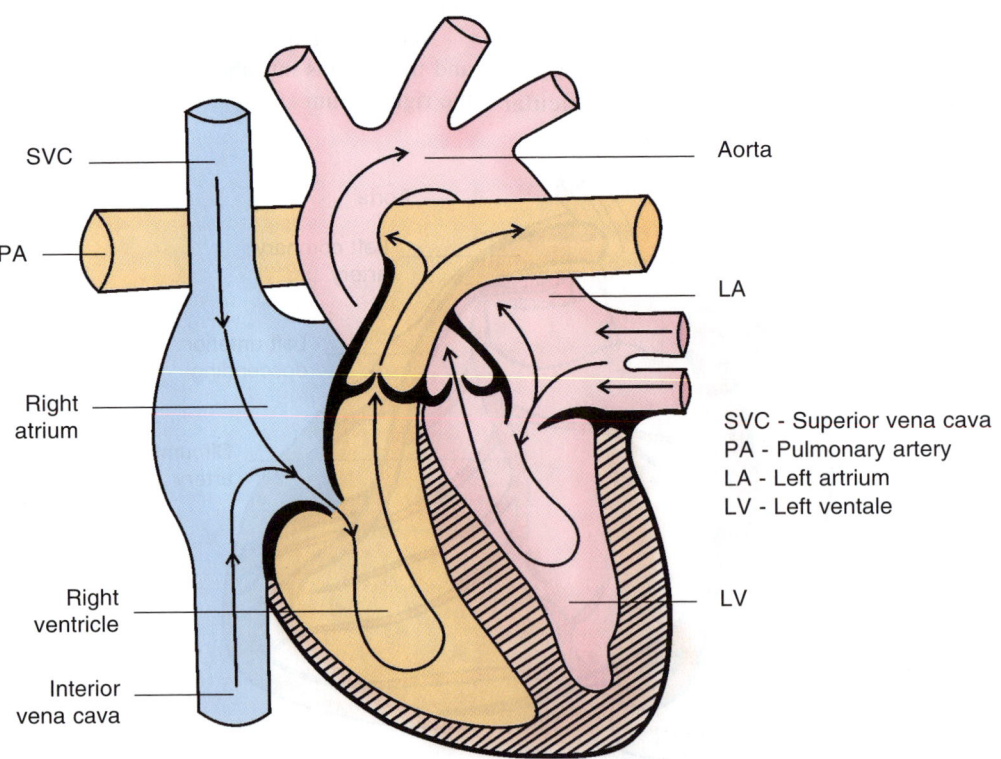

SVC

PA

Right atrium

Right ventricle

Interior vena cava

Aorta

LA

SVC - Superior vena cava
PA - Pulmonary artery
LA - Left artrium
LV - Left ventale

LV

Fig. 3.34 Blood flow inside the heart

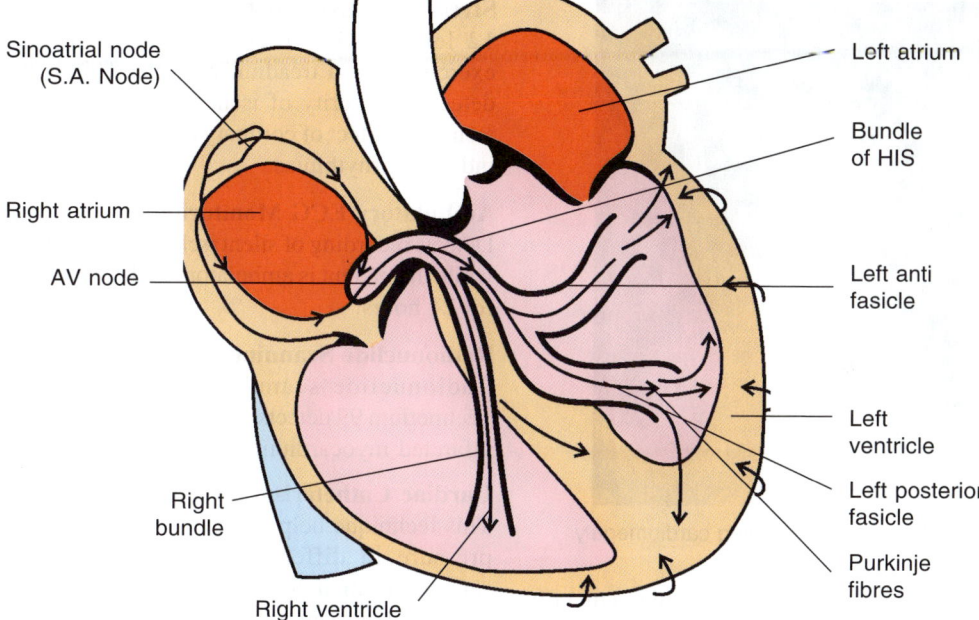

Fig. 3.35 Conduction system of the heart

* Normal systolic blood pressure = 120 mm of Hg.

Diastolic Blood Pressure

* Maximum pressure in the arteries during the diastole of the heart.
* Normal diastolic blood pressure = 60–80 mms of Hg.

Pulse Pressure

Pulse pressure is the difference between systolic and diastolic blood pressure.

Electrical Activity of the Heart (Fig. 3.35)

The electrical impulse of the heart under normal conditions starts at the sino atrial node (SA node) which is situated at the junction of superior vena cava and right atrium.

Depolarisation of sino atrial node causes a wave front which travels through the atrium up to the AV NODE (Atrioventricular node). AV node regulates the impulse and conducts slowly to the ventricles.

From AV node electrical impulse reaches the ventricle and activates the ventricle through 'bundle of His' which divides into right and left bundle and then radiates as Purkinje net work. Electrical activity of the heart can be recorded as electro cardiogram.

Investigations of Cardiovascular Disorders

Radiology

Chest X–ray will help in determining the cardiac size, shape of the heart, pulmonary blood vessels and lung fields (Fig. 3.36).

Cardiomegaly

Cardiomegaly is made out by measuring the cardiac size and comparing the cardiac size with the maximum intrathoracic diameter. If the ratio is >0.5 there is evidence of cardiomegaly.

Left atrial enlargement: Produces straightening of left cardiac border.

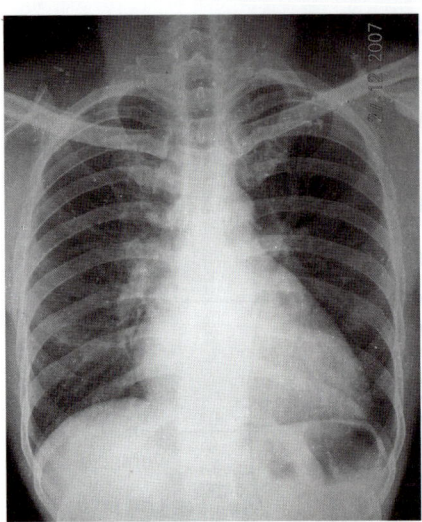

Fig. 3.36 Chest X-ray showing cardiomegaly

Right atrial enlargement: Produces enlargement of right cardiac border >5cm from the mid sternal line.

Left ventricular enlargement: Causes enlargement of cardiac size with rounding of left heart border.

Right ventricular enlargement: Causes enlargement of cardiac size with up ward movement of apex.

Oblique and lateral views of heart are useful in detecting definite chamber enlargement and valve calcification.

ECHO Cardiogram

Useful in detecting cardiac abnormalities, function of the ventricles, thrombus inside the heart, vegetations of infective endocarditis, tumors of the heart and congenital cardiac lesions.

CT Scan and MRI

Useful in imaging the chambers of the heart, blood vessels, ventricular and surrounding structures.

Electrocardiogram (ECG)

Detects the electrical activity of the heart. ECG can detect myocardial ischaemia, infarction, conduction defect in the heart, arrhythmias, chamber enlargement, electrolyte and drug effect on the heart and pericardial diseases.

Stress Test (Exercise ECG)

12 lead ECG is recorded while the person is exercising on a treadmill\tricycle. This is useful in detecting severity of ischemic heart disease, silent ischemia, effect of coronary angioplasty and exercise induced arrhythmias.

Ambulatory ECG Monitoring

Detects recording of silent ischaemia and arrhythmias while the patient is ambulatory and records the events for 24 hours.

Radionuclide Scanning

Radionuclide scanning with thallium 201 or Technetium 99 detects viable myocardium\scarred or infarcted myocardium respectively.

Cardiac Catheterisation

This technique helps in measuring the intra cardiac pressure in different cardiac chambers. Blood samples from individual cardiac chambers can be taken and angiogram can be performed in different parts of the heart. A catheter which has been specially designed is inserted into the artery/vein and then advanced into the chambers of heart under fluoroscopic guidance for measurement of cardiac parameters.

Causes and Different Types of Cardiovascular diseases

Depending on the aetiology
1. Congenital heart disease
2. Rheumatic heart disease
3. Hypertensive heart disease
4. Ischemic heart disease (coronary artery disease)
5. Cardiomyopathies

Due to infection of the endocardium
1. Infective endocarditis

Due to diseases of pericardium
1. Pericarditis
2. Pericardial effusion

Due to abnormal cardiac rhythm
1. Bradycardia
2. Tachycardia
3. Dysarrhythmias

Due to alteration in the circulating blood volume
1. Due to decrease blood volume- Hypovolemic shock.
2. Due to increase blood volume- Hypervolemic-circulatory overload.
3. Pregnancy with heart disease

Due to extracardiac factors affecting the heart:
1. Thyrotoxicosis
2. Anemia
3. Chronic respiratory disease - Cor pulmonale
4. Beriberi

Acute Rheumatic Fever

Common cause of valvular diseases in tropical countries. Results in chronic rheumatic valvular disease due to fibrosis and distortion of valve leaflets.

Aetiology and Pathogenesis

Due to pharyngitis caused by group A-Beta hemolytic streptococci (strains-1, 3, 5, 6, 18, etc.). There is formation of antibodies against the streptococcal antigens which cross react with the myocardial cells and other connective tissues of humans.

There may be genetic factors influencing the abnormal immunological response by the human host against the group A streptococcal infection of the upper respiratory tract.

Pathology

Antibodies produced against the streptococcal antigen produces inflammatory changes in the endocardium, myocardium, pericardium, skin and joints.

Connective tissue of rheumatic fever undergo fibrinoid degeneration including the cardiac connective tissues.

Pathognomonic lesion is the Aschoff body consists of macrophages and lymphocytes and multinucleated giant cells. Aschoff bodies are found in the myocardium.

Clinical Features

Patient presents with history of pharyngitis (sore throat) 2–3 weeks prior to the onset of systemic symptoms.

Important clinical manifestations of rheumatic fever (Fig. 3.37)
- Arthritis
- Carditis
- Chorea
- Subcutaneous nodules
- Erythema marginatum
- Fever
- Joint pain (Arthralgia)

Arthritis

Extremely painful involvement of large (major) joints (knee, ankle, elbows) and joint pain migrates from one joint to the other. Joints are swollen, red and tender. Joint pain usually subsides in at least 3 weeks without residual deformity.

Carditis

Rheumatic carditis is a form of pancarditis involving all 3 layers of heart (endocardium, myocardium and pericardium).

Symptoms
Chest pain, dyspnea and palpitation

Signs
- Tachycardia, cardiomegaly, Carrey Coomb's murmur due to mitral valvulitis (mid diastolic murmur) and systolic murmur due to mitral regurgitation and cardiac failure.
- Mitral and aortic valve is commonly involved.

Other Features
- Characteristic skin rash - Erythema marginatum - rounded bordered macular lesion present on the trunk.
- Cerebral involvement causes involuntary movement of hands - Sydenham's chorea (Saint vitus dance).
- Chorea usually occurs after a latent period of several months after the initial attack of rheumatic fever.
- Subcutaneous nodules - Around elbow and occiput (firm, non tender 1 to 2 cms in size associated with severe rheumatic fever).

- Pleural and pulmonary involvement in the form of pleuropneumonitis.

Investigations
- WBC count- increased
- C- Reactive protein (CRP) is raised
- ESR is elevated
- ASO (anti streptolysin O) titer >200 units
- ECG changes- prolonged PR interval
- Chest X-ray: Cardiomegaly and pleuropneumonitis
- ECHO cardiogram for evidence of cardiac involvement

Criteria for Diagnosis of Rheumatic Fever

Jones criteria

Major criteria	Minor criteria
Polyarthritis	Fever
Carditis	Arthralgia
Chorea	ESR is increased
Subcutaneous nodules	CRP is increased
Erythema marginatum	Prolonged PR interval

Essential (supporting) Criteria
Evidence of recent streptococcal infection, e.g. Increased ASO titer

Diagnosis of Rheumatic Fever
- One major and two minor criteria + essential criteria or two major criteria + essential criteria.

Sequelae of Rheumatic Fever
- Acute
  - Cardiac failure
  - Valvular regurgitation
- Chronic
  - Rheumatic valvular disease involving mitral, aortic, pulmonary and tricuspid valves.
  - Chronic rheumatic myocarditis with cardiac failure

Treatment

General Measures
- Absolute bed rest till symptoms, signs and ESR decrease.
- Good nutritious diet

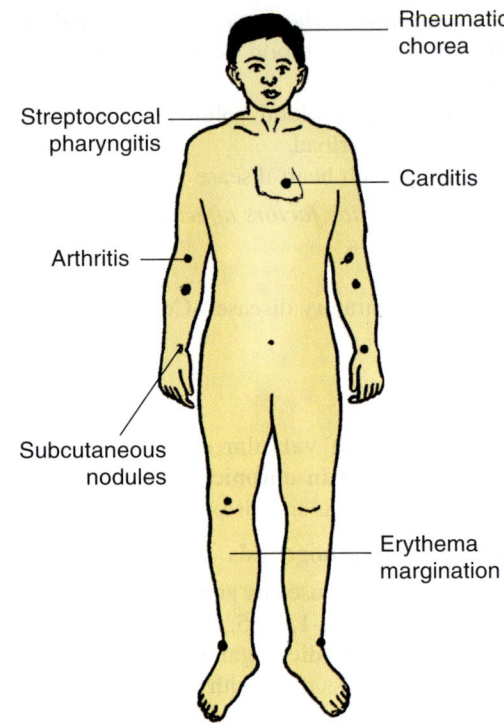

Fig. 3.37 Signs of acute rheumatic fever

- For Streptococcal infection - benzathine penicillin 1–2 million units I.M. or oral phenoxy methylpenicillin 500 mg qid ×10 days. In patients with Penicillin allergy: Erythromycin 250 QID × 10 days.

Specific Measures
- For joint pain: Aspirin 60–100 mg/kg after food in divided doses. Aspirin should be continued till ESR is normal and then tapered and stopped.
- For carditis: Corticosteroids - Tab prednisolone 1mg\kg till ESR is normal and tapered and stopped.
- Cardiac failure is treated with diuretics and digoxin.
- If severe valvular damage occurs, surgical repair is required.

Prophylaxis

To prevent recurrent attacks of streptococcal infection and rheumatic fever:

Inj. Benzjathine penicillin - 1.2 million units I.M. once in 3 weeks upto the age of 25 years/ for at least 5 yrs after the first attack.

Persons with documented evidence for rheumatic valvular disease/recurrence of rheumatic fever, lifelong prophylaxis is recommended.

If allergic to penicillin, erythromycin or sulphadiazine can be used.

Dental Aspects of Rheumatic Fever
- Dental treatment is less likely required during an acute attack of rheumatic fever.
- If dental treatment is required, prefer local anesthesia.
- Avoid general anesthesia as patient may be having myocarditis

CHRONIC RHEUMATIC HEART DISEASE

- Acute rheumatic fever may result in chronic rheumatic heart disease.
- Chronic rheumatic activity results in abnormality of valvular cusps and chordae tendinae resulting in valvular lesions.
- Mitral valve is commonly involved and results in mitral stenosis and regurgitation
- Aortic value involvement results in aortic stenosis and Aortic regurgitation.
- Infective endocarditis may complicate valvular lesions.

Pathology of Chronic Rheumatic Disease
Valve cusps are damaged due to fibrosis and cusps are also involved due to shortening of chordae tendinae. These pathological changes result in valvular stenosis and regurgitation, Fibrosis of myocardium and pericardium may result in cardiac failure and conduction defects.

Mitral Stenosis (MS)

Mitral stenosis occurs due to narrowing of mitral valve.

Main Causes
- Rheumatic fever

- Congenital
- Calcified valve
- Collagen vascular disease.

Features

Symptoms
- Dyspnea and paroxysmal nocturnal dyspnea (PND)
- Haemoptysis
- Palpitation
- Easy fatiguability
- Symptoms due to systemic arterial embolisation, e.g. cerebrovascular accident (stroke).

Signs
- Mitral facies
- Tapping apical impulse
- Diastolic thrill at the apex
- Mid diastolic rumbling murmur at the apex with an opening snap and loud 1st heart sound.

Investigations
- ECG: Demonstrable left atrial enlargement- wide P wave in lead II. Right atrial and right ventricular hypertrophy.
- Chest X-ray: Cardiomegaly, left atrial enlargement causing straightening of left heart border (mitralisation).
- ECHO cardiogram: Demonstrates mitral valve orifice size, other valvular involvement and left atrial enlargement and calcification of cusps and left atral thrombus.

Treatment

Medical
- Prophylaxis for rheumatic fever
- Treatment of cardiac failure
- Anticoagulation in patients with atrial fibrillation and embolism

Surgical
- Mitral valvotomy/balloon valvuloplasty/valve replacement

Complications
- Left side cardiac failure

- Atrial fibrillation with systemic embolisation
- Pulmonary hypertension
- Right ventricular failure
- Haemoptysis

Mitral Regurgitation (MR)

Causes

- Rheumatic fever
- Mitral valve prolapse
- Ischemic heart disease

Features

Symptoms

- May not have any symptom
- Easy fatigability
- Palpitation
- Dyspnea and PND

Signs

- Hyper dynamic apical impulse (apex - shifted out and down)
- Systolic thrill at the apex
- Muffled 1st heart sound
- Pan systolic murmur radiating to the axilla at the apex
- Left sided 3rd heart sound.

Investigation

- ECG: Left atrial enlargement, left ventricular hypertrophy and right atrial enlargement and atrial fibrillation
- Chest X-ray: Left atrial and left ventricular enlargement, pulmonary venous congestion.
- ECHO cardiogram: Estimation of regurgitation, other valvular lesions, condition of the valve and vegetations of endocarditis

Treatment

Medical

- Avoid severe exertion
- Treatment of cardiac failure
- Vasodilators like ACE inhibitors
- Anti infective endocarditis prophylaxis before dental procedures.

Surgical

- Mitral valve replacement

Aortic Regurgitation (AR)

Causes

- Rheumatic fever
- Infective endocarditis
- Marfan's syndrome, syphilis
- Ankylosing spoudylitis

Features

Symptoms

- Easy fatigability
- Exertional dyspnea
- Palpitation
- Chest pain

Signs

- High volume collapsing pulse
- Peripheral signs of AR (refer clinical examination)
- Hyper dynamic apex
- Early diastolic murmur in the aortic area.
- Austinflint mid diastolic murmur at the apex.

Investigations

- ECG: Left ventricular hypertrophy with ST, T changes.
- X-ray: Left ventricular hypertrophy, massive cardiomegaly, dilatation of aorta.
- ECHO: Nature of aortic valve (bicuspid or tricuspid), valvular calcification and chamber hypertrophy.

Treatment

Medical

- Treatment of cardiac failure
- Vasodilators like ACE inhibitors
- Treatment of the cause like syphilis

Surgical

- Aortic valve replacement

Aortic Stenosis (AS)

Causes

- Rheumatic fever

- Congenital bicuspid valve
- Calcified aortic valve

Features

Symptoms
- Exertional syncope
- Chest pain
- Palpitation
- Dyspnea

Signs
- Low volume pulse
- Heaving apical impulse
- Systolic thrill in the aortic area.
- Ejection systolic murmur in the aortic area conducted to carotids.
- Muffled aortic component of 2nd heart sound.

Investigation
- ECG: LV hypertrophy with ST, T changes LA hypertrophy
- X-ray: LVH, aortic calcification and post stenotic dilatation of aorta
- ECHO: Nature of aortic valve (bicuspid or tricuspid), valvular calcification and chamber hypertrophy.

Treatment
- Avoidance of severe exertion
- Treatment of cardiac failure
- Aortic valve replacement

Complications of Rheumatic Valvular Heart Disease
- Left sided cardiac failure
- Pulmonary arterial hypertension
- Right sided cardiac failure
- Atrial fibrillation
- Systemic embolisation
- Infective endocarditis
- Haemoptysis

Dental Aspects of Chronic Rheumatic Valvular Diseases
- Infective endocarditis may follow after dental procedure if antibiotic prophylaxis cover is not given before the procedure (see endocarditis).

- Obtain the history of rheumatic fever in the past and do a cardiac evaluation before the dental procedure in suspected cases of valvular heart disease.
- Give prophylactic antibiotic in suspected patients of heart murmurs before dental procedure.
- Risk of endocarditis is not related to the severity of valvular lesion.

CONGENITAL HEART DISEASE

Congenital heart diseases present at birth affecting the heart and great vessels.

Classification
Acyanotic (without intracardiac shunt)
- Dextrocardia
- Complete heart block
- Obstructive lesions
  - Coarctation of aorta
  - Congenital aortic stenosis
  - Congenital pulmonary stenosis

Acyanotic (with intracardiac shunt)
- Left to right shunt
  - Arial sepal defect (ASD)
  - Ventricular sepal defect (VSD)
  - Patent ductus arteriosus (PDA)

Cyanotic (right to left shunt)
- Tetralogy of Fallot
- Eisenmenger syndrome
- Tricuspid artesia
- Ebstein's anomaly
- Transposition of great arteries
- Total anomalous pulmonary venous connection

Clinical Aspects of Congenital Heart Disease
- Severe congenital heart disease manifests in early childhood but minor defects may pass unnoticed and may be detectable only in adult life.
- Congenital heart diseases can be associated with birth oral anomalies like cleft palate.
- Some types of congenital heart diseases present with cyanosis at birth or in early childhood due to deoxygenated blood from right ventricle entering into the aorta, e.g. Fallot's Tetralogy.

- Congenital shunt lesions (shunting of blood from left to right through the sepal defects) cause recirculation of cardiac output through the pulmonary circulation resulting in pulmonary hypertension, right ventricular hypertrophy (RVH) and right ventricular failure (CCF).
- Chronic hypoxemia can lead to clubbing, impaired growth, polycythaemia (excess Hb% and RBC mass) with haemorrhagic/ thrombotic features.
- Patients with congenital heart diseases have got susceptibility to infective endocarditis and heart failure and these may complicate dental procedures.

Aetiology of Congenital Heart Disease

Following aetiological factors may be responsible for the development of congenital heart diseases.

- Rubella virus infection in the mother in the 1st 3 months of pregnancy can cause - PDA, pulmonary stenosis, ASD.
- Alcohol abuse in the mother during pregnancy can cause septal defects.
- Chromosomal defects (genetic abnormalities) can be associated with congenital heart disease, e.g. Down's syndrome (Trisomy -21) with septal defects.
- Exposure to drugs/toxins during 1st trimester of pregnancy can result in congenital heart disease.

General Features of Severe Congenital Heart Disease

- Growth retardation in childhood and learning difficulties.
- Central cyanosis and clubbing
- Recurrent childhood respiratory infection.
- Severe congenital pulmonary stenosis, aortic stenosis and pulmonary hypertension can be associated with syncopal attacks.
- Reversal of shunt lesions occur in patients with ASD, PDA and VSD due to pulmonary hypertension causing cyanosis and clubbing. This is called Eisenmenger syndrome.

IMPORTANT TYPES OF CONGENITAL HEART DISEASES

Ventricular Sepal Defect (VSD)

Congenital VSD occurs as a result of defective ventricular septation.

Most common type of VSD is of perimembranous type.

Clinical Features

- Pan systolic murmur at the left sternal border.
- Small defect can produce a loud murmur (maladie de Roger).
- Development of pulmonary hypertension, RVH and CCF

Investigations

- ECG: shows biventricular hypertrophy.
- Chest X ray: shows pulmonary plethora (increased vascularity of pulmonary arteries).
- ECHO: Reveals the defect and confirms the diagnosis

Management

- Smaller defect: no treatment is required
- Larger defect: closure of the defect

Dental aspects

Shunting of blood occurs from left ventricle to right ventricle. Flow of blood impinging on the part of the right ventricle or margin of the septal defect can be the site of infective endocarditis. Requires prophylaxis against endocarditis before dental extraction.

Atrial Sepal Defect (ASD)

One of the most common form of congenital heart disease.

Females are affected more common than males.

Types of ASD

- Ostium secundum defect
  - Common type of ASD
  - Involves fossa ovalis
- Ostium primum defect
  - Due to defect in the atrioventricular septum
  - Usually associated with cleft mitral valve

Because of the shunt between the left atrium and the right atrium, large amount of blood enters into the right heart (right atrium to right ventricle and to the pulmonary artery and to the lungs). There will be gradual development of pulmonary artery hypertension later in life.

Features

Symptoms
- May be asymptomatic/detected on routine examination.
- May present with chest pain, palpitation and dyspnea.

Signs
- Wide and fixed splitting of second heart sound and ejection systolic murmur at the pulmonary area.
- Pulmonary hypertension, RVH and CCF are late features.

Investigations
- ECG: Presence of RBBB pattern
- Chest X-ray: Reveals pulmonary plethoric appearance
- ECHO cardiogram: Detects the size of the defect and right atrial and right ventricular hypertrophy.

Management
- Closure of the defect—surgical/during cardiac catheterisation

Dental Aspects
Venous embolus can pass from right to left heart through the septal defect into the systemic circulation. This is called paradoxical embolism.
- Infective endocarditis risk is small in patients with ASD.
- Uncorrected ASD patients should receive antibiotic prophylaxis before dental procedure.

Patent Ductus Arteriosus (PDA)

Features
- Persistence of communication between aorta and pulmonary artery.
- A loud continuous machinery murmur is heard in the left infra clavicular area
- Pulmonary hypertension can develop causing right ventricular failure.
- Infective endarteritis may be a complication.
- Uncorrected defects should receive antibiotic prophylaxis before dental procedure.

Coarctation of Aorta

Features
- Narrowing of aorta beyond the origin of left subclavian artery.
- There is restricted supply of blood to the lower limbs with upper part of the body receiving normal blood supply.
- There is severe hypertension in the upper part of the body.
- Femoral pulse is delayed from the radial pulse. This is called radio femoral delay.
- Bicuspid aortic valve, aneurysm of aorta can be associated with coarctation of aorta.
- LV failure and infective endocarditis can complicate the lesion.

Fallot's Tetralogy

Components
VSD, infundibular pulmonary stenosis, over riding of aorta over the inter ventricular septum and RVH.

Features
- Cyanosis, clubbing
- Syncope, dyspnea, squatting episodes in children.
- Respiratory infection, cerebral abscess and rarely infective endocarditis can occur.

Mitral Valve Prolapse (MVP)

Features
- Prolapse of mitral valve into the left atrium
- Can result in mitral regurgitation.
- Can predispose to endocarditis
- Should receive antibiotic prophylaxis before dental procedure if associated with mitral regurgitation.

Bicuspid Aortic Valve

Features
- Aortic valve is having two leaflets instead of normal 3 leaflets.
- Totally asymptomatic throught life
- May develop aortic stenosis
- High risk for infective endocarditis

Dental Aspects of Congenital Heart Disease

Congenital heart diseases can be associated with the following oral abnormalities

- Enamel hyperplasia
- Positional anomalies and delayed eruption of teeth.
- Gross vasodilatation of pulps
- Cleft palate
- Because of lack of proper oral hygiene there is more risk of dental caries and periodontal disease.
- There is greater risk of cerebral abscess in patients with Fallot's tetralogy may be due to dental sepsis or occasionally following endodontic treatment.

HYPERTENSION

High blood pressure is defined as persistently elevated blood pressure above the normal level for that corresponding age.

As age advances systolic blood pressure also increases and ischemic heart disease and stroke incidence is directly proportional to the average blood pressure at all ages.

Stress including dental treatment can raise the blood pressure and may result in complications.

Causes and Classification of Hypertension

- Primary/essential hypertension
- Secondary hypertension

KEY POINTS 3.6

To be remembered in patients with congenital heart disease.

- Administer general anaesthesia for dental procedures only after specialist consultation (in patients with congenital heart disease).

- There is increased risk of infective endocarditis after dental procedures in patients (with congenital heart disease).

- Platelet dysfunction and increased fibrinolysis can lead onto tendency for bleeding after dental procedures in patients with congenital heart disease.

Causes of Secondary Hypertension

1. Renal
- Renal parenchymal disease
  - Acute and chronic glomerulonephritis
  - Chronic pyelonephritis
  - Polycystic kidney disease
- Renal artery stenosis
2. Endocrinal
- Cushing's syndrome
- Conn's syndrome
- Acromegaly
- Myxedema
- Phaeochromocytoma
- Hypercalcemia
3. Vascular
- Coarctation of aorta
- Polyarteritis nodosa
4. Miscellaneous
- Glucocorticoid therapy
- Pregnancy induced hypertension
- Oral contraceptive pills therapy.

Primary (Essential) Hypertension

- Accounts for 95% of cases of hypertension
- No definite aetiological factors can be identified.
- Genetic factors may be responsible.

Kidneys, peripheral vascular system and sympathetic nervous system (adrenaline and noradrenaline) appear to play roles in the pathogenesis of essential hypertension. Anger, anxiety and emotion can also raise the blood pressure.

Secondary Hypertension

- Constitutes about 5% of all cases of hypertension.
- Specific aetiological factors can be identified.
- Treatment of specific aetiology can cure hypertension.

Technique of recording of blood pressure (see under clinical examination of cardiovascular system)

- *Isolated systolic hypertension:* Systolic blood pressure equal to or above 140 mm of Hg with diastolic blood pressure less than 90 mm of Hg.
- *Diastolic hypertension:* Diastolic blood pressure equal to or above 90 mm of Hg.

- *Accelerated hypertension:* Sudden rise of blood pressure above the previous recordings with fundal hemorrhages but without papilledema.
- *Malignant hypertension:* Recording of diastolic blood pressure above 140 mm of Hg associated with papilledema.

Pathogenesis of Essential Hypertension

Essential Hypertension
- Constitutes about 95% of hypertension.
- Pathogenesis is not clearly understood.
- Hypertension results due to interplay of factors like renal, sympathetic nervous system and peripheral arterial system.
- Genetic factor plays an important role in the genesis of hypertension. Black rays are more likely to develop hypertension.
- Environmental factors like increased salt intake, excessive consumption of alcohol, over weight, lack of exercise and intrauterine growth retardation are important factors in the pathogenesis of essential hypertension.

Clinical Aspects of Hypertension
- Many hypertensives are asymptomatic and are only detected on routine measurement or may present for the first time with complications.
- Enquire the details of smoking, alcoholism, dietary habits (high salt intake), exercise and drug intake (NSAIDS, steroids, oral contraceptives) in all patients of hypertension.
- Obtain the history of renal disease (puffiness of face, pedal edema, and decrease urine output), cardiac symptoms like (chest pain, palpitation, and dyspnea) and for secondary causes of hypertension.
- Correctly measure the blood pressure twice under basal conditions before establishing hypertension.
- Examine the patient for secondary causes of hypertension and for target organ involvement.

Examination of a Patient of Hypertension
- Record the pulse and blood pressure
- Do specific examination for following signs to ruleout secondary causes of hypertension.

Abnormalities	Corresponding disorders
Radio femoral delay	Coarctation of aorta
Moon face	Cushing's syndrome
Puffiness of face, pedal edema	Renal parenchymal disease
Enlarged and palpable kidneys	Polycystic kidney disease
Renal artery bruit	Renal artery stenosis

Examine the patient also for target organ involvement like
- Optic fundus for retinopathy
- Cardiac examination: Heaving cardiac apex suggests LVH.
  – Loud aortic component of 2nd heart sound
  – Ejection systolic murmur in the aortic area.
- Nervous system examination for neurological deficit.

Target organ involvement in patients with Hypertension
- Blood vessels - Widespread atherosclerosis of vessels including coronary vessels.
- Cardiac - Left ventricular hypertrophy
- Retina - Retinal vascular damage
- Renal - Renal vascular damage
- Cerebral vessels - Cerebrovascular damage.

Complications of Hypertension
- Cardio vascular
  – Epistaxis
  – Left ventricular failure
  – Acute myocardial infarction
  – Aortic aneurysm
  – Aortic dissection
- Retina
  – Hypertensive retinopathy
- Renal
  – Renal vascular thickening and renal failure
- Blood vessels
  – Peripheral vascular disease
- Central nervous system
  – Hypertensive encephalopathy
  – Intracranial hemorrhage
  – Cerebral thrombosis
  – Subarachnoid hemorrhage

Investigations of a Patient of Hypertension

Routine investigations
- Blood sugar estimation
- Fasting lipid profile
- Urine for protein, blood and sugar and microscopy
- Blood urea, creatinine and electrolytes
- Electrocardiogram
- Chest X-Ray for cardiomegaly and cardiac failure

Specific Investigations in Suspected Cases of Secondary Hypertension
- Abdominal ultrasound for renal disease, e.g. polycystic kidney
- Renal artery Doppler for renal artery stenosis
- Echo cardiogram for left ventricular size and function and coarctation of aorta.
- Thyroid function tests for thyroid disease.
- Serum calcium level for hyperparathyroidism
- 24 hours urinary catecholamine and VMA (vanilyl mandolic acid for phaeochromocytoma.
- Serum cortisole and dexamethasone suppression test for Cushing's syndrome
- Plasma renin activity and aldosterone level for possible primary aldosteronism (Conn's syndrome).
- ANA (Antinuclear antibody) and ANCA (anti neutrophil cytoplasmic antibody) for vasculitis and collegen diseases.

Management of Hypertension
- Life long treatment is required in patients with primary (essential) hypertension.
- In patients with secondary hypertension if the cause is treated hypertension can be cured.

Indications for Treatment of Hypertension
- Patients with repeated systolic blood pressure > 140 mm of Hg. and diastolic blood pressure of > 90 mm of Hg.
- Isolated systolic blood pressure of >160 mm of Hg above 65 years of age.
- Patients with diabetes mellitus and evidence of atherosclerosis with diastolic blood pressure of 85 to 90 mm of Hg.

Non pharmacological measures in the treatment of Hypertension
- Weight reduction in obese patients
- Decrease alcohol intake
- Restricted salt intake (less than 5 g/day)
- Regular aerobic exercise
- Increase intake of vegetables and fruits
- Stop smoking
- Relief of stress, treatment of other risk factors of atherosclerosis.

Steps in the Management of Hypertension
- VMA - vanilyl mandolic acid
- Try non pharmacological measures in all patients of hypertension (see above).
- Try to achieve the target blood pressure (see above) with the drug therapy if the non drug therapy is not effective.
- Find out and treat the cause in a patient of secondary hypertension.

Drug Therapy (Table 3.11)
- Start with a single drug and increase the dose to the maximum level till the BP is controlled which can be tolerated by the patient and long term compliance is mandatory.
- Add another class of drug if the initial single drug fails to control the blood pressure.
- Adding a diuretic is recommended whenever two drugs are required.
- After the full doses of initial two drugs are tried and if the BP is not controlled, try to add the 3rd drug. Mean while look for the salt intake, compliance of drug and secondary causes of hypertension.

Examples of Drug Combinations in Patients with Hypertension
- Beta blockers + diuretics
- ACE inhibitors + diuretics
- ACE inhibitors + calcium channel blockers
- Calcium channel blockers + beta blockers
  Selection of the drug depends on the patient's co existing clinical condition. For example
- Diuretics in hypertension with cardiac failure
- ACE inhibitors in diabetic nephropathy/CCF with hypertension

Table 3.11 Drug therapy of hypertension

Drugs Used	Dose / day	Side effects
Diuretics		
Thiazide		
E.g.: Bendro flumethiazide	2.5 mg	Electrolyte imbalance
Loop diuretic		
E.g.: Frusemide	40 mg	Hyperuricemia, hyperglycemia
B-blockers		
Atenalol	25–100 mg	Bradycardia
Metoprolol	100–200 mg	Bronchospasm
ACE inhibitors		
Captopril	25–75 mg	
Enalapril	20 mg	Hypotension
Ramipril	5–20 mg	Cough
Angiotensin II-receptor blockers		
Losartan	50–100 mg	Cough, hypotension
Calcium channel blockers		
Amlodepin	5–20 mg	Gum hyperplasia
Nifedipine	30–90 mg	Pedal edema
Alpha blockers		
Prazosin	0.5–20 mg	Dizziness
Alpha and Beta blockers		
Labetalol	100–600 mg	Hypotension
Carvedilol	12.5–50 mg	
Vasodilators		
Hydralazine	25–100 mg	Head ache
Minoxidil	10–50 mg	Palpitation
Diazoxide	1–3 mg/kg	Hyperglycemia
Nitroprusside	0.5–8 mg/kg/min	Anxiety, sweating
Centrally acting drugs		
Clonidine	150–900 mg	Dry mouth
Methyldopa	750 mg	Postural hypotension

- Calcium channel blockers- elderly hypertensives and angina with hypertension
- Beta blockers-hypertension with angina/tachyarrhythmias

  Regular once in 3 months follow up is required for BP monitoring, for the drug side effects and life style modification in all patients with hypertension.

Emergency Drugs in Accelerated Hypertension
- IV Labetalol
- IV Nitroglycerin
- IM Hydralazine
- IV Sodium Nitroprusside
- IV Furosemide

Dental Aspects of Hypertension
- Hypertension as such may not cause any oral manifestation.
- Severe hypertension can cause cerebrovascular accident and may result in facial and hypoglossal nerve paralysis and can cause facial and lingual abnormalities.
- Anti hypertensive drugs can cause significant oral side effects.

- Adequate control of blood pressure is required before dental treatment and before general anesthesia.
- Sudden stoppage of antihypertensive drugs should not be done as it can cause rebound hypertension.
- It is preferable to use local anaesthesia for dental treatment in patients with hypertension.

Oral Side Effects of Anti Hypertensive Medications

Drugs	Oral manifestations
Beta - blockers	Lichenoid lesions
Calcium channel blockers	Gingival hyperplasia
ACE inhibitors	Oral ulcers and sore mouth
Clonidine	Dry mouth
Methyldopa	Lichenoid lesions and oral ulcers
Adrenergic neuron blockade	Dry mouth parotid pain

General anesthetics can potentiate the action of antihypertensive drugs and can result in hypotension. This can cause decrease blood supply to vital organs (kidney, heart and brain) especially in patients with vascular disease and can cause complications.

Note
- Intravenous barbiturates potentiate the action of anti hypertensive drugs
- Halothane, isoflurane etc can potentiate the action of Beta - blockers causing hypotension.
- Diuretics like frusemide cause hypokalemia (decreased serum potassium level) causing cardiac arrhythmias and can potentiate the action of muscle relaxants like curare and pancuronium during anesthesia.

Dental Treatment in Patients with Hypertension
- Reassure and sedate (with diazepam) the patient if required before dental treatment and surgery as anxiety can increase the blood pressure.
- Avoid using adrenaline while giving local anesthesia in patients with hypertension as it can raise the blood pressure and can cause cardiac arrhythmias.

- Do the dental procedures in the morning after control of BP.
- Cardiac and renal failures caused by hypertension can complicate the dental procedures.
- Corticosteroids should be administered carefully if required as they can raise the blood pressure.

Calcium Channel Blockers in Cardiovascular Disorders
3 subclasses of calcium channel blockers:
1. Dihydropyridines, e.g. amlodipine
2. Benzothiazepines, e.g. diltiazem
3. Phenylalkylamines, e.g. verapamil

Amlodipine group of drugs produce vasodilatation with tachycardia.

Diltiazem and Verapamil group of drugs cause decrease in the heart rate.

Longer acting calcium channel agents are preferred for treatment of hypertension.

Uses of Calcium Channel Blockers
- Hypertension
- Peripheral vascular disease
- Angina pectoris
- Pulmonary hypertension

Side effects of Calcium Channel Blockers
- Head ache
- Pedal edema
- Gum hyperplasia

Contraindications for the Uses of Calcium Channel Blockers
- Complete heart block
- CCF

CORONARY ARTERY DISEASE (ISCHEMIC HEART DISEASE)

Clinical Aspects of Coronary Artery Disease
Coronary artery disease or ischemic heart disease (IHD) is the most common form of heart disease.
- Coronary artery disease (CAD) is usually due to coronary atherosclerosis causing progressive decrease of blood flow resulting in myocardial ischemia.

- Coronary atherosclerosis and its complications is the most common form of coronary artery disease.
- Coronary arteries can also be involved in aortic valve disease, vasculitic syndromes and aortitis.

Risk Factors for the Development of Coronary Artery Disease

- Diabetes mellitus
- Hypertension
- Hypothyroidism
- Familial hyperlipidemia
- Smoking
- Lack of exercise
- Obesity

Different Clinical Presentation of Coronary Artery Disease

- Angina pectoris
  - Stable angina
  - Unstable angina
- Myocardial infarction
- Heart failure
- Cardiac arrhythmias
- Sudden death

ANGINA PECTORIS (STABLE ANGINA)

Angina pectoris is characterised by pain in the retrosternal area usually precipitated by exertion and pain is relieved by rest or by sublingual nitroglycerin.

Pathophysiology of Angina Pectoris

- Clinical syndrome occurs due to transient myocardial ischemia.
- Atheroma formation in the coronary artery with fixed obstruction is the most common cause of stable angina pectoris.
- Aortic valve disease, vasculitis and obstructive cardiomyopathy can also cause angina pectoris.

Others Factors Contributing for Angina

- Coronary artery spasm
- Decrease filling of coronary arteries.

Note: Angina pectoris can also occur due to left ventricular hypertrophy which causes increased oxygen demand and narrowed coronary arteries may not be able to supply adequate oxygen to the myocardium.

Clinical Description of Angina Pectoris

- *Site of pain:* Precordium/retrosternal
- *Character:* Feeling of heaviness/pain in the retrosternal area
- *Radiation:* Left side of the neck, angle of the jaw on the left side, medial border of the left upper limb till the little finger and interscapular area.
- *Duration of pain:* Usually 5 to 15 minutes
- *Precipitating factors:* Exertion, anxiety, emotion, cold exposure exertion in cold weather after heavy meals.
- *Relieving factors:* Rest, sublingual nitroglycerin tablets
- *Associated symptoms:* Nausea, vomiting, sweating
- *Decubitus angina:* Angina occurs on lying down.
- *Nocturnal angina:* Angina occurs during sleep.

Examination of a Patient of Angina Pectoris

- May not have any clinical signs even during the attack of angina.
- Look for evidence of cardiac involvement like cardiomegaly, 3rd and 4th heart sound and murmurs.
- Rule out other causes of angina like aortic valve disease.
- Look for evidence of vascular disease like peripheral vascular occlusion, and carotid bruit.
- Search for risk factors like hypertension, diabetes mellitus, obesity and hyperlipidemia.
- Rule out severe anemia and thyrotoxicosis as they can increase myocardial oxygen demand and precipitate angina.

  Patients of angina pectoris can develop repeated attacks of chest pain and may progress to myocardial infarction.

Investigations of Angina Pectoris

- *Resting ECG:* May be normal in between the attack or may show ST segment and T wave abnormalities.
- *Exercise ECG:* Stress test may detect evidence of ischemia to the myocardium.

Myocardial Perfusion Scanning
- Thallium 201 scan: Viable and healthy myo-cardium takes up thallium.

Dobutamine echocardiography: To detect healthy and diseased myocardium.

Coronary arteriography: Gives details of severity and nature of coronary artery disease. Usually performed before coronary artery bypass graft (CABG) and coronary angioplasty.

Investigations for Risk Factors
Hb%, packed cell volume, blood sugar, lipid profile and thyroid function tests.

Management of Angina Pectoris
Management of risk factors
- Reduction of weight, if obese
- Regular exercise depending on the patient's tolerance and avoid severe exertion.
- Stoppage of smoking, treatment of hypertension, diabetes mellitus and hyperlipedemia

Symptomatic Treatment of Angina

Nitrates
Produces coronary vasodilatation and increases myocardial oxygen supply and decreases myocardial oxygen demand by causing peripheral vasodilatation.

Short Acting Nitrates
For immediate relief sublingual nitrates 300–500 microgram, can cause severe headache.

Long Acting Nitrates
- Iso sorbide dinitrate 10–20 mg 8th hrly.
- Iso sorbide mononitrates: 20–60 mg once/twice daily.

Beta-blockers
These decrease heart rate, blood pressure and myocardial contractility and decreases oxygen demand of the myocardium, e.g.
> Cardioselective Beta - blockers.
> T. Atenolol 50–100 mg/day or T. Metoprolol 200 mg/day.

Calcium Channel Blockers
These decrease the myocardial oxygen demand by decrease of blood pressure and contractility of myocardium, e.g.
> Verapamil - 40 mg 8th hrly
> Diltiazem 90–120 mg/day

Potassium Channel Activators
Cause arterial and venous dilatation
E.g.: Nicorandil 10–30 mg BD

Anti platelet drugs
Aspirin 75-150mg/day or Clopidogrel 75mg/day. Aspirin or clopidogrel should be given to all patients with IHD life long to reduce the risk of myocardial infarction.

Invasive Therapy

Percutaneous Coronary Angioplasty (PTCA) with Stenting
Dilating the narrowed coronary artery by a balloon which is positioned at the site of narrowing with the help of a guidewire which is passed under radiographic guidance. A metallic stent can be put to maintain the dilatation of graft or site of dilation.

Coronary Artery by Pass Graft (CABG)
Surgically by passing the stenosed coronary artery by using a graft (Graft is made of patient's own internal mammary artery or saphanous vein).

UNSTABLE ANGINA

Unstable angina constitutes one of the acute coronary syndromes along with acute myocardial infarction.

Characteristics
1. Angina which occurs at rest
2. Angina occurring on minimal exertion
3. Rapid worsening of angina.

Unstable angina suggests significant and may be sudden reduction in the myocardial blood supply either due to
- Local spasm of coronary artery
- Platelet rich thrombus
- Ulcerated atheromatous plaque.

Above pathology occurs in the coronary artery in a patient who is already having coronary atherosclerosis and angina pectoris. There is significant risk of acute myocardial infarction and unstable angina pectoris should be treated in the same way as acute myocardial infarction (see below).

Dental Aspects of Angina Pectoris

- Reassure the patient of angina pectoris before dental treatment and if required sedate with diazepam.
- Angina can cause pain in the mandible, teeth or oral tissues.
- Give the daily medication which the patient is taking before the dental procedure.
- Glyceryl trinitrate (nitroglycerin) should be available for immediate use if chest pain occurs.

If angina occurs during dental procedure, stop the procedure and give sublingual glyceryl trinitrate 0.5mg. Pain usually gets relieved within 2–3 minutes. If not consult the physician.

- Except for minor dental procedures which can be performed under local anesthesia - all patients with chest pain should undergo detail medical examination before major dental procedures.
- Avoid dental surgery and general anesthesia in patients with recent onset angina and unstable angina.
- Prophylaxis against infective endocarditis is not required for patients who have undergone CABG.

ACUTE MYOCARDIAL INFARCTION (MI)

Most severe and dangerous form of coronary artery disease due to acute decrease in the blood supply to the myocardium.

Myocardial infarction is invariably due to the development of a thrombus occluding at the site of erosion or rupture of an atheromatous plaque in the coronary artery. Myocardial infarction results in ischemic necrosis of the myocardium.

Mortality rate (death) is highest within the 1st hour after myocardial infarction.

Patients of acute myocardial infarction may give history of recurrent attacks of angina.

Clinical Features

Symptoms

Chest pain: Severe uncontrollable and prolonged pain typical of angina. Pain is not relieved by rest or nitrates.

Myocardial infarction may be painless in patients with diabetes mellitus and elderly patients called silent myocardial infarction.

Myocardial infarction may also present with following symptoms apart from chest pain due to its complications.

- *Syncope:* Due to arrhythmias or hypotension.
- *Breathlessness:* Due to cardiac failure
- *Nausea vomiting:* Due to vagal stimulation or drug (opiate) induced.
- Anxiety, restlessness, sweating and fear of death.
- *Sudden death:* Due to arrhythymias or cardiac asystole (usually within 1st hour of myocardial infarction).

Signs

- May not have any clinical sign.
- Non specific signs: Pallor, sweating and fever

Specific Signs

Cardiovascular

- *Bradycardia:* Due to vagal stimulation/conduction defect
- *Tachycardia:* Due to sympathetic stimulation, due to tachyarrhymias.
- *Irregular pulse:* Due to arrhythmias.
- *Cold extremities and hypotension:* Due to cardiogenic shock
- Diffuse apical impulse
- Muffled 1st heart sound

Signs due to Cardiac Complications

Cardiac failure and myocardial damage

- Raised JVP
- 3rd heart sound
- Bilateral crepitations in the lung base
- Mitral regurgitation murmur
- Pericardial rub

Investigations

ECG shows characteristic ST and T changes and Q waves. (ST elevation, T inversion and prominent Q waves) (Figs 3.38 and 3.39).

Cardiac Enzymes
- CK and CKMB - Cardiac specific isoenzyme
- Raise occurs within 4–6 hrs.
- Cardiac troponin T and I - Raise within 4–6 hrs and remain elevated up to 2 weeks.

Other Investigations
- Raised WBC count, ESR, and CRP
- *Chest X-Ray*: May demonstrate pulmonary edema
- *ECHO:* Detects LV and RV function. Detects complications such as VSD, cardiac rupture, mitral regurgitation and pericardial effusion.

Complications of Acute Myocardial Infarction

Acute
- Left ventricular failure
- Cardiogenic shock
- Arrhythmias
  - Sinus bradycardia
  - Supra ventricular arrhythmias
  - Ventricular premature beats, tachycardia and fibrillation
  - Conduction blocks
- Pericarditis
- Recurrent chest pain
- Left ventricular rupture and ventricular septal defect
- Papillary muscle dysfunction and mitral regurgitation
- Thromboembolism

Chronic
- Ischemic dilated cardiomyopathy
- Chronic cardiac failure
- Ventricular aneuryrm
- Thromboembolism

Treatment of Myocardial Infarction

Immediate Measures
- Admission to intensive coronary care unit.
- Absolute rest and reassurance
- Intra venous access
- ECG and cardiac monitoring
- High flow oxygen, if required

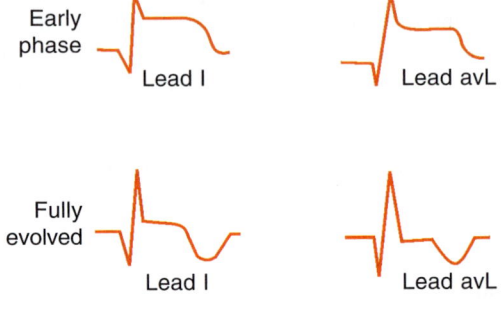

Fig. 3.38 ECG sequence with anterior wall Q wave infarction

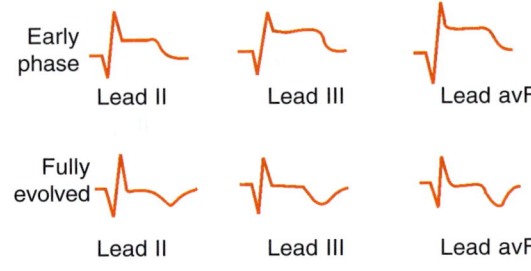

Fig. 3.39 ECG sequence with inferior wall Q wave infarction

- IV analgesics: IV opiates - IV morphine sulphate 10mg + cyclizine 50mg (to prevent vomiting)

Coronary Reperfusion
1. Aspirin 75–300 mg/day - 1st tablet to be chewed and then orally every day
2. Thrombolysis: (if not contraindicated) IV streptokinase 1.5million units in 100ml of saline over 1 hour or human tissue plasminogen activator.
3. Immediate percutaneous coronary angioplasty

Other Drug Therapy in Myocardial Infarction
Subcutaneous heparin to prevent reinfarction and thromboembolism.

β-blockers

Atenalol 5–10 mg or Metoprolol 5–25 mg (it not contraindicated) - Reduce pain and arrhythmias.

Nitrates

Sublingual and IV Nitrate
* To relieve pain and cardiac failure
* Sublingual gleceryl trinitrate: 300–500 microgram
* Isosorbide dinitrate 1–2 mg/ hr or IV. Nitroglecyrin 0.6–1.2 mg/hr for relief of repeated attacks of chest pain and severe left ventricular failure.

ACE Inhibitors

Beneficial if given within 24 hrs after acute MI with systolic blood pressure > 100 mms Hg. Reduces the risk of congestive cardiac failure and recurrent infarction.

General Measures

* *Bed rest:* Absolute bed rest is recommended for the 1st 12 hours and then allow the physical activity depending on the clinical situation.
* *Diet:* Patient is kept nil orally till the vomiting subsides and then liquid diet is allowed for the 1st 12 hours. Later patient is allowed to take adequate calories with complex carbohydrates with less of saturated fat.
* *Bowel:* Usage of diet with fibres, laxatives and stool softeners is beneficial in patients with acute myocardial infarction.
* *Sedation:* Minimal sedation with diazepam 5 mg 3 or 4 times is recommended in patients with acute MI.

HEART FAILURE

Definition

A condition when the heart can not maintain adequate cardiac output or can maintain the cardiac output only with an elevated filling pressure.

Pathogenesis of Heart Failure

Impaired left ventricular function leads to decreased cardiac output which in turn gives rise to activation of sympathetic and rennin Angiotensin system.

Activation of renin angiotensin system leads to vasoconstriction and retention of sodium and water aggravating cardiac failure.

Different Types of Heart Failure

Left sided Cardiac Failure

Left side of the heart includes left ventricle, left atrium, aorta, mitral and aortic valves.

Features
* There is decrease in the left ventricular output.
* There will be increase in the left atrial pressure and pulmonary venous congestion and edema.

Right sided Cardiac Failure (CCF)
* Right heart comprises right atrium, right ventricle, tricuspid valve and pulmonary valve.
* There is decrease in the right ventricular output
* There is increase in the right atrial and systemic venous pressure and congestion, causing edema of feet and enlargement of liver.

Biventricular failure

Diseases which affect both sides of the heart (left and right heart) can cause biventricular failure, e.g. cardiomyopathy, IHD.

Precipitating factors of Cardiac Failure
1. Infection, e.g. Pulmonary infection
2. Onset of atrial fibrillation
3. Myocardial infarction
4. Therapy with Beta-blockers, steroids and NSAIDS
5. Pulmonary thromboembolism
6. Anemia, thyrotoxicosis, pregnancy

Different mechanisms of Heart Failure
1. Mitral stenosis, tricuspid stenosis and constrictive pericarditis cause obstruction to the inflow tract to the ventricle and cause heart failure
2. Pressure overload of the ventricle
   * Obstruction to the outflow tract of the ventricle
   * Hypertension, aortic stenosis cause left sided cardiac failure.
   * Pulmonary hypertension and pulmonary stenosis cause right sided cardiac failure.

3. Volume overload of the ventricle, e.g. MR, AR, ASD and VSD
4. Cardiac arrhythmias: cause defective filling of the ventricle.
5. Cardiac muscle dysfunction causing defective contraction of the ventricle, e.g. IHD, myocardial infarction, cardiomyopathy.

> **Note**
> * Volume overload indicates the amount/volume of blood in the ventricle at the end of diastole of the ventricle.
> * Pressure overload indicates pressure developed in the ventricle at the end of diastole.

Acute Heart Failure

Sudden onset of left heart failure
E.g. Myocardial infarction

Sudden onset of right heart failure
E.g. Massive pulmonary embolism

Chronic Heart Failure

In patients with slow development of heart disease chronic heart failure causes relapsing and remitting course.

High Output Cardiac Failure

Disorders like severe anemia, thyrotoxicosis, beriberi are associated with very high cardiac output and can cause cardiac failure.

Clinical Features of Cardiac Failure
Cardiac failure causes decrease in the cardiac output and decrease blood supply to the muscle and hypoxia to the tissues and can cause following symptoms.

Symptoms in General
* Fatigue
* Decreased urine output
* Syncope
* Cold extremities
* Hypotension

Causes of Left Ventricular Failure
* Due to increased load on the left ventricle
  – Hypertension

  – MR, AR and AS
  – Cardiac arrhythmias
  – Circulatory overload
* Due to damage to the myocardium: Ischemic heart disease
  – Cardiomyopathy
  – Myocarditis

In patients with mitral stenosis person develops left atrial failure.

Features of Left Heart (left ventricular) Failure or Pulmonary Edema

Symptoms
* Restless, apprehension, sweating
* Dyspnea, PND and orthopnea
* Cough, pink frothy sputum

Signs
* Left sided 3rd heart sound
* Bilateral basal crepitations in the lungs
* Central cyanosis, low volume pulse

Causes of Right Ventricular Failure
* Pulmonary hypertension
  – Primary
  – Secondary: Left sided heart disease, corpulmonale, left to right cardiac shunt, pulmonary embolism
* Pulmonary and tricuspid value disease
* IHD

Features of Right Heart Failure

Symptoms
* Dyspnea, right hypochondriac pain
* Swelling of feet, abdominal distention

Signs
* Raised JVP
* Enlarged tender liver
* Pedal edema
* Ascites, pleural effusion

Investigations of Heart Failure

Routine Investigations
* Hb%, renal function tests

- Blood sugar, lipid profile
- Thyroid function tests
- For evidence of heart disease and abnormal cardiac function (ECG, chest X-ray, ECHO cardiogram)

Complications of Heart Failure

Due to heart failure itself
- Atrial and ventricular arrhythmias
- Pulmonary and systemic embolism
- Renal failure due to decreased perfusion to the kidney
- Liver dysfunction due to congestion of liver

Due to diuretic therapy
- Hypokalemia
- Hyponatremia

Hyperkalemia due to ACE inhibitors
- Spironolactone due to renal failure

Treatment of Cardiac Failure

General measures
- Salt and fluid restriction
- Stop smoking
- Reduction of body weight in obese
- To carry out minimal tolerable exercise
- Treatment of hyperlipedemia

Treatment of acute pulmonary edema (Acute left ventricular failure)

1. *Position of the patient:* Since the patient is orthopneic keep the patient in the sitting/semi reclining position with lower limbs below on side of the bed.
2. *Oxygen inhalation:* 100% oxygen inhalation is required in patients with acute pulmonary edema
3. *Morphine:* Reduces anxiety, tachycardia and can cause venous dilatation dose - IV 2 to 4 mg.
4. *Diuretics:* IV Frusemide 40 to 60 mg.
5. *Vasodilatation:*
   - Nitrates: Sublingual/IV can cause vasodilatation and decrease pulmonary edema.
   - Sodium Nitro prusside: Arterial dilatation. IV nitroprusside can decrease pulmonary edema, careful monitoring is required.
6. *ACE inhibitors:* Especially in hypertensives

7. *Digitalis:* Helpful in patients with left ventricular dysfunction and atrial fibrillation with rapid ventricular rate.

Other Measures
IV dopamine/dobutamine, intra-aortic balloon pump and positive pressure ventilation.

Drug Therapy of Chronic Cardiac Failure

Diuretics
They cause urinary sodium and water loss causing decrease of blood volume, e.g.
- Loop diuretics-oral/IV Frusemide 40–80mg
- Thiazides - Bendroflumethiazide 5mg/day
- Spironolactone - Potassium sparing diuretic- 50 mg/day (can be added with other diuretics)

Dilators

Vasodilators
- Arterial reduce after load, e.g.
  ACE inhibitors, Enalapril: 5–20 mg/day, angiotensin II receptor antagonists, losartan: 50–100 mg/day
- Venodilators, e.g. nitrates/IV Nitroglycerin

Digoxin
Useful in patients with heart failure with atrial fibrillation with fast ventricular rate.
Dose: 0.25–0.5mg/day.

Digoxin itself can cause dangerous cardiac arrhythmias in patients with hypokalemia.

Beta-Blockers in heart failure
Beta blockers are not as such indicated in cardiac failure and may aggravate cardiac failure.

Beta-blockers like Carvedilol block the dangerous effects of increased sympathetic activity in patients with cardiac failure. Carvedilol may decrease the incidence of dangerous arrhythmias, sudden death and improve cardiac performance. But they should be avoided in patients with bradycardia and hypotension, e.g. carvedilol 3.125 mg to 6.25 mg/day.

Treatment of the Cause

- Coronary artery disease - coronary bypass or angioplasty.
- Valvular heart disease - valve replacement/valvular plasty
- Treatment of hypertension, diabetes mellitus and hyperlipedemia and correction of congenital cardiac defects.

Cardiac Transplantation

In patients with severe heart failure, heart transplantation may be tried and can be successful.

For example, in patients with cardiomyopathy and ischemic heart disease.

Dental Aspects of Heart Failure

- Surgery under general anesthesia is contraindicated if heart failure is present.
- While performing dental procedure patients with heart disease and heart failure cannot be asked to lie supine.
- Some patients may develop venous thrombosis and pulmonary embolism.
- Digitalis can cause vomiting

INFECTIVE ENDOCARDITIS

Infective endocarditis is characterized by infection of the heart valves, sepal defects, and prosthetic valves by microbial organisms.
Infective endocarditic may be
- Acute
- Sub acute
- Chronic

Infective endocarditis can cause damage to the heart valves, valve abscesses and systemic embolisation to brain, kidney, etc.

Prerequisites for Development of Infective Endocarditis

Occurrence of Bacteremia

After dental extraction or genitourinary instrumentation.

Streptococcus viridians group bacteria are normal commensals in the upper respiratory tract. It can enter the blood stream during chewing, brushing of teeth or at the time of dental extraction. In susceptible individuals it can cause endocarditis.

Bacteremia and entry of organisms can occur due to
- Dental procedures including dental extraction
- Genito urinary instrumentation
- Intra venous injections and IV drug addicts.
- Cardiac surgery and presence of prosthetic valves.

HOST FACTORS AND PRESENCE OF CARDIAC LESIONS (More vulnerable to endocarditis)

Impaired Host Immunity
- Cytotoxic drugs
- Steroid treatment
- Alcoholism

Presence of Cardiac Lesions
- Valvular lesions
- Congenital lesions
- Prosthetic valves
- Occasionally normal valves

Factors which can Prevent Endocarditis
- Prophylactic antibiotic before dental procedures.

Pathophysiology of Infective Endocarditis
- Infective endocarditis usually occurs over the abnormal valves.
- *Staphylococcus aureus* can affect normal heart valves (common in intravenous drug addicts).
- High risk cardiac lesions for endocarditis - AR, MR, VSD, PDA
- Low risk for endocarditis - ASD, severe stenotic lesions.

Pathological Lesions of Infective Endocarditis

Vegetations over the heart valves are the characteristic pathological lesions of infective endocarditis.

Vegetation consists of
- Fibrin, platelets along with microbes

Vegetation can cause
- Valvular destruction and abscess formation
- Valve obstruction
- Systemic embolisation
- Vasculitic lesions

Microbiological Aspects of Infective Endocarditis

Common organisms responsible for infective endocarditis
- *Streptococcus viridans*
- Enterococcus
- *Staphylococcus aureus*
- Coagulase negative staphylococcus
- Gram negative bacilli
- *Hemophilus influenza*
- Anaerobes

Rarer causes: Fungi, anaerobes, coxiella

Clinical Features

Suspect endocarditis in all patients which cardiac lesions if they develop fever especially after 2–3 weeks of dental extraction or genitourinary instrumentation or after cardiac surgery.

Acute Endocarditis

Features
- High grade fever
- Occurrence of new murmurs
- Systemic embolisation
- Valve abscesses
- Cardiac failure

Sub-acute Endocarditis

Features
- Insidious onset of low grade fever
- Fatigability
- Weight loss
- Occurrence of new murmurs
- Cardiac failure
- Systemic embolisation causing cerebrovascular accident may be the presenting feature of infective endocarditis.

Other Important Physical Signs of Infective Endocarditis (Fig. 3.40)
- Pallor

- Osler's nodes - Tender nodules beneath the nail
- Clubbing
- Petechial hemorrhages
- Roth's spots - In ophthalmic fundus (pale centered hemorrhagic spot).
- Splinter hemorrhage beneath the nail

Right Sided Endocarditis

Common in drug addicts. Involves the tricuspid valve. Can cause pulmonary embolism.

Post-operative/prosthetic Valve Endocarditis

Features
- Fever after cardiac surgery
- Can cause valve ring abscesses
- Coagulase negative staphylococcus can cause post operative endocarditis.

Investigations
- Blood culture and sensitivity: 3 samples at different sites and times (10 ml of blood each).
- Echocardiogram: Diagnostic investigation can detect
  – Vegetation on the valves
  – Valve lesion
  – Cardiac disease
- Non specific investigations:
  – ESR and CRP is raised
  – Leucocytosis
  – Noromocytic anemia
  – Thrombocytopenia
  – ECG can detect conduction defect

Diagnosis of Infective Endocarditis

Criteria for the diagnosis (Dukes criteria)

Major criteria
1. ECHO cardiogram (transthoracic/oesophageal): Presence of mass over the valve leaflets.
2. Positive blood culture (two positive cultures for common organisms and single culture positivity for the uncommon organism)

Minor criteria
1. Fever
2. Preexisting heart disease / IV drug addicts

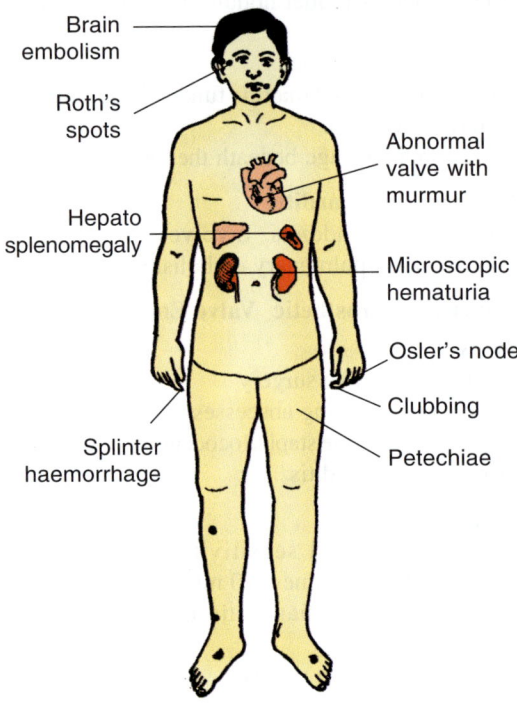

Brain embolism

Roth's spots

Hepato splenomegaly

Abnormal valve with murmur

Microscopic hematuria

Osler's node

Clubbing

Splinter haemorrhage

Petechiae

Fig. 3.40 Clinical signs of endocarditis

3. Evidence of arterial embolisation
4. Evidence of immunological phenomena (Roth's spots, Osler's node/ glomerulonephritis.
5. Positive blood culture (not as mentioned for major criteria)

Diagnosis
1. By two major criteria or one major + 3 minor criteria or 5 minor criteria.

Treatment (Table 3.12)
- Remove the source of infection, e.g. tooth with apical abscess
- Identify the organism and select the correct antibiotic of choice with proper dosage.
- Penicillin plus gentamycin one of the preferred drugs for empirical therapy (organism not known).
- Watch (varicomycin and gentamycin can cause renal toxicity).
- In patients with penicillin allergy varicomycin/ Teicoplanin can be used.
- Surgical treatment of the valve may be required for staphylococcal/fungal endocarditis.
- Take care of nutrition and give symptomatic therapy and treat complications.

Table 3.12 Antibiotic therapy		
Pathogens	*Antibiotic dosage*	*Duration*
Streptococci Penicillin sensitive	Inj. cry. Penicillin 2–3 million units IV 4th hrly	2–4 weeks
Penicillin resistant	Inj. cry. Penicillin 3 million units	4–6 weeks
	IV 4th hrly + Inj. Gentamycin 1 mg/kg 8th hrly	2 weeks
Enterococcus	Inj. cry. Penicillin 3–4 million units	4–6 weeks
	IV 4th hrly + Inj. Gentamycin 1 mg/kg 8th hrly	
Sraphylococcus penicillin sensitive	Inj. Cryst. Penicillin 2–3 million units	4–6 weeks
	IV 4th hrly. + Inj. Gentamycin 1mg/kg 8th hrly	1 week
Staphylococcus (penicillin resistant) and methicillin resistant	Inj. Vancomycin 1grIV 12th hrly	4–6 weeks
	+	
	Inj. Gentamycin 1mg/kg 8th hrly	1 week

Note: Anaerobes, gram negative pathogens, coxiella and HACEK group of organisms and fungal endocarditis require specific antomicrobial therapy.

Surgical Treatment of Infective Endocarditis

Indications
- Severe valve damage
- Formation of valve abscess
- Large vegetation with embolisation not responding to treatment

Chemoprophylaxis Against Endocarditis
(Table 3.13)

Following categories of patients with cardiac disease require medical evaluation and hospital reference before dental procedures
- Persons with penicillin allergy.
- Person has received penicillin within the past 1 month.
- Patients with artificial (prosthetic) heart valves requiring general anesthesia .
- Patients with previous history of infective endocarditis

Following cardiac lesions have high risk of developing infective endocarditis
- Rheumatic heart disease
- Congenital heart disease
- Mitral valve prolapse
- Prosthetic valves
- Hypertrophic obstructive cardiomyopathy
- Previous infective endocarditis

Persons with lowest risk of developing infective endocarditis
- MVP without mitral regurgitation
- Prior coronary artery bypass graft
- Septum secundum ASD
- Pacemaker implantation
- Repaired intracardiac shunts.

Measures to prevent the development of infective endocarditis
Enquire all persons before dental extractions, the following history
- Previous history of rheumatic fever
- Congenital heart disease
- Previous cardiac surgery
- Presence of cardiac murmur
- Previous history of infective endocarditis
- Prosthetic cardiac valve
  Above category of patients require antibiotic prophylaxis before dental procedures.

Dental Procedures Requiring Antibiotic Prophylaxis in Susceptible Patients
- Dental extraction
- Incision of dental abscesses
- Sub gingival procedures causing gingival bleed
- Surgery of periodontal tissues
- Avulsed teeth implantation
- Tooth reposition following trauma
- Scaling of teeth

Table 3.13 Chemoprophylaxis against endocarditis

Procedures to be performed	Antibiotics
Dental/upper respiratory / oesophageal (local anaesthesia)	Oral Amoxycillin 2–3 gms one hour before the procedure
Under general anaesthesia (G.A.)	Inj. Amoxycillin 1gm/30 mins before G.A. + 500 mg 6 hours after the procedure.
Genitourinary and gastrointestinal procedures (apart from oesophagus)	Inj. Amoxycillin 1gm/IV+ Inj. Gentamycin (upto 120 mm) at induction of anaesthesia and oral amoxycillin 500 mg after 6 hours
In patients with penicillin allergy	Oral Clindamycin 600 mg/hr before the procedure or IV 30 mins. before the procedure
In high risk patients	Inj. Vancomycin 1 gr infused over 1 to 2 hours - 30 minutes before the procedures. + Inj. Gentamycin 120 mg IV before the procedure

Measures which may help to prevent the development of infective endocarditis

1. Apply chlorhexidine (0.5%) to the gingival margins before preparing the dental procedures. This will help in decreasing the severity of bacteremia.
2. Maintain good dental health and hygiene and keep periodontal infection least.
3. To look for fever after dental extraction especially in patients with cardiac lesion even as late as 2 months after extraction.
4. All patients with cardiac lesion should carry the card showing the details of cardiac lesion and antibiotic prophylaxis.

CARDIAC ARRHYTHMIAS

Abnormal Cardiac Rhythm

Disturbance in the rhythm of heart leads to alteration in the heart rate. Abnormalities of cardiac rhythm may occur due to disease of SA node, AV node or abnormality of conduction system. Cardiac arrhythmias decrease the efficiency of cardiac contraction and decrease the cardiac output. Cardiac arrhythmias occur usually secondary to IHD, hypertension, valvular heart disease, congenital heart disease, drug induced and electrolyte imbalance like hyperkalemia.

Tachyarrhythmias (associated with increase in the heart rate)

- Supra ventricular tachyarrhythmias
  - Atrial and junctional complexes
  - Paroxysmal and junctional tachycardias
  - Atrial flutter
  - Atrial fibrillation
- Ventricular Tachyarrhythmias
  - Ventricular premature complexes
  - Ventricular tachycardia
  - Ventricular flutter and fibrillation
- Bradyarrhythmias (associated with decrease in the heart rate)
  - Sinus node dysfunction
  - AV conduction block
  - AV dissociation

Tachycardia

Heart rate more than 100/minute

Sinus Tachycardia

- Fever
- Cardiac failure
- Anemia
- Thyrotoxicosis
- Anxiety neurosis
- Beta stimulants
- Pregnancy

Tachy Arrhythmias

- Supraventricular tachycardia
- Atrial fibrillation
- Ventricular tachycardia

Extra Systole

- Ectopic impulse arising in the atrium causing extra systolic contraction of the atrium with irregular heart beat.
- Person may feel as though there is sudden stoppage of heart beating.
- Extra systoles may be atrial or ventricular. Most of the extra systoles are benign and may not require treatment. Multiple ventricular ectopics can progress to ventricular fibrillation and cardiac arrest.

Paroxysmal Atrial Tachycardia

Paroxysmal increase in the heart rate and causes palpitation. Severe increase in the heart rate causes decrease in the ventricular filling and can precipitate cardiac failure in the presence of heart disease.

Atrial Fibrillation

Arrhythmia characterised by uncontrolled and ineffective contraction of the atrium.

Causes of Atria Fibrillation

- Rheumatic heart disease
- Congenital heart disease
- Hypertensive heart disease
- Ischemic heart disease
- Thyrotoxicosis
- Digitalis

Atrial fibrillation causes defective ventricular filling due to irregular and rapid ventricular rate.

There may be formation of thrombus in the left atrium and can result in systemic embolisation including stroke.

Atrial fibrillation can precipitate heart failure.

Ventricular Tachycardia

Ventricular tachycardia is usually due to ischemic heart disease, digitalis, and ventricular muscle disease. It can cause cardiac failure or can result in ventricular fibrillation and can cause cardiac arrest.

Ventricular Fibrillation (VF)

- Most serious form of arrhythmia
- Can cause sudden cardiac death
- There is complete failure of ventricular contraction and cardiac output.

Ventricular fibrillation can occur due to
- Acute myocardial infarction
- Adrenaline administration
- Thyrotoxicosis
- Digitalis
- Halothane anesthesia

BRADYCARDIA

Heart rate is less than 60/min

Causes
- Physiological: Athlets with high vagal tone
- Pathological
  – Cholestatic jaundice
  – Raised intracranial pressure
  – Sick sinus syndrome
  – Hypothermia
  – Hypothyroidism
  – Complete heart block

Drugs: Beta blockers, verapamil, digoxin

Severe bradycardia in elderly can cause syncope and loss of consciousness.

Sick Sinus Syndrome
- Severe disturbance in the functioning of sino atrial node.
- Occurs due to ischemia/fibrosis or degenerative changes of the sinus node.
- Presents as bradycardia/tachycardia or pauses
- It can cause syncope and may require artificial pacemaker implantation.

Complete Heart Block
- There is complete blocking of the conduction of impulse through the conduction system of the heart.
- There is severe bradycardia (heart rate-30–40/ minute due to intrinsic ventricular rate) causing loss of consciousness (Stokes-Adams attack).

Causes of Complete Heart Block
- Myocardial infarction
- Digitalis intoxication
- Excess of beta and calcium channel blockers
- Viral myocarditis
- Infiltrative disorders: Amyloidosis, sarcoidosis
- Degenerative disorders: Lev's and Lenegre's disease

Complete heart block requires permanent pacemaker implantation.

SUDDEN CARDIAC DEATH AND CARDIAC ARREST

In persons who develop cardiac arrest there will be sudden and total loss of functioning of the heart. There will be loss of pulse, stoppage of respiration loss of consciousness and death if not intervened immediately. Most common cause of sudden cardiac death is ventricular fibrillation.

Causes of Sudden Cardiac Death
- Ischemic heart disease
  – Acute myocardial infarction
  – Myocardial ischemia
- Valvular heart disease
- Severe aortic stenosis
- Cardiomyopathy
- Congenital heart disease
- Prolonged QT interval and WPW syndrome.
- Hyperkalemia
- Adverse drug reaction

Cardiomyopathy

Cardiomyopathy is a disease of the cardiac muscle.

Causes
- Primary

– Idiopathic
– Endomyocardial fibrosis
• Secondary
– Connective tissue disorders
– Amyloidosis
– Muscular dystrophy
– Myocarditis
– Hemochromatosis
– Nutritional deficiency
– Alcohol/drug induced
– Peripartum state

Different Types of Cardiomyopathy

1. **Dilated cardiomyopathy:** There will be dilatation and impaired functioning of left and right ventricles.
2. **Hypertrophic cardiomyopathy:** There will be inappropriate hypertrophy of inter ventricular septum and myocardial fibrosis.
3. **Restrictive cardiomyopathy:** There will be impaired ventricular filling due to stiff ventricle.

All causes of cardiomyopathies result in cardiac failure, cardiac arrhythmias. There will be regurgitant murmurs in dilated cardiomyopathy. Hypertrophic obstructive cardiomyopathy can result in sudden cardiac death. There is risk of infective endocarditis.

COR PULMONALE

Cor pulmonale is the term given to a condition characterised by right ventricular hypertrophy or dilatation with or without cardiac failure due to pulmonary artery hypertension secondary to primary respiratory/lung disease. There is no preexisting heart disease.

Types

• Acute, e.g. massive pulmonary embolism
• Subacute, e.g. miniature pulmonary embolism
• Chronic, e.g. COPD

Features

• Right ventricular hypertrophy
• Pulmonary artery hypertension
• May develop right sided cardiac failure

• Evidence of respiratory/lung disease, e.g. COPD

Note
General anesthesia, IV barbiturates, diazepam, cause respiratory depression and are contra indicated in patients with corpulmonale.

Deep Vein Thrombosis and Pulmonary Embolism

Deep vein thrombosis is common in patients with
• Elderly persons
• Bed ridden states
• Postoperative states
• Oral contraceptive therapy
• Hyper coagulable states

Features

• Sudden onset of pain in the lower limb.
• Common site of involvement:
– Deep veins of calf
– Pelvic veins
• Calf becomes swollen and tender may get infected

Deep vein thrombosis can cause pulmonary embolism and sudden cardiac death.

Pulmonary Embolism

Pulmonary embolism usually occurs secondary to deep vein thrombosis and can cause sudden cardiac death.

It presents with sudden onset of chest pain, dyspnea and haemoptysis.

Small recurrent pulmonary embolisation occurring over a long period of time can result in pulmonary artery hypertension and right sided cardiac failure.

Treatment

• Deep vein thrombosis can be treated by IV Heparin (anticoagulation) followed by oral antocoagulation with warfarin.
• Deep vein thrombosis can be prevented by active contraction of calf muscles in bed ridden/post operative patients and by using prophylactic anticoagulation.
• Pulmonary embolism is treated by intravenous heparin and thrombolysis.

Scheme of History Taking

Symptoms and History of Present Illness
- Cough with expectoration
- Haemoptysis
- Dyspnoea
- Chest pain
- Fever
- Symptoms of upper respiratory illness
- Syncope
- Pedal oedema and puffiness of face
- Bones and joint pain and muscle weakness
- Headache, altered mental status
- Personality changes and other neurological symptoms.
- Symptoms of other systemic illness

Past History
- Tuberculosis
- Recurrent attacks of pleurisy and pneumonia since childhood
- Previous chest trauma and surgery
- History of altered consciousness and vomiting
- Previous history of allergy
- Risk factors for embolism

Family History
Tuberculosis, bronchial asthma, bronchiectasis etc.

Personal History
- Loss of weight and appetite
- Smoking
- Alcoholism
- High risk behavior

Occupational and Environmental Exposure
Exposure to organic/inorganic dust

Treatment History

COUGH

Definition
Sudden expulsion of irritant material and secretions from the lower respiratory tract through the glottis.

Symptom of Cough is Analysed as Follows
1. Onset and duration
2. Type and nature
3. Dry or associated with expectoration
4. Aggravating factors

Onset and Duration

Causes of sudden onset of cough
- Acute pulmonary oedema
- Pulmonary infarction
- Pneumothorax
- Aspiration into the lungs

Causes of short duration (2–3 weeks) of cough
- Infection of the upper respiratory tract
- Acute bronchitis
- Pneumonia
- Pneumothorax
- Pulmonary embolism
- Pulmonary edema

Causes of longer duration of cough (weeks to months)
- Pulmonary tuberculosis
- Bronchogenic carcinoma
- Interstitial lung disease

Causes of cough (months to years)
- COPD

- Bronchial asthma
- Bronchiectasis

Type and Nature of Cough

Brassy Cough
- Attacks of cough associated with production of metallic sound.
- Occasionally harsh and barking type, e.g. tracheo bronchitis, mediastinal mass.
- Tumour or aortic aneurysm compressing the trachea can cause brassy cough.

Bovine Cough
- Present in patients with vocal cord paralysis.
- Non explosive cough associated with low-pitched sound.
- Usually accompanied by hoarseness of voice
- Less effective in clearing secretions, e.g. vocal cord paralysis (usually left).

Whooping Cough
- Severe attack of prolonged cough.
- Characteristic sound (whoop) is produced due to inspired air entering through a narrow glottis, e.g. Pertussis

Aggravating Factors
Dust, pollen, and cold air can aggravate cough in patients with bronchial asthma.

Cough with expectoration: Cough may be dry or may be associated with expectoration (discussed below).

Analysis of Cough Depending on the Other Associated Symptoms

Cough Associated with Chest Pain

Causes
- Pleuritis
- Diseases of the chest wall
- Tracheobronchitis
- Root pain due to dorsal spine disease

Cough which is Predominantly Nocturnal and may also be paroxysmal
- Left side cardiac failure

- Bronchial asthma
- Gastric contents aspirated into the lungs
- Cough associated with Hoarseness of voice

Causes
- Infection: Viral/ bacterial laryngitis
- TB larynx
- Neoplastic: Laryngeal tumors
- Neurological: Paralysis of larynx

Note: Corticosteroid inhalation can also cause hoarseness of voice.

Cough with Diurnal Variation

Predominantly in the morning
- Bronchiectasis
- Chronic bronchitis
- Common in smokers

Predominantly in the evening
- Day time exposure to irritants

Occurrence of cough during the act of eating and swallowing: Due to
- Aspiration into the lungs
- Defective swallowing mechanism
- Tracheo-oesophageal fistula

Recent Change in the Nature of Cough
Recent change in the nature of cough in a chronic smoker may suggest the possibility of bronchial malignancy.

Complications of Severe Cough
- Vomiting
- Syncope
- Cough fracture in elderly person with osteoporosis.

Causes of recurrent attacks of cough since childhood
- Childhood onset asthma
- Bronchiectasis (e.g. cystic fibrosis, ciliary abnormality)
- Cystic disease of the lung
- Congenital left to right shunts
- Hypogammaglobulinemia

Cough with Expectoration
Most of the times cough is associated with

expectoration except in the following situations where in it may be dry.

Causes of Dry Cough
- Viral infection of the respiratory tract
- Interstitial lung disease
- Radiation injury to lungs
- Tumors in the lung
- Irritant gas inhalation
- Occasionally if may be difficult to differentiate sputum from saliva. Presence of alveolar macrophages on microscopy indicates the presence of sputum sample rather than saliva.

Clinical Evaluation of Expectoration is as Follows

Quantity

Conditions associated with minimal sputum
1. Viral infection of the respiratory tract.
2. Bronchial asthma

Large quantity of sputum 100 ml/day
- Bronchiectasis
- Lung abscess
- Broncho pleural communication.
- Bronchorrhea is the term used for expectoration of large (>100 ml/day) quantity of watery sputum, e.g. Bronchoalveolar carcinoma, chronic bronchitis.

Quality of sputum
- *Mucoid:* Gelatinous/sticky and colorless/white. For example, chronic bronchitis, chronic bronchial asthma
- *Serous:* Colourless and watery and occasionally frothy. For example, left heart failure, bronchoalveolar carcinoma
- *Purulent:* Yellow coloured, usually thick and viscous, may be foul smelling and indicates pyogenic infection
  Occasionally bronchial asthmatics can bring out casts of bronchial tree with mucus in the sputum.

Color of sputum
- *Yellow:* Indicates infection with pus forming organisms, e.g. streptococcal/staphylococcal infection.
- Occasionally green color of the sputum may be due to the enzyme verdoperoxidase liberated by disintegrating cells.
- *Rusty coloured:* Pneumococcal pneumonia. Rusty color is due to dispersion of blood evenly in the sputum.

Note: Patients of bronchial asthma may bring out green colored sputum even without infection due to the sputum containing excess eosinophills.

- Red currant jelly sputum (bright red, and viscid), e.g. *Klebsiella pneumonia.*
- Black coloured sputum (malanoptysis): Found in coal miner patients and due to coal dust inhalation.
  Patients with infection due to Mycoplasma like organisms will not have colored sputum.

Odour of sputum: Foul-smelling sputum is usually due to infection with anaerobic organisms, e.g. bronchiectasis and lung abscess.

Postural variation of sputum: Quantity of sputum expectorated is more in certain body postures.

Conditions associated with postural variation of sputum
- Bronchiectasis
- Lung abscess
- Broncho-pleural communication
- Gastro-oesophageal reflux and aspiration into the lungs
- Post nasal drip

Haemoptysis

Coughing out of blood from the lower respiratory tract.

Clinical evaluation and approach to a patient of haemoptysis

True haemoptysis should be differentiated from
1. *Spurious haemoptysis:* Bleeding from the upper respiratory tract trickling into the lower tract and coughed out.
2. *Pseudohaemoptysis:* Due to infection with organism like *Serratia marcescens* producing a red pigment.

Common causes of Haemoptysis
- Pulmonary causes

– Tuberculosis
– Necrotising pneumonia/lung abscess
– Bronchogenic carcinoma
– Acute bronchitis
– Bronchiectasis
• Cardiac cause
  – Mitral stenosis

Haemoptysis should be differentiated from haemetemesis.

Following are the differences between haemoptysis and haemetemesis

Differences between haemoptysis and haemetemesis

	Haemoptysis	Haemetemesis
History	coughing	Nausea and vomiting
Food particles	absent (contains) sputum	present in the vomitus
Colour	bright red	coffee ground.
pH	alkaline	acidic
History of malena	absent	present.

Differential diagnosis of Haemoptysis

• Enquire frequency, amount and duration of haemoptysis in all patients with haemoptysis.
• Massive haemoptysis without severe coughing can occur (> 600 ml/day) in patients with pulmonary cavity and tumours.
• Repeated expectoration of 2–3 ml of blood especially in a chronic smoker may suggest the possibility of bronchogenic carcinoma.
• Recent onset of cough, wheeze and purulent blood streaked sputum is common in patients with acute bronchitis.
• Recurrent episodes of haemoptysis over many years with purulent sputum are usually found in patients with bronchiectasis.
• Patients with bronchiectasis may have massive haemoptysis (bright red) due to varicosity of bronchial vessels.
• High grade fever, chills, rigors and haemoptysis is a common manifestation of pneumonia.
• Mild to moderate fever, weight loss, cough and haemoptysis signifies pulmonary tuberculosis.

• Acute onset of dyspnoea with chest pain and haemoptysis may suggest pulmonary infarction especially with predisposing factors (acute heart failure may also have such a presentation).
• Consider Goodpasteur's syndrome and collagen vascular disease in patients with haemoptysis associated with renal disease.

Rare Clinical Circumstances

• Direct chest trauma causing lung damage can cause haemoptysis.
• Amoebic liver abscess: Rupture of amoebic abscess into the tracheobronchial tree can produce chocolate colored (Anchovy sauce) sputum.
• Occasionally anti coagulant therapy may be a cause for haemoptysis.
• Patients with upper respiratory tract bleed may localise the site of bleed and describe it as spitting or hawking of blood rather than coughing.

Causes of haemoptysis in a patient of tuberculosis

• Endobronchial lesion
• Cavitory lesion (Rasmussen's aneurysm - rupture of a dilated vessel in a cavity).
• Secondary bacterial infection.
• Post tubercular bronchiectasis (bronchiectasis sicca)
• Erosion of a fully patent vessel located in the wall of a cavity.

DYSPNOEA

Respiratory Causes of Dyspnoea

Acute (hours to days) may be sudden onset
• Bronchial asthma (acute attack)
• Pneumothorax
• Acute pneumonia
• Pulmonary embolism
• Laryngeal oedema or foreign body
• ARDS

Subacute (days to weeks)
• Pleural effusion
• Pneumonias
• Guillian Barre syndrome
• Bronchial carcinoma

Chronic (months to years)
- COPD
- Bronchial asthma
- Interstitial lung disease

Approach to a patient of dyspnoea with respiratory disease

Exertional dyspnoea of respiratory origin may be due to COPD, interstitial lung disease and bronchial asthma

Wheeze

When air passes through narrowed airways (bronchi) a musical sound is produced called wheeze.

Causes of episodic attacks of respiratory dyspnoea with wheeze
- Bronchial asthma
- Pulmonary eosinophilia
- Bronchopulmonary aspergillosis

Orthopnoea

Following respiratory disorders may be associated with orthopnoea
- Severe attack of asthma
- Massive pleural effusion
- Tension pneumothorax

Platypnoea

Respiratory Causes
- Occasionally mass lesion in the upper airway
- Pulmonary A-V fistula

> *Note*
> - Patients with bronchial asthma can have an attack of dyspnoea after exposure to allergens.
> - Dyspnoea on returning to work after a day of rest, e.g. 'Byssinosis' (monday morning chest tightness).

STRIDOR

Characteristics
- High pitched inspiratory sound
- May be associated with cough and dyspnoea

Suggests: Obstruction to the airflow during inspiration.

Site of Obstruction
- Region of glottis (larynx or trachea predominantly upper airway)
- May be due to narrowing, exudate or oedema of upper airways.

Causes of Sudden Onset of Stridor
- Laryngeal oedema due to anaphylaxis
- Foreign body inhalation
- Inhalation of toxic gases

Causes of stridor (may not be of sudden onset)

In children
- Foreign body in the upper respiratory tract
- Diphtheria
- Croup (acute laryngotracheobronchitis)

Adults
- Oedema of larynx/laryngeal tumours
- Tracheal compression by lymph node
- Vocal cord paralysis-bilateral.
- Tracheal malignancy

APNOEA

Suggests sudden stoppage of breathing.

Definition: 10 seconds pause of breathing is called apnoea.

Types
Obstructive: Oropharyngeal airway obstruction

Causes
- Obesity, acromegaly, hypothyroidism
- Alcohol can aggravate obstructive apneas

Central: Neuronal stimulation to the respiratory muscle is suddenly stopped.

Mixed: Obstructive with central component

CHEST PAIN

Important symptom of respiratory disease

Respiratory Causes of Chest Pain
Pleuritic pain - pleural involvement due to

- Pneumonia
- Tuberculosis
- Malignancy
- Pulmonary infarction

Pain due to chest wall disease
- Inter costal myalgia
- Costochondritis
- Rib fracture
- Herpes zoster - spinal root involvement
- Tumor invasion of the chest wall

Pain predominantly central
- Tracheobronchitis
- Inflammatory and neoplastic disease of mediastinum.

Chest pain of respiratory disease is analysed as follows

Chest wall disorder and musculoskeletal pain
- Chest pain increases with respiratory movement and chest movement.
- Intensity is less compared to pleuritic pain
- Associated with local tenderness.
- Pain in the distribution of C8 T1 root is common in patients with Pancost' tumour. There will be local tenderness over the first and second ribs associated with atrophy of hand muscles.

Pulmonary and Pleural Disorder

Tracheitis and Tracheobronchitis
- Retrosternal or central chest pain
- Increases after coughing

Pulmonary Hypertension
- Retrosternal pain
- Exercise and stress precipitates pain
- Pain is not present at rest
- Dyspnoea may be associated with the pain

Pulmonary Mass Lesion
- Pain may be localised to an area of chest or may be diffuse.
- Present continuously
- Dull aching/sharp pain
- Pain is due to tumor invading the parietal pleura/chest wall

Pleuritic Pain

Characteristics of pleuritic pain
- Severe catching type of pain
- Increases on coughing and inspiration
- Pain is due to stretch of inflamed parietal pleura
- Visceral pleura is insensitive to pain
- Pain originates in the parietal pleura
- On inspiration parietal pleura gets stretched giving rise to pain.
- Inflammation of diaphragmatic pleura gives rise to the pain which may be referred to the tip of the shoulder and hypochondrium.

FEVER

Fever is a common manifestation of respiratory infection. Occasionally fever may also be due to bronchogenic malignancy.

Significance of fever in a respiratory disorder is as discussed below
- Moderate fever: URTI and tracheobronchitis.
- Fever with chills, rigors - Pneumonia, lung abscess, empyema thoracis.
- Fever associated with night sweats- Soaking of bedclothes at night. For example pulmonary tuberculosis.
- Fever in a patient of bronchogenic carcinoma may be due to necrosis of tumour or secondary infection.
- Mesothelioma of pleura may present with febrile illness.

Fever is not a dominant symptom in following respiratory disorders
- Pneumoconiosis
- Idiopathic pulmonary fibrosis
- Sarcoidosis - unless extensive
- Multiple pulmonary secondaries

Symptoms of Upper Respiratory Illness

Disorders of Nose and Nasopharynx
- Discharge from the nose
- Nasal obstruction

- Epistaxis
- Repeated sneezing, e.g. allergic rhinitis
- Headache due to recurrent sinusitis

Symptoms of Laryngeal Disease and Associated Disorders

- Hoarseness of voice and throat pain due to laryngeal infection or growth
- Harsh, barking and dry cough due to laryngitis
- Bovine cough due to laryngeal paralysis
- Stridor due to laryngeal obstruction

Symptoms of Tracheal Disease

Tracheitis: Retrosternal chest pain more on coughing.
Tracheal obstruction: Dyspnoea and stridor

Miscellaneous Symptoms of Respiratory Disease

Syncope
Respiratory causes
- Severe and prolonged coughing
- Severe pulmonary hypertension
- Massive pulmonary embolism

Oedema and Puffiness of Face
Puffiness of face: Pancoast's tumour with superior venacaval obstruction can produce puffiness of face.
Pedal oedema: Common in patients with cor pulmonale and CCF.

Occasionally long standing bronchiectasis can result in amyloid deposition in the kidney causing nephrotic syndrome and oedema.

Bone and Joint Pain and Muscle Weakness
Bony pain can be due to hypertrophic pulmonary osteoarthropathy or hypercalcemia associated with bronchogenic carcinoma.
- Bony pain in the region of Ist and 2nd rib may be due to tumour invasion (Pancoast's tumour).
  - Myasthenic type of muscle weakness may be associated with paraneoplastic manifestation of bronchogenic carcinoma.

Neurological Symptoms

- Headache, personality changes and mental state alteration
- Hypoxia and hypercapnea associated with respiratory failure can manifest with headache altered mentation and personality changes.
- Convulsions and focal neurological deficits may be due to tuberculosis and cerebral abscess which may be associated with pulmonary tuberculosis and lung abscess or bronchiectasis respectively.
- Bronchogenic carcinoma can cause neurological disturbances either due to metastasis or due to non-metastatic manifestation.

Systemic Symptoms

Primary disorder of liver, cardiovascular system, gastrointestinal or musculoskeletal system can involve the respiratory system. A detailed enquiry about the symptoms of system illness is essential in patients with respiratory disease.

Past History
1. *Importance of previous history of pulmonary tuberculosis*
   - Childhood tuberculosis can become reactivated in the adult.
   - Prior pulmonary tuberculosis may cause bronchiectasis later.
   - Extensive pulmonary fibrosis due to tuberculosis can result in significant alteration in the lung function and hypoxia.
   - Details of prior treatment of tuberculosis, duration, drugs used, etc. should be elicited in detail as it will help in deciding the effectiveness of therapy.
2. *Haemoptysis may occur due to formation of Aspergilloma in an old TB cavity*
3. *Recurrent attacks of pleurisy and pneumonia (may be since childhood) are common in patients with:*
   - Cystic fibrosis
   - Bronchiectasis
   - Hypogammaglobulinemia
4. *Childhood measles and whooping cough may be responsible for adult bronchiectasis.*

5. *Previous chest trauma and surgery:* Haemothorax caused by previous chest trauma can cause pleural thickening with diminished chest expansion. Previous chest surgery can cause chest deformity.
6. *Recent history of altered consciousness, general anaesthesia, vomiting or oropharyngeal surgery-* may suggest aspiration of septic material from URT and development of lung abscess.
7. *Previous history of eczema, urticaria and exacerbation of symptoms after exposure to pollens and dusts* common with atopic asthma.
8. *Long standing history of cough with sputum wheeze and breathlessness with recurrent exacerbations* - common in patients of COPD, bronchial asthma and bronchiectasis
9. *Recent surgery, severe illness, or prolonged bed ridden states are important risk factors for pulmonary embolism.*

It is beneficial to obtain the previous chest radiographs with dates for comparison of the present radiological status and also for previous evidence of respiratory pathology.

Family History

Respiratory disorders with familial occurrence
• Bronchial asthma
• Cystic fibrosis (bronchiectasis)
• Ciliary dyskinesia
• Alpha-1antitrypsyn deficiency (emphysema)
Pulmonary tuberculosis can manifest in several members of a family as it can get transmitted due to close contact and over crowding.

Personal History

Loss of Weight and Appetite
• Most of the acute and chronic respiratory disorders can manifest with loss of appetite.
• Significant weight loss occurs with pulmonary tuberculosis, malignant disorders of lung, emphysema and chronic suppurative lung diseases.
• Infection with human immunodeficiency virus should always be considered in all patients with extreme weight loss and respiratory symptoms.

Extreme Obesity
• Predisposes for hypoventilation and obstructive sleep apnoea syndrome.
• They are more likely to develop hypoxic pulmonary hypertension.

Smoking
• Smoking 20 cigarettes per day for 1 year constitutes a pack year and number of pack years smoked should be enquired. This has got direct relationship with disorders like COPD and bronchogenic carcinoma. Smokers are more predisposed for the development of pulmonary tuberculosis.
• 5% of bronchogenic carcinoma may also be due to passive smoking.

Alcoholism
• Aspiration pneumonia is common in alcoholics specially with altered sensorium.
• Alcoholics have decreased immunity predisposing them for respiratory infection.

High Risk Behaviour
Intravenous drug abusers and persons having multiple sexual partners can contact HIV infection and associated respiratory diseases.

Occupational and Environmental Exposure
1. Prolonged exposure to inorganic dusts results in the development of pneumoconiosis and can exacerbate also asthma.
2. Chronic exposure to asbestos can cause asbestos related lung disease and mesothelioma of pleura.
3. Exposure to organic substances like moulds, animal products may cause extrinsic allergic alveolitis or precipitate an attack of asthma.
4. Contact with pet animals may be responsible for conditions like ornithosis. Hanta virus pneumonia can occur secondary to exposure to mouse droppings.
Persons from coastal areas of India are more chance of developing tropical pulmonary eosinophilia.

Treatment History
Details of prior treatment with ATT duration, combination of the drugs used and their dosage

should be enquired. This is important in the treatment of reactivation or resistant pulmonary tuberculosis.

All patients with recent onset of cough - enquire about ACE inhibitor therapy.

Anti hypertensive like beta blockers can precipitate an attack of asthma.

Treatment with methotrexate, bleomycin can cause pulmonary fibrosis.

Chronic nitrofurantoin therapy can rarely result in interstitial pulmonary fibrosis.

EXAMINATION OF THE RESPIRATORY SYSTEM

General Physical Examination
- Build and nourishment
- Vital signs: Pulse, BP, temperature, respiratory rate, pallor, jaundice, cyanosis, lymphadenopathy, clubbing, pedal oedema
- Examination of eyes, oral cavity, neck and skin

Examination of the Upper Respiratory Tract

Nose and Paranasal Sinuses
- Nostril
- Nasal septum
- Sinus tenderness
- Pharynx
- Tonsil

Examination of the Lower Respiratory Tract

Inspection
- Shape and symmetry of chest
- Position of trachea and apical impulse
- Respiratory movement
- Visible pulsations
- Visible veins and scar mark
- Spine

Palpation
- Position of trachea and apical impulse
- Respiratory movements and measurements
- Vocal fremitus
- Intercostal and rib tenderness

- Palpable respiratory sounds (fremitus)
- Rib crowding

Percussion
- Normal lung resonance, abnormal percussion notes
- Liver dullness, cardiac dullness

Percussion in Specific Circumstances
- Shifting dullness
- Tidal percussion
- Traube's area

Auscultation
- Breath sound intensity
- Type of breathing and alteration of inspiration and expiration, added sounds, vocal resonance.

Examination of Other Systems
- CVS
- GIT
- CNS
- Other related systems

EXAMINATION OF RESPIRATORY SYSTEM

Build and Nourishment
Respiratory causes of severe emaciation and weight loss
- Pulmonary tuberculosis
- Bronchogenic malignancy
- Emphysema
- Suppurative lung disease
- Respiratory disorders associated with HIV infection

Recording of weight is important as
- It is required for calculating the dose of medication.
- For monitoring the benefit of therapy
- Extreme degree of obesity may be associated with hypoxia and pulmonary hypertension, e.g. Pickwickian syndrome

Vital Signs

Pulse
- Record the rate, rhythm, volume and character of the pulse.

Important pulse abnormalities related to respiratory disorders:

Tachycardia (Rate may be > 120/min): Severe form of pneumonia, severe airflow obstruction.

High volume bounding pulse: CO_2 retention. (Type 2 respiratory failure).

Pulsus paradoxus: Severe airflow obstruction (acute severe asthma).

Respiration

- Rate - Normal rate 16–20 /min.
- Normal ratio of pulse to respiration 4:1.
- Tachypnoea - Respiratory rate > 20/min.

Causes of Tachypnoea

Physiological

- Anxiety neurosis (hysterical hyperventilation)
- Exertion

Pathological

- Diseases of the chest wall and lungs
- Hypoxic conditions
- Metabolic acidosis

Bradypnea - Respiratory rate < 12/min

Causes

- Narcotic overdosage
- Head trauma
- Hypothermia

Counting the Respiratory Rate

Observe and count the chest or abdominal movement while counting the pulse rate.

Normal Breathing Pattern and Muscles of Respiration

Muscles of Inspiration

Main group of muscles: External intercostals, diaphragm.

Accessory muscles: Strap muscles of neck, muscles of pharynx and face.

Muscles of Expiration

Main group of muscles: Abdominals

Accessory muscles: Internal intercostals

Breathing Pattern in Males

- Predominantly abdominothoracic
- Abdomen moves outward during inspiration

In females: More of chest wall movement than diaphragm (thoracoabdominal).

Causes of Purely Thoracic Breathing

- Peritonitis
- Pregnancy
- Ascites, ovarian cyst

Causes of Purely Abdominal Breathing

- Paralysis of intercostal muscles
- Pleuritic pain
- Defective chest expansion due to ankylosing spondylitis

Abnormal Patterns and Rhythm of Respiration

1. Increased depth of breathing (hyperapnoea)
   - Kussmaul breathing (metabolic acidosis)
2. *Stertorous breathing:* Due to vibrations of soft tissues of the nasopharynx, larynx and cheeks resulting from loss of muscle tone.
   Causes: Coma from any cause during snoring.
3. *Abnormal rhythm of respiration:* See under examination of an unconscious patient.
4. *Prolonged inspiration:* Obstruction to the upper airways. Patient will have stridor.
5. *Prolonged expiration:* Obstruction to the intra thoracic airways.

Abdominal paradox: Due to fatigue of the Diaphragm

During inspiration: Abdomen moves inwards (Opposite to normal), e.g. severe COPD

Blood pressure: Recording of blood pressure is important in monitoring of the patient for noting hypotension and recording of pulsus paradoxus.

Temperature: For making out febrile respiratory disorders.

Pallor

Significant pallor may be found in patients with pulmonary tuberculosis, bronchogenic carcinoma and chronic suppurative lung disease. Patient with chronic hypoxic states like COPD, bronchial asthma can have suffused conjunctiva due to polycythemia.

Icterus

Following respiratory conditions may be associated with icterus

- Hepatitis due to anti tuberculous drugs
- Disseminated tuberculosis
- Bronchogenic carcinoma with secondaries in the liver
- Pneumonia with toxic hepatitis
- Pulmonary infarction

Cyanosis

Respiratory disorders which cause type II respiratory failure (Acute or chronic) cause central cyanosis, for example

Acute: Foreign body inhalation, acute severe asthma, respiratory muscle paralysis

Chronic: COPD, ankylosing spondylitis, kypho-scoliosis

Clubbing

Causes of respiratory disorders associated with clubbing

1. Suppurative lung diseases - lung abscess and bronchiectasis.
2. Pleural diseases like empyema thoracis and mesothelioma of pleura
3. Malignant disease - bronchogenic carcinoma
4. Secondaries in the lung
5. Interstitial lung disease

Bronchogenic carcinoma and bronchiectasis may also be associated with hypertrophic pulmonary osteoarthropathy (see general physical examination).

Oedema

Oedema of feet can occur in following respiratory conditions

- Cor pulmonale with CCF
- Bronchiectasis with nephrotic syndrome due to amyloidosis.
- Hypoproteinemia associated with respiratory diseases
- Puffiness of face can occur in patients with Bronchogenic carcinoma due to SVC obstruction.

Lymphadenopathy

Respiratory disorders may be associated with localised lymphadenopathy like cervical or axillary lymphadenopathy.

Respiratory diseases associated with cervical lymphadenopathy

1. Bronchogenic carcinoma with secondaries in the neck
2. Hodgkin's lymphoma with cervical and mediastinal lymphadenopathy.

Lungs can also be involved in conditions like Sarcoidosis, tuberculosis, etc. which may cause generalised lymphadenopathy (right supra clavicular lymph node is involved in malignancies of right lung and left lower lobe. Left upper lobe malignancy may involve the left supraclavicular node).

Pathology in the chest wall may cause enlargement of the axillary node.

Scalene node significance (see general physical examination).

Examination of Skin, Neck and Eyes in Relation to Respiratory Disorders

Eyes

Eye should be inspected for the following abnormalities

Abnormalities	Conditions associated
Papilloedema	SVC obstruction CO_2 retention
Conjunctival suffusion	CO_2 retention polycythemia
Scleritis	TB, sarcoidosis (Lung involvement)
Uveitis	due to collagen disease
Choroid tubercles phlycten	Pulmonary TB
Ptosis (Horner's syndrome)	Pancoast's tumour

Neck

Neck should be examined for the following abnormalities

- Cervical lymphadenopathy (see above).
- Previous lymph node biopsy scar- tuberculosis/ malignancy

- Excessive contraction of neck muscles- Dyspnoeic patient.

Distended neck veins: Cor pulmonale with CCF, SVC obstruction.

Severe emphysema: Neck vein distend during expiration and collapse during inspiration.

Thyroid enlargement: May cause tracheal shift.

Tracheal descent with respiration: Severe airflow obstruction.

Examination of skin reveal several abnormalities in patients with respiratory disease as mentioned below (Table 4.1).

Systemic Examination of the Respiratory System

Upper Respiratory Tract (URT)

Upper respiratory tract extends from external nostril to the junction of larynx and trachea (glottis).

Examination of the different parts of the URT with related abnormalities

Nose and nasopharynx

Abnormalities	Conditions
Nasal discharge Post nasal drip	Rhinitis
Deviated nasal septum	Produces nasal obstruction
Hypertrophied turbinates	
Nasal polyps	Allergic rhinitis

Paranasal sinuses and ear

- Paranasal sinus tenderness - suggestive of acute/chronic sinusitis.

Table 4.1 Examination of skin reveal several abnormalities in patients with respiratory disease

Abnormalities	Disorder associated
Butterfly rash of SLE	SLE with pleural and pulmonary involvement.
Herpes labialis	Pneumonia.
Herpes zoster	Can cause unilateral chest pain
Metastatic tumour nodules	Secondary from bronchogenic carcinoma
Erythema nodosum	TB/Collagen disease/sarcoidosis

- Recurrent sinusitis and otitis media are associated with ciliary dyskinesia syndrome and bronchiectasis.
- Necrotising granuloma of nasal passage: Rule out Wegener's granulomatosis
- Tonsils and pharynx: Look for tonsillar infection.
- Posterior pharyngeal wall congestion suggests Pharyngitis
- Oral cavity: check for gingival suppuration. Aspiration may lead onto acquired lung abscess

EXAMINATION OF THE LOWER RESPIRATORY TRACT

Important Anatomical Landmarks
- *Sternal angle or angle of Louis:* Bony ridge corresponds to the junction of 2nd rib with the sternum.

Tracheal Bifurcation
- Anteriorly at the level of angle of Louis.
- Posteriorly at the lower border of T4 vertebra.

Midclavicular Line
Line drawn from the mid point of the left and right clavicles.

Hilum or root of the lung: Corresponds to 4th, 5th, 6th thoracic spines.

Apices of upper lobe: Lie 2 to 3 cms above the clavicles.

Spine of the scapula corresponds to the level of 2nd thoracic vertebra and angle of the scapula corresponds to the T7 vertebra.

Major Interlobar Fissure (Oblique fissure)
Draw a line from T2 spine along the scapular border through the 5th rib in the mid axillary line so as to meet the 6th rib anteriorly in the mid clavicular line.

Minor Fissure (Horizontal fissure)
Draw a Horizontal line on the right side from the 4th rib at the sternal border to meet the major fissure at 5th rib in the mid axillary line.

Lung Borders (Lower border)
- Normally on the right side (lower border)

– Mammary line-at 6th rib
– Mid axillary line at 8th rib
– Scapular line at 10th rib
• Left side almost like the right side.

Bronchopulmonary Segments (Fig. 4.1)

Part of the lung tissue correspondingly supplied by a single bronchus, corresponding artery and vein.

Distributions of Bronchopulmonary segments are as follows

Right lung	Left lung
Right upper lobe	Left upper lobe
Apical (1)	Apicoposterior (1) and (2)
Posterior (2)	Anterior (3)
Anterior (3)	
Right middle lobe	Lingula
Lateral (4)	Superior (4)
Medial (5)	Inferior (5)
Right lower lobe	Left lower lobe
Apical (6)	Apical (6)
Medial basal (7)	Anteromedial basal (7) and (8)
Anterior basal (8)	Lateral basal (9)
Lateral basal (9)	Posterior basal (10)
Posterior basal (10)	

Respiratory disorders like consolidation or atelectasis may correspond to bronchopulmonary segments.

Inspection of the Chest

Position of the Patient

For anterior and posterior aspect: Patient sitting upright.

Note: Semi reclining position may also be used for inspection of the respiratory system.

In case of bed ridden patients, inspection can be carried out from the foot end of the bed.

Normal Chest in Healthy Adults

• Elliptical in cross section
• Bilaterally symmetrical
• Transverse diameter is more than anteroposterior diameter in the ration of 7:5
• Subcostal angle is 90° or less than 90°

Abnormalities of Shape of the Chest

Barrel Shaped Chest

Characteristic Features

• Ribs are more horizontal with flaring upwards of lower ribs
• Prominent angle of Louis
• Anteroposterior diameters has increased
• Upper thoracic spine is kyphotic
• Subcostal angle becomes obtuse (> 90)

Causes

• Long standing airflow obstruction, e.g. emphysema

Pectus Excavatum

• Lower or all parts of the sternum is depressed.

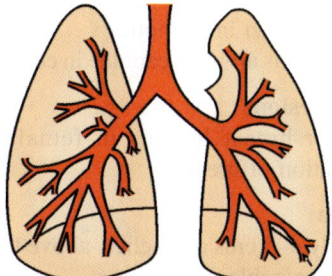

Bronchial tree on the right side (lateral view)

Bronchial tree on the left side (left lateral view)

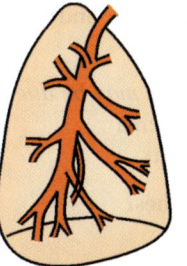
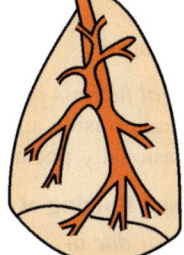

Anterior view of bronchial bifurcations

Fig. 4.1 Bronchopulmonary segments

- Costal cartilages attached to sternum may also be depressed.

    Severe pectus excavatum can cause shift of cardiac apex and restriction of lung expansion.

Condition associated
- Congenital
- Rickets

Pectus Carinatum
Prominent anterior protrusion of sternum and costal cartilages attached to it. For example, rickets and chronic respiratory disease since childhood (e.g. childhood asthma).

Harrison's Sulcus
- Sulci or depressions on either side of the xiphisternum and the groove corresponds to the diaphragmatic attachment to the ribs.
- It is due to the pulling in of the softened ribs at their attachments by the diaphragm, (e.g. rickets).

Symmetry of the Chest
Normal chest is bilaterally symmetrical.

Asymmetry of the chest may be due to
- Previous thoracic surgery
- Kyphoscoliosis
- Chest trauma
- Lung/pleural disease

Pathological causes of Chest Asymmetry
Unilateral flattening and shoulder droop suggests volume loss on the same side.
For example, pulmonary collapse and fibrosis and pleural fibrosis.

Unilateral fullness of the chest may be due to
- Pleural effusion and empyema
- Occasionally pneumothorax

Localised Bulging of the Chest

Can occur due to
- Empyema necessitans (empyema pointing through chest wall).
- Aortic aneurysm
- Malignancy of the lung and chest wall

Lesions of the Chest Wall
Superficial skin lesions and their significance
- *Bleeding spots over the chest wall:* Bleeding disorder with haemoptysis
- *Vesicles over the chest wall:* Herpes zoster with root pain
- *Scar over the chest wall* may be suggestive of previous surgery.
- *Deeper skin lesions:* Look for
    - Axillary lymphadenopathy
    - Metastatic deposits
    - Neurofibromas/lipomas

Subcutaneous Emphysema
Feel for the cracking sensation (produced by the air) when the subcutaneous tissues are palpated.

Causes
- Severe asthma with air leaking into the mediastinum.
- Leaking of air from intercostal tube drainage for pneumothorax/empyema

Local Tenderness

Causes
- *Intercostal tenderness:* Empyema/pleuritis
- *Bony tenderness:* Fracture/secondaries/tumour invasion of the chest wall.
- *Venous engorgement:* Due to prominent chest wall veins in SVC obstruction

Arterial Lesions over the Chest Wall

Causes
- Spider naevi in cirrhotics
- Collaterals around scapulae in coarctation of aorta

Breast Lesions
Look for breast lesions in female patient (see examination of breast).

Trachea
Normally 4–5 cms of trachea above the suprasternal notch is palpable.

Trails Sign (sternomastoid sign)
Tracheal shift to one-side results in sternomastoid on that side to become prominent called Trail's sign.

Apex Beat

Note the position of apical impulse. Shift of the apex may be indicative of mediastinal shift.

Apical impulse may be difficult to be visualized in patients with:

- Thick chest wall
- Pleural effusion
- Emphysema
- Pericardial effusion

Respiratory Movement

Observe the movements of the different parts of the chest.

Different Areas of Chest

- Supraclavicular
- Axillary (upto 4th rib)
- Suprascapular
- Clavicular
- Infraaxillary
- Interscapular
- Infraclavicular (upto 2nd rib)
- Infrascapular (up to 11th rib)
- Mammary (2nd to 6th rib)

Localised decrease of movements or decrease of movement on one side localises the site of the disease to that side.

Flail Chest

Occurs due to multiple rib fractures

Characteristics of flail chest

- **On inspiration** affected area moves inwards.
- **On expiration** affected area moves outwards.

Abnormal Respiratory Movements

Excessive contraction of sternomastoid and scalene muscles:

- Advanced COPD
- Acute severe asthma
- Laryngeal and tracheal obstruction

Indrawing of intercostal spaces, suprasternal space and supraclavicular fossae occurs in conditions like

- COPD
- Bronchial asthma
- Severe upper airway obstruction

Unilateral intercostal retraction occurs in patients with pulmonary fibrosis or collapse.

Breathing Pattern in Patients with Advanced Emphysema

- Person is breathless
- Person tries to increase the effort of expiration by sitting upright and catching the edge of the bed or chair.
- Above manoeuvre fixes the shoulder girdle and allows latissimus dorsi to help in expiration.

Pursed Lip Breathing

- Observed in patients with advanced emphysema.
- Expiration is carried through the mouth with pursing of lips.
- In persons with advanced air flow obstruction high intraalveolar pressure (due to air trapping) tends to collapse the intrathoracic airways. Purse lip breathing prevents the airway collapse by keeping intra airway pressure above the intra alveolar pressure.

Litten's Sign

Sign for observing the movement of diaphragm.

Elicitation of Litten's Sign

- Patient lies down supine with lower part of the chest wall exposed to light.
- Examiner sits on the side of the patient
- Movement of diaphragm is made out as a waveform (phrenic wave) moving up and down in the lower part of the chest with each respiration.
- Persons who are obese or with shallow breathing it may be difficult to make out abnormal movement.

Significance

Unilateral absence of movement suggests defective movement of diaphragm on that side.

Note: Bilateral diaphragm paralysis will be associated with thoracoabdominal discoordination of respiratory movement.

Hoover's Sign

- Found in patients with advanced COPD.
- There will be indrawing of intercostals during inspiration.

Spine

It is preferable to ask the patient to stand while examining the spine.

Kyphosis suggests backward bending of the spine.

Scoliosis: Lateral bending of the spine (convexity determines the side of scoliosis)

Kyphoscoliosis can cause change in the position of the mediastinum.

Scar Mark

* Look for previous surgery scar (lobectomy/pneumonectomy)
* Mark of pleural aspiration/biopsy

PALPATION

Schematic Approach to the Palpation of the Chest

Trachea

* Normal length of the trachea above the suprasternal notch is 4–5 cms.
* Thyroid enlargement may occasionally be responsible for tracheal shift.

Technique of Palpation for Position of Trachea

(Fig. 4.2)

* Introduce the tip of the index finger into the suprasternal notch in the midline and note the relationship of the trachea and sternomastoid.
* Observe the resistance offered on each side of the

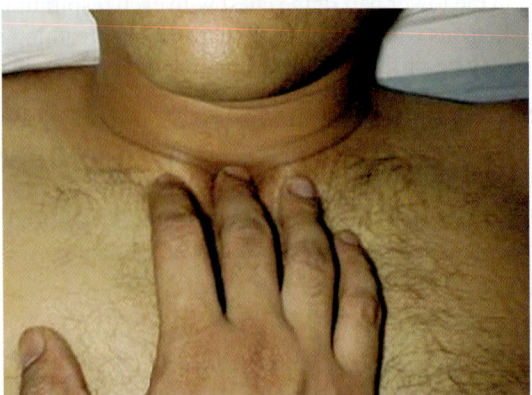

Fig. 4.2 Technique of tracheal palpation

trachea by introducing the finger in between the trachea and sternomastoid.

* Deviation of trachea to one side will offer more resistance to palpation on that side. Normally trachea is central or minimally deviated to right side.

Position of the Apical Impulse

* Palpate for the position of the apical impulse and observe for any shift.
* Diseases of the lung and pleura may cause shift of the mediastinum.
* Only shift of trachea can occur with pathology of the upper lobe and pathology involving only the lower lobe can cause only shift of cardiac apex.

Respiratory Disorders Causing Shift of Trachea and Apex (mediastinum)

* Shift of mediastinum to the same side of pathology
  – Pulmonary fibrosis
  – Pulmonary collapse
* Shift of mediastinum to the opposite side of pathology
  – Pleural effusion
  – Empyema thoracis
  – Pneumothorax
  – Upper lobe pulmonary mass
* Respiratory disorders usually without mediastinal shift
  – COPD
  – Bronchial asthma
  – Bronchiectasis
  – Interstitial lung disease
  – Consolidation
* Non-respiratory causes of shift of cardiac apex
  – Scoliosis
  – Cardiomegaly
  – Pectus excavatum

Respiratory Movements

Movement of different areas of chest:

1. Infraclavicular Area Movement

Technique of Palpation

* Patient is either sitting up or in supine position.

- Look tangentially at the infraclavicular area on both sides of chest.
- While patient is breathing steadily note for any difference in movement.
- Movement can also be made out by the movement of two hands, which are kept in the infraclavicular area on either side.

2. Movement of Mammary and Lower Part of the Chest (Fig. 4.3)

Technique of Palpation

- Sides of the chest are grasped with fingers so as to approximate the tips of out stretched thumbs in the region of

  1. Mammary area

  2. Xiphoid process (for lower part of chest)

- A loose fold of skin in between the two thumbs is produced by the adjustment of the hands and with each chest expansion hands move apart.
- Degree of movement on the two sides of the chest can be estimated by the relative movements of two thumbs with each respiration.

3. Posterior Movement (Fig. 4.4)

Chest is grasped from behind as mentioned above in the region of the lower thoracic spine (10th). Degree of movement of two thumbs on either side is noted.

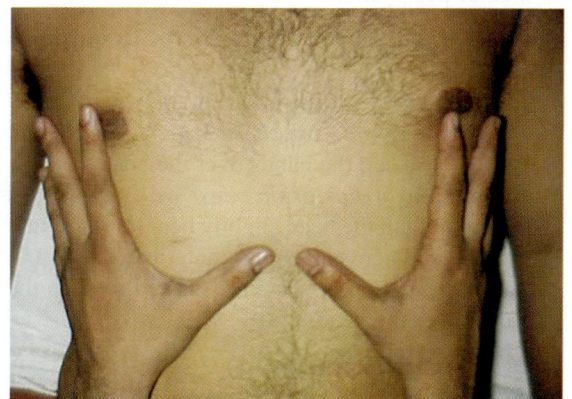

Fig. 4.3 Demonstration of respiratory movement - anterior lower part of chest

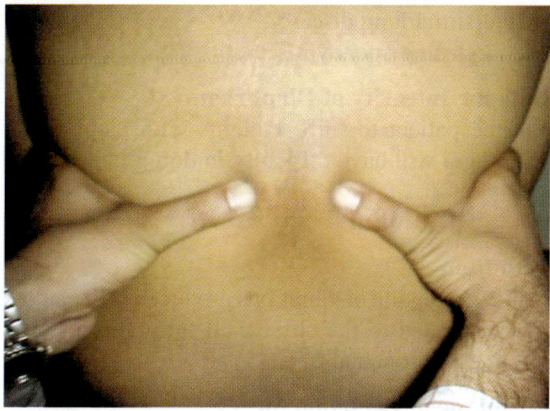

Fig. 4.4 Technique for movement of infrascapular area

Localised Impairment of Respiratory Movement (unilateral decrease of chest movement)

1. Empyema and pleural effusion
2. Consolidation
3. Pulmonary collapse
4. Pneumothorax
5. Pleural and pulmonary fibrosis

Bilateral Decrease of Chest Movement

- Airflow obstruction (COPD, bronchial asthma).
- Diffuse pulmonary fibrosis

Chest Expansion

- Place a measuring tape around the chest at the lower part of the chest (xiphoid process/ T8 vertebrae).
- Record the maximum inspiratory/expiratory difference in the chest circumference which indicates chest expansion.
- Normal chest expansion: 3–5 cm and above. Expansion of less than 2 cm is suggestive of diminished expansion.

Causes of Diminished Chest Expansion

Unilateral diseases of lungs, pleura and chest wall decrease the chest expansion on the affected side.

Causes of Bilateral Diminution of Chest Expansion

- Bronchial asthma
- Emphysema

- Interstitial lung disease
- Ankylosing spondylitis

Tests for Integrity of Diaphragm

Ask the patient to sniff. Patients with paralysis of diaphragm will have difficulty in doing it.

Vocal Fremitus (VF)

Definition

Tactile perception of vibrations produced in the larynx communicated to the chest wall through the lungs and tracheobronchial tree.

Technique of Palpation for VF

Keep the ulnar border of the palpating hand on identical areas of both sides of the chest while the patient is repeating 'one-one'. Compare the 2 sides of the chest for the intensity of vibrations felt by the palpating hand.

Normally VF is equally felt on both sides of the chest.

Unilateral increase of Vocal Fremitus

- Pneumonic consolidation
- Pulmonary cavity

Unilateral decrease of VF

- Fibrosis
- Pleural effusion
- Collapse
- Pneumothorax

Measurement of anteroposterior (AP) and transverse (Tr) diameter

- *AP diameter:* measure the distance between the sternum and thoracic spine at the mammary level.
- *Transverse diameter:* measure the distance between the 2 sides of the chest at the mammary level.
- *Normal Transverse:* AP diameter is 7:5. In emphysema ratio becomes almost equal.

Other Palpable Sounds over the Chest (Tactile Fremitus)

- Crepitations
- Rhonchi
- Pleural rub

Tenderness over the Chest Wall

- Intercostal tenderness
  - Acute pleurisy
  - Empyema
- Rib tenderness
  - Fracture rib
  - Malignant deposit

Examination of the Spine

- Evidence of kyphoscoliosis can be made out with palpation of spine.
- Extreme degree of kyphoscoliosis may cause hypoxia and pulmonary hypertension.

PERCUSSION

Rules of Percussion

- Middle finger (Pleximeter finger) of the left hand is placed firmly on the part to be percussed.
- Strike the middle phalanx of the left middle finger with the tip of middle finger of the right hand (percussing finger).
- Movement should be at the wrist joint
- Striking should be perpendicular and repeated heavy striking should be avoided.
- Sound and feel of percussion should be felt.
- Percuss directly over the bones and percuss from resonance to dull area.
- It is ideal to percuss only 2 to 3 times over each area of percussion.

Position of patient for percussion of Respiratory system

- *Ideal position:* Patient is sitting up.
- *Percussion of anterior chest:* Patient upright and is asked to keep the hands over the head.
- *Percussion of posterior chest wall:* Patient is sitting up with the head slightly bent forwards and arms folded across the chest anteriorly.
- *Axillary percussion:* Patient is asked to keep the hands over the head.

Areas of Percussion (Fig. 4.5)

- Anteriorly
  - Supraclavicular area
  - Clavicles

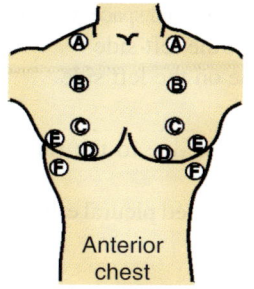 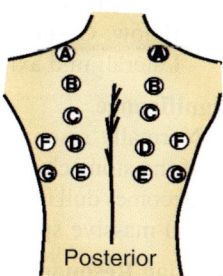

Fig. 4.5 Area of percussion and auscultation of chest

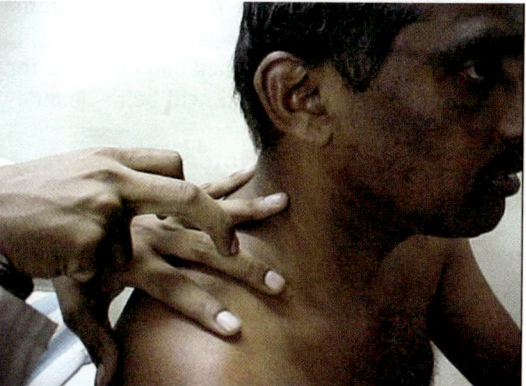

Fig. 4.6 Percussion of the apex of the lung

KEY POINTS 4.1

- Percussion over the normal lung should be learnt by practice.
- It is ideal to percuss identical areas of chest for comparison.
- Percuss the normal side first.
- Use light percussion while percussing clavicles and anterior chest (with less depth of tissues).
- Use heavy percussion while percussing the posterior chest (greater depth of tissues).

  – Infraclavicular region up to 5th Intercostal space.
- Laterally
  – Apex of axilla up to 7th intercostal space.
- Posteriorly
  – Chest wall above the scapula (above the spine of scapula).
  – Interscapular region (in between scapulae)
  – Infrascapular up to 10th Intercostal space (below the angle of scapula upto the 11th rib.)

Percussion of Lung Apex (Fig. 4.6)

Corresponds roughly to the supraclavicular area. Keep the middle finger of the left hand over the trapezius from behind and percuss with downward movement.

Main Causes of Dullness over the Apex

- Upper lobe pneumonia
- Tuberculosis
- Pancoast's tumour

Cardiac Dullness

Percuss the cardiac borders.

Obliteration or diminished cardiac dullness-indicates emphysema.

Clavicular Percussion

Percuss the medial 1/3 of the clavicle.

- Percussion of the lateral part of the clavicle normally produces dull note due to lateral muscle mass.
- A lesion of the upper lobe produces abnormal percussion note over clavicle.

Normal Percussion of the Lung

- Normal lung is resonant to percuss.
- Percussion note is moderately low in pitch and heard easily.
- Anterior aspect of the chest is more resonant than the back. Lesions 5 cm deeper to the chest wall or smaller than 2–3 cm in diameter may not alter the percussion note.

Genesis of Normal Percussion Note

- Vibrations of the pleximeter fingers, chest wall and underlying tissues together produce composite notes, which is felt or heard when the chest is percussed. Selective resonating action of the thorax reinforces the percussion note.
- Density of the medium through which the sounds travel determines the quality of the percussion

note. Quieter notes are produced by denser medium.

- If vibrations are undampened and continue for a longer time percussion note will be resonant.

Abnormal Percussion Notes

Hyperresonant Note

Increase of Normal Resonance
For example, unilateral pneumothorax, compensatory emphysema and large thin walled cavity.

- Hyper-resonance over localised area of chest: Obstructive emphysema
- Bilateral hyper-resonance: Emphysema of the lung.
- Tympanitic note: Abnormally low-pitched. (loudest note): Drum like note and heard over the hollow viscus

   Hyper-resonance and tympanitic notes are due to the vibrations produced by percussion which are undampened, continue for significant time due to large acoustic mismatch of the conducting media. For example Tissues overlying the air filled space.

Decrease or Absence of Resonance
- Impaired Note: Decrease of resonance due to airless lung.
- Percussion note is shorter in duration with low in intensity, e.g. consolidation, pulmonary collapse, pulmonary fibrosis.
- Dull note: Significant or total decrease of resonance, e.g. consolidation, pulmonary collapse/ fibrosis, pleural thickening.
- Stony dull note: Absolute decrease of resonance (quietest note) with resistance felt by the percussing finger (as though percussion over muscles), e.g. pleural effusion.

Mechanism of Impaired or Dull Note
- Due to rapid decrease of vibrations
- Underlying tissue is similar to the surface tissues and vibrations decay quickly.

Traube's Area
- A semilunar area
- Boundaries

- Above: Lower part of 5th intercostal space (6th rib)
- Below: Costal margin on the left side
- Lateral: mid axillary line on the left side

Significance
- Normally resonant to percuss due to the fundus of the stomach.
- Becomes dull in cases of left sided pleural effusion and massive splenomegaly.

Skodiac Resonance
Resonant percussion note heard above the level of pleural effusion (when the underlying lung is compressed by the fluid).

Shifting Dullness
Significance: Indicates the presence of air and fluid in the pleural space (hydropneumothorax)

   If the pleural cavity contains fluid and air upper border of the dullness will be horizontal.

   Percussion can detect change in the level of fluid if the patient's position is changed.

Elicitation of Shifting Dull Note
- Keep the patient upright
- Percuss the chest from above downwards and detect the upper border of dull note (upper part will be hyper resonant due to associated pneumo-thorax).
- Patient is asked to lie down and if necessary turn, while keeping the pleximeter finger in the same area of previous dull note.
- Observe for resonant note while percussing the previously dull area after changing the patient's position.
- Note the degree of shift of fluid by percussing downwards in the newer position of the patient.

Myotatic Irritability
Percussion over the front of the chest close to the sternum may produce transient flickering of the neighbouring muscle, e.g. in case of extreme emaciation in diseases like pulmonary tuberculosis.

Percussion for Movement of Diaphragm (Tidal Percussion)
Significance to make out the lower border of lung resonance and lung expansion.

Decreased movement of lower border of lung resonance

For example, pulmonary fibrosis, pleural effusion.

Conditions associated with decreased movement of diaphragm.

In patients with emphysema on tidal percussion there is no change in the lower border of the lung resonance as the lung is already fully expanded.

Technique of Tidal Percussion

- Percuss the upper border of the liver dullness normally in the right 5th intercostal space.
- Ask the patient to take deep inspiration
- Percuss for the liver dullness at the height of inspiration.
- Normally liver dullness moves down by 1–2 intercostal spaces.

> *Note*
> - In patient's with pushed up diaphragm due to infra-diaphragmatic causes upper border of dullness moves down on deep inspiration.
> - Tidal percussion can also be carried out posteriorly by noting the change in the level of lower border of lung resonance on inspiration and expiration.

AUSCULTATION

Key points for Auscultating the Respiratory System

- Ideal position for auscultation is either the patient sitting up/standing.
- Corresponding areas on either side of the chest should be auscultated and compared.
- Avoid deep breathing as it may produce dizziness and tetany (occasionally).

Auscultate the Following Areas of Chest

- Anteriorly from supraclavicular area upto the liver dullness (5th intercostal space).
- Lateral sides from apex of axilla to the 8th rib.
- Posteriorly from suprascapular area to the 11th rib.
- Avoid auscultation within 2–3 cm of midline.
- Auscultation after coughing is helpful in detection

of crepitations and post-tussive suction (avoid coughing in patient with severe pleuritic pain).

- Auscultation of upper lobe supra and infra-clavicular area.
- Auscultation of lower lobe infrascapular area.
- Right mid lobe and lingula anteriorly on either side of lower 1/3rd of sternum.
- All lobes auscultatory events of all lobes can be heard in the axilla.

Schematic Auscultation of the Respiratory System

Check for

1. Intensity of breath sounds
2. Type of breathing
3. Comparison of inspiratory and expiratory element of breathing.
4. Added sounds
   - Crackles
   - Rhonchi
   - Pleural rub
5. Voice sounds
   - Vocal resonance
   - Bronchophony
   - Aegophony
   - Whispering pectoriloqusy

Breath Sounds

Genesis of Normal Breath Sounds

Normal breathing pattern is vesicular which resembles rustling of trees.

Predominantly produced in the major airways (200–2000 Hz) and is heard at the chest wall with low frequency (200–400Hz) due to filtering of high frequency sounds by the lung and chest wall.

- Inspiration is of longer duration (3 times) than expiration.
- Inspiratory sound is due to the gas turbulence in the major airways.
- Expiratory sound is due to elastic recoil of the lung and produced by central airways and at their bifurcations due to convergence of airflow, maximal at the onset of expiration.
- Expiration contains predominantly low frequency sounds and ear is less sensitive to low frequency

sounds (falls below the threshold of audibility early in expiration).

Characteristics of Vesicular Breathing (Fig. 4.7)

Normally heard over the chest except over the larynx, trachea, upper part of sternum, lower cervical vertebra and 3rd and 4th dorsal vertebra.
- Rustling in quality
- Inspiration is longer than expiration
- There is no gap between inspiration and expiration.

Intensity (loudness) of Breath Sounds

- Normal intensity depends on the acoustic density of the conducting medium of the sound.
- Normally breath sounds are of equal intensity on both sides of the chest (normally inflated lung).

Diminished Intensity of Breath Sounds

Impedance and resistance to transmission of sound can occur as the sound waves propagate through tissues of different acoustic density resulting in sound reflection results in decreased intensity of sound.

The sound reflection can occur at boundaries between gas—liquid (alveoli), lung—pleura and pleura—chest wall with different acoustic properties due to the underlying pathology.

Conditions Associated with Diminished Breath Sounds

Bilaterally diminished breath sounds (hyperinflated chest).

For example, emphysema, attack of bronchial asthma.

Chest wall and hyperinflated lung will have different acoustic property resulting in reflection of sound at the pleural surface causing decreased intensity of breath sound.

Bilaterally, breath sounds can also be decreased due to respiratory muscle paralysis.

Unilateral Decrease of Breath Sounds

1. Pleural effusion
2. Pneumothorax
3. Pleural thickening
4. Pulmonary collapse (breath sounds absent)

Decreased intensity of breath sound is due to sounds getting reflected at the pleural surface because of the different acoustic density of the conducting media.

Causes of Prolonged Inspiration

- Upper airway obstruction
- Produces stridor

Causes of Prolonged Expiration

- Smaller airway obstruction, e.g. bronchial asthma, COPD

Bronchial Breathing (Fig. 4.8)

Characteristics

- Greater in intensity
- Harsh blowing in quality
- Sound is of higher frequencies
- Expiratory sound is of equal duration and louder as that of inspiration.

Genesis of Bronchial Breathing

Diseased lung does not filter the higher frequency sounds produced in the central airways. Tracheal sounds are transmitted to the periphery without attenuation.

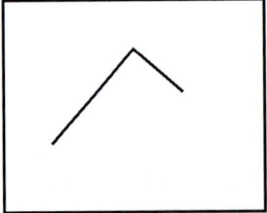

Fig. 4.7 Vesicular breathing

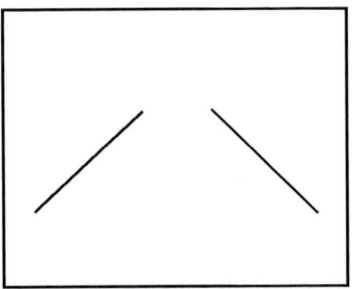

Fig. 4.8 Bronchial breathing

Different Types and Causes of Bronchial Breathing

1. Tubular breathing: Resembles tracheal breathing, e.g. pneumonic consolidation

Occasionally upper lobe fibrosis with tracheal shift. Sometimes direct transmission of the sound from the trachea can occur as mediastinal surface of right upper lobe is in direct contact with the trachea (irrespective of patency of right upper lobe bronchus).

In patients with right upper lobe fibrosis tracheal shift to right side can cause bronchial breathing in the infraclavicular area (not heard in the axilla).

2. Cavernous breathing: For example, cavity

Cavity acts as a resonating chamber producing a hollow quality cavernous breathing.

3. Amphoric breathing: High pitched metallic quality bronchial breathing as though blowing through a top of a bottle. For example, large cavity and tension pneumothorax (with bronchopleural communication).

Broncho-vesicular Breathing

- Type of breathing which is intermediate between bronchial and vesicular in its character.
- Inspiration and expiration are almost of equal duration and character.
- There is no gap between inspiration and expiration.
- Normally heard over upper interscapular and suprascapular areas.

Adventitious Sounds

Classification

a. Continuous sounds wheeze (rhonchi)/stridor
b. Discontinuous sounds–crackles (crepitations)

Continuous Sounds

Even though rhonchi are relatively lower pitched than wheeze (high pitched) two terms can be used interchangeably.

Characteristics of Rhonchi/Wheeze

- Musical sounds lasting longer than 250 milli seconds.
- Due to the vibrations of an airway at the point of closure.
- Expiration is prolonged.

Genesis of Rhonchi

- Produced in the medium sized airways
- Acceleration of airflow through a narrowing airway will decrease the pressure in that airway (Bernoulli effect) and then tends to close it. This in turn decreases flow and airway opens producing rapid vibrations of airways generating wheeze/rhonchi.

Narrowing of airways may be due to

- Mucosal oedema
- Spasm of bronchial musculature
- Partial obstruction

Different Types of Rhonchi

1. Monophonic: Single musical note

Generated from single airway with partial obstruction.

Fixed monophonic wheeze, i.e. localised wheeze which does not change on coughing.

Suggests fixed partial obstruction to single bronchus. Evidence of associated obstructive emphysema may be present. For example, tumour, foreign body, rarely stricture.

2. Polyphonic wheeze

Multiple varieties of musical notes.

Suggests-widespread narrowing of airways (multiple or diffuse).

Always associated with airway disease with prolonged expiration. For example, COPD, bronchial asthma, acute bronchitis.

Causes of Rhonchi

- Inspiratory and expiratory: Bronchial asthma, (predominantly expiratory)
- COPD (both inspiratory and expiratory)
- Pulmonary eosinophilia
- Bronchopulmonary aspergillosis
- Pulmonary oedema

Significance of Absence of Wheeze in an Asthmatic

Severe attack of asthma - Flow rate decreases below the critical level necessary to generate oscillations of airways.

It will be associated with severe airflow obstruction.

Stridor

Inspiratory sound can be heard to a distance, best heard over the neck.

Suggests upper airway obstruction (larynx/trachea), e.g. foreign body, carcinoma.

Crepitations (crackles)

Fine crepitations: Non musical discontinuous sounds

Higher in pitch and less louder than coarse crepitations

Genesis of Fine Crepitations

Occurs due to sudden reopening of closed airways during inspiration, which were closed during previous expiration.

When two areas of lung contain gas at widely different pressures, if the pressure becomes suddenly equalised airways reopen and gas is set into oscillations producing crepitations.

Examples of Fine Crepitations

- Early inspiratory: Produced at proximal bronchi. For example, chronic bronchitis, bronchial asthma
- Late inspiratory crepitations: Generated at the distal airways and alveolar level. For example, pulmonary oedema, fibrosing alveolitis and early pneumonia.

Coarse Crepitations

- Non musical discontinuous sounds
- Low pitched and of longer duration.
- Bubbling sounds produced due to air passing through liquids/secretions.
- May be palpable over the chest wall
- May be heard in both inspiration and expiration.
- Crepitations can decrease after coughing, e.g. bronchiectasis, pulmonary cavity, resolving pneumonia.

Post Tussive Crepitations

- Crepitations appear after coughing.
- Characteristically found in patients with early pulmonary tuberculosis in the apical region.

Leathery Crepitations

- Coarse crepitations: Characteristic of bronchiectasis.

Velcrocrepitations

End inspiratory crepitations: Sound resembles that produced when adhered two strips of velcro tapes are separated apart.

Found in patients with interstitial lung disease.

VOICE SOUNDS

Voice resonance (VR): Sounds auscultated over the various parts of the chest during phonation.

Technique of Auscultation for Vocal Resonance

- Patient is asked to repeat words like one-one-one.
- Auscultate symmetrical areas on either sides of chest and compare the intensity of sounds.

Normal Regional Variations of VR

Suprasternal and interscapular areas have increased intensity of VR.

Pathological Variations of VR

- Increased VR
  - Consolidation (increased intensity of breath sounds)
  - Cavity
- Decreased VR
  - Unilateral: Pleural effusion, pneumothorax, pulmonary collapse, pulmonary fibrosis
  - Bilateral: Emphysema, diffuse airflow obstruction

Bronchophony

Voice sounds which are spoken are heard with greater clarity (e.g. one-one-one) (distinction between individual syllabus is not possible).

Bronchophony is due to the better transmission of higher frequency sounds. For example, consolidation, cavity.

Aegophony

Voice sounds heard by the stethoscope over the chest with nasal quality (bleating of a goat), e.g. consolidation, cavity, above the level of pleural effusion.

Aegophony may be an extreme degree of bronchophony. It is due to better transmission of amplified higher frequency sound.

Whispering Pectoriloquy (WP)

Characterised by better appreciation of whispered voice sounds by the stethoscope.

Technique of Auscultation of WP

- Patient is asked to repeat with whispered voice sounds (one-one-one).
- Auscultate symmetrical areas of chest.
- Whispered voice sounds are better heard with clarity and each syllabus can be distinguished. For example, cavity, consolidation.
- These higher frequency sounds are better transmitted through airless lung (consolidation and cavity). Whispered voice sounds are not transmitted by normal lung as it transmits predominantly low frequency sounds.
- Whispering pectoriloquy is a confirmatory sign of consolidation.

Pleural Rub

Sound generated by the movement of inflamed layers of pleura.

Characteristics

1. Superficial coarse scratching sound
2. Present on both phases of respiration
3. Sound does not alter by coughing
4. Associated with pleural pain
5. Intensified by pressure of diaphragm

Usually heard at infrascapular and infra-axillary area (due to maximum movement of pleural layers).

Causes

Pleuritis due to:

- Viral infection
- Tuberculosis
- Pneumonias
- Malignant disorder
- Collagen disorder

Distinguishing features between Coarse Crepitations and Pleural Rub

Crepitations

- Present only on one phase of respiration
- Altered by coughing

- Not associated with pleuritic pain

Pleural Rub

- Both phases of respiration
- Does not change on coughing
- Associated with pleuritic pain

Succussion Splash (Hippocratic splash)

Apply the stethoscope over the area of chest at the level of fluid and air and shake the patient. A splashing sound is heard, classically heard in a patient of hydropneumothorax.

Causes of succussion splash heard over the chest apart from hydropneumothorax are

- Hydro/pyopneumothorax
- Large cavity with fluid
- Herniation of stomach into the thorax

Coin Test

- Tap a coin, which is held flat against the chest with another coin.
- Auscultate the opposite chest wall for a metallic sound.
- Heard in patients with pneumothorax.

Post tussive Suction

- Ask the patient to cough and take a deep inspiration.
- Auscultate for the suction sound

Suggests

- Thin walled collapsible cavity communicating with the bronchus.
- Sucking sound is heard due to entry of air into an empty cavity during inspiration.

D'Espine's sign

Whispered voice sounds, which are heard below the T3 vertebra in adults.

Suggests: Posterior mediastinal mass.

Note: Normally whispered voice sounds are heard only up to T3 vertebra.

Pneumothorax click (Hamman's sign)

Rhythmical sound which is heard synchronous with cardiac systole.

Suggests: Pneumomediastinum

COMMON RESPIRATORY CONDITIONS IN CLINICAL PRACTICE

Pleurisy

Suggests inflammation of the pleura - also called dry pleurisy (there is no accumulation of fluid in the pleural cavity).

Signs
- Audible pleural rub
- Intercostal tenderness

Important Causes
- Viral infection
- Bacterial pneumonia
- Tuberculosis

Pleural Effusion

Suggests presence of fluid in the pleural cavity.

Signs
- Mediastinal shift to opposite side.
- Decreased chest movement and expansion on the affected side.
- Stony dull note on percussion
- Decreased or absent breath sound

Causes
- Transudates
- Exudates
- Cirrhosis of liver
- Tuberculosis
- Nephrotic syndrome
- Malignant effusion
- CCF
- Syn. pneumonic

Empyema

Signs
- All signs of pleural effusion
- Toxemia
- Clubbing
- Inter costal tenderness

Pneumothorax

Presence of air in the pleural cavity

Signs
- Mediastinal shift to opposite side
- Decreased chest expansion and movement on the affected side.
- Hyper resonant note on percussion
- Absence of breath sounds

Causes
- Tuberculosis
- Rupture of emphysematous bulla
- Rupture of pulmonary cavity

Types of Pneumothorax
- Open type
- Closed type
- Tension type

Hydropneumothorax

Presence of air and fluid in the pleural cavity.

Causes
- Tuberculosis
- After aspiration of pleural fluid
- Trauma
- Rupture of lung abscess cavity into pleural cavity.

Signs
- Horizontal level of dullness
- Shifting dullness
- Succusion splash
- Mediastinum shifted to opposite side

Pneumonic Consolidation

Signs
- Mediastinum not shifted.
- Movement is decreased on the affected side (due to associated pleuritis).
- Dull percussion note.
- Tubular bronchial breathing and presence of crepitations.

Classification of Pneumonia
- Depending on the host condition
  - Primary (no pre-existing lung disease)
  - Secondary (pre-existing lung disease)
- Depending on the aetiology
  - Bacterial

– Fungal
– Viral
– Chemical
– Parasitic
- Depending on the anatomical site involved
  – Lobar
  – Segmental
  – Bronchopneumonia

Lung Abscess

Causes
- Community acquired
- Septic embolisation into the lungs
- Aspiration of septic material from the URT/ Oral cavity

Signs
- Toxemia
- Clubbing
- Signs of consolidation/cavity

Bronchial Asthma

Signs During an Acute Attack
- Dyspnoeic patient
- Diminished chest expansion
- Hyper resonant percussion note
- Diminished intensity of breath sounds
- Rhonchi and prolonged expiration

Signs of Acute Severe Asthma
- Dyspnoeic patient
- Presence of central cyanosis
- Tachycardia and pulses paradoxus
- Hyper resonant chest percussion
- Silent chest on auscultation

Pulmonary Fibrosis

Signs
- Signs of volume loss on the affected side.
- Mediastinum is shifted to same side of pathology.
- Movements and expansion is decreased on the affected side.
- Impaired percussion note.
- Breath sound is diminished with presence of crepitations.

Causes
- Pulmonary TB
- Lung abscess
- Interstitial lung disease
- Pneumoconiosis

Note: Upper lobe fibrosis can result in bronchial breathing in the infraclavicular area on the affected side due to tracheal shift.

Cavity in the Lung

Signs
- Cavernous type of bronchial breathing
- Presence of crepitations
- Presence of post tussive suction in a thin-walled collapsible cavity

Causes
- Pulmonary tuberculosis
- Lung abscess
- Malignancy undergoing cavitation

Pulmonary Collapse

Signs
- Decreased movement and expansion on the affected side.
- Signs of volume loss on the affected side.
- Mediastinum shifted to the same side of pathology
- Impaired or dull percussion note
- Absence of breath sounds

Causes
- Bronchial obstruction due to foreign body
- Intra-bronchial growth
- Extrinsic compression of the bronchus

Bronchiectasis

Signs
- Halitosis
- Clubbing
- Coarse leathery crepitations

Causes
- Congenital
  – Ciliary abnormality
  – Cystic fibrosis

- Acquired
  - Necrotising pneumonia
  - Pulmonary tuberculosis
  - Obstruction to the bronchus

Bronchiectasis sicca: Secondary to pulmonary tuberculosis.
- Patient will have haemoptysis
- Affects the upper lobe

COPD Signs
- Only chronic bronchitis — presence of rhonchi and crepitations.
- Signs of airflow obstructions — rhonchi, prolonged expiration.

Signs of Emphysema
- Barrel shaped chest
- Decreased chest expansion
- Hyper resonant percussion note
- Cardiac dullness obliterated
- Liver dullness pushed down
- Decreased breath sounds

Causes of Chronic Bronchitis
- Chronic smoking
- Atmospheric pollution
- Occupational exposure to dust and minerals
- Repeated respiratory infection

Causes of Emphysema
- Chronic bronchitis
- Pneumoconiosis
- Alpha - 1antitrypsin deficiency

Different Types of Emphysema
- Pulmonary emphysema (secondary to COPD)
- Obstructive emphysema
- Surgical emphysema
- Compensatory emphysema.
- Mediastinal emphysema

Table 4.2 gives differences between compensatory emphysema and emphysema secondary to COPD

Obstructive Emphysema

Causes
- Fixed partial intra bronchial obstruction
- Foreign body/ Tumour

Table 4.2 Difference between compensatory emphysema and emphysema secondary to COPD

Emphysema sec. to COPD	Compensatory emphysema
Bilateral	Unilateral
Cardiac dullness obliterated	Cardiac dullness is not obliterated
Breath sounds decreased	Breath sound intensity normal
Expiration is prolonged	Expiration is not prolonged. Evidence of significant lung disease on the opposite side

Signs
- Fixed monophonic wheeze
- Localised hyper resonance

Bronchial Carcinoma

May present with
- Pleural effusion
- SVC obstruction
- Mass lesion
- Mediastinal mass
- Pulmonary collapse

Mass Lesion

Signs
- Dull note
- Diminished breath breath sounds

Note: Occasionally mass lesion can result in bronchial breathing due to better conduction of breath sounds.

Upper lobe bronchial carcinoma
(Pancoast's tumor)
Signs
- Wasting of small muscles of hand
- 1st and 2nd rib tenderness
- Horner's syndrome
- Signs of mass in the upper lobe

Evidences of Mediastinal Mass
- SVC obstruction

- Horner's syndrome
- Hoarseness of voice
- Diaphragm paralysis
- Dullness on percussion over the sternum/either side of the sternum
- D'Espine's sign

Differential diagnosis of dullness at right lung base

Due to conditions above the diaphragm

- Pulmonary causes: Lower lobe consolidation, collapse and fibrosis
- Pleural causes: Pleural effusion, pleural fibrosis

Due to conditions below the diaphragm

- Elevated diaphragm due to massive ascites
- Upward enlargement of liver
- Subdiaphragmatic abscess

Features of SVC Obstruction

Above the Joining of Azygos

- Chest wall veins are not prominent
- Main collaterals: Superior intercostal veins

SVC Obstruction Involving Azygos

- Collaterals: Veins inside and outside the chest carrying the blood to inferior vena cava.
- There will be prominent veins over the chest.
- Patients with SVC obstruction will also have facial puffiness, non pulsatile and engorged veins over the neck and oedema of upper limbs.

Causes of SVC Obstruction

- Carcinoma bronchus
- Lymphoma
- Mediastinal secondaries (e.g. testicular tumor, carcinoma breast)
- Retrosternal goiter
- Aortic aneurysm
- Fibrosing mediastinitis

4b Respiratory System II

Anatomy of Respiratory System

Anatomically respiratory system can be divided into upper and lower respiratory tract.

Upper Respiratory Tract (URT)
- Upper respiratory tract consists of nose, nasopharynx and larynx. URT is lined by ciliated epithelium and covered by mucus.

Lower Respiratory Tract (LRT)
- Lower respiratory tract consists of trachea and bronchi. Main bronchi divide into many generation of bronchi ending in terminal bronchioles. Terminal bronchioles end in acini which consist of alveoli. Lower respiratory tract is lined by ciliated epithelium.

Gas Exchange Unit of the Lung
- Respiratory bronchioles with groups of alveoli form an acinus which is the gas exchange unit of the lung. Pneumocytes type I and type II form the lining of alveoli.

Blood and Nerve Supply of Lungs
- Lung is supplied by autonomic nervous system and vascular supply is both by pulmonary arteries and bronchial arteries.
- Pulmonary artery pumps un-oxygenated blood into the lungs, with a rich capillary network which helps in gas exchange.

Defence Mechanisms of the lung

Physical Barriers
- Nose and larynx act as protective barriers. Ciliated columnar epithelium of the nose removes the large particles contained in the inspired air.
- Larynx with the mechanism of cough and expectoration protect the lower airways from foreign particles.

Mucociliary Defence
- Trachea and bronchi are lined by mucus and cilia which trap the particles entering through the inspired air and then clear it.

Defensive Proteins of the Lung
- Lining layers of the lung contain protease inhibitors, bactericidal proteins, immunoglobulins and compliments which can counteract inflammation. Surfactant protein has also got bactericidal property.

Alveolar Macrophages

Functions
- Can destroy foreign substance and bacteria
- Can attract neutrophils and monocytes.
- Generate immune response by liberating lymphokines
- Clearing the inflammatory end products.

Investigations of Respiratory Disease

Radiology

X-ray chest
Chest X-ray is helpful in detecting parenchymal and pleural diseases. Serial X-rays after treatment are helpful in determining the response to treatment/ progression of the disease.

CT Scan of the Chest

Helpful in Detecting
- Pulmonary nodule

- Mass lesion in the lung
- Hilar lymphadenopathy
- For staging of bronchogenic carcinoma

CT guided needle biopsy helps in histopathological diagnosis of the disease. High resolution CT scan helps in diagnosing interstitial lung disease and bronchiectasis.

Pulmonary Angiogram
Pulmonary angiogram is helpful in the early diagnosis of pulmonary embolism.

Ventilation Perfusion Scan
Ventilation perfusion scan helps in the detection of pulmonary embolism. This is also helpful in detection of functional effects of bronchogenic carcinoma and emphysematous bullae.

Radiolabelled Technetium 99 is used for diagnosis of pulmonary embolism.

Lung Function Testing:
Following lung function tests are helpful in the diagnosis of pulmonary diseases
- Forced expiratory volume in 1st second: (FEV1): FEV1 is reduced in bronchial asthma and COPD.
- Vital capacity: Vital capacity is low in-bronchial asthma, COPD and pulmonary fibrosis.
- Carbon monoxide diffusion capacity: Carbon monoxide diffusion capacity is low in patients with: Emphysema, pulmonary fibrosis.
- Total lung capacity (TLC) and residual volume (RV)
  – TLC and RV is increased in patients with bronchial asthma and emphysema.
  – TLC and RV is decreased in patients with pulmonary fibrosis.

Arterial Blood Gas (ABG) and Pulse Oximetry
Arterial blood gas is helpful in the diagnosis of respiratory failure by measuring arterial oxygen and carbon dioxide levels.

Hypoxia
Hypoxia indicates decreased level of oxygen in the blood ($PaO_2 < 60$ m Hg)

Causes
- Pulmonary oedema

- Emphysema
- Bronchial asthma
- Pneumonic consolidation

Hypercapnia
Hypercapnia indicates increased level of arterial CO_2 in the blood. It is usually caused by alveolar hypoventilation or ventilation perfusion mismatch.

Causes of Hypercapnia
- Chronic obstructive pulmonary disease
- Kyphoscoliosis
- Ankylosing spondylitis
- Myasthenia gravis
- Brainstem disease

Microbiological Investigations
- Blood, sputum, throat swab, pleural fluid and bronchial washing can be examined for bacteria, fungus. Sputum and bronchial washing may yield mycobacterium tuberculosis.

Endoscopic Examination
- Laryngoscopy, bronchoscopy and media-stinoscopy can be used to visualise the pathological status in the respiratory tract and if necessary materials can be taken for histopathological examination.

Cytology and Histopathology
- Sputum, pleural fluid and bronchial washings can be examined for malignant cells.
- Biopsy materials from bronchoscopy, laryngo-scopy, pleural biopsy and CT guided biopsy material are examined for histopathological examination.

CHRONIC OBSTRUCTIVE PULMONARY DISEASE

Chronic Bronchitis
Definition: Cough with expectoration on most of the days of at least 3 consecutive months for more than 2 successive years.

Emphysema
Definition: Permanent enlargement of air spaces distal to the terminal bronchioles.
Chronic obstructive pulmonary disease is a slowly

progressive disorder of the lung characterised by chronic airflow obstruction. It comprises both chronic bronchitis and emphysema.

Aetiology of Chronic Bronchitis
- *Smoking:* Cigarette smoking for long duration.
- Exposure to occupational dusts
- Exposure to smoke, dust, fuel, etc.
- Recurrent respiratory infection
- Alpha-1-antitrypsin deficiency
- Smoking causes constant airway inflammation. It increases the lung damage by unbalanced action of oxidants and proteinases.

Causes of Emphysema
- All causes of chronic bronchitis
- Alpha-1-antitrypsin deficiency

Pathology
Pathological changes in chronic bronchitis

a. Airway inflammation

b. Increase in the number of goblet cells with excess mucus production.

c. Decrease in the number of ciliated cells.

   Above pathological changes lead on to irreversible airflow obstruction.

Pathological Changes in Emphysema
- Enlargement of air spaces
- Destruction of interalveolar septa
- Reduction in the alveolar surface area for gas exchange.

Clinical Features
- Cough with expectoration with recurrent exacerbations after upper respiratory infection especially during winter months.
- Sputum is usually streaky and may have hemoptysis.
- Recurrent respiratory infection can cause purulent sputum.
- Gradually progressive dyspnoea with wheeze and dyspnoea increases with respiratory infection, exposure to smoke and adverse atmospheric conditions.

Signs: May not have clinical signs. Following signs may be present
- Bilateral rhonchi
- Bilateral crepitations
- Evidence of emphysema
- Polycythemia
- Later stages - Evidence of pulmonary hypertension and CCF.

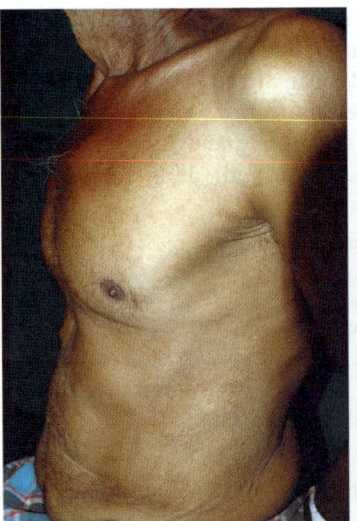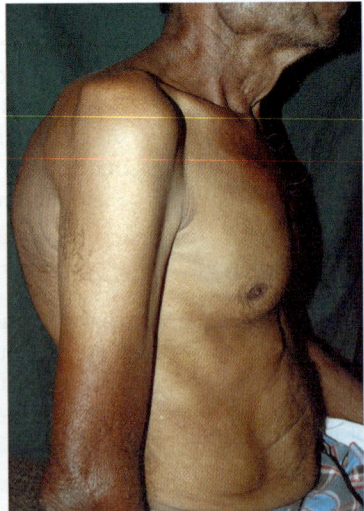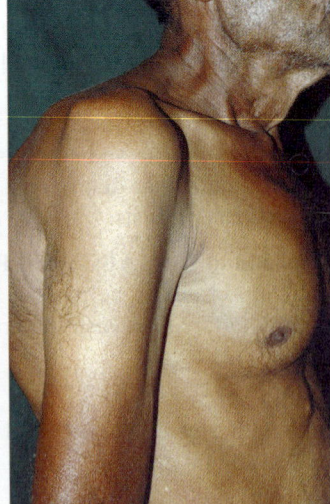

Fig. 4.9 Barrel-shaped chest in patients with emphysema

- Signs of airway obstruction: Rhonchi and prolonged expiration
- Signs of emphysema
  - Barrel-shaped chest (Fig. 4.9)
  - Decreased chest expansion
  - Hyperresonant percussion note
  - Bilateral breath sound intensity decreased

Complications
- Pneumothorax
- Pulmonary hypertension
- Right ventricular failure
- Polycythemia

Investigations
- Polycythemia = Hb% > 17 g/dl
- Chest X-ray shows evidence of air trapping and hyperinflation.
- Pulmonary function test
  - Shows evidence of airflow obstruction and air trapping.
  - CT scan can demonstrate emphysema along with emphysematous bullae
- ECG and echocardiogram: May demonstrate right ventricular hypertrophy

Complications of COPD
- Pulmonary hypertension, corpulmonale and CCF
- Respiratory failure
- Polycythemia
- Pneumothorax due to rupture of emphysematous bulla
- Recurrent respiratory infection
- Bronchogenic carcinoma

Management
- Stop smoking, avoid exposure to dust and smoke.
- Treatment of respiratory infection (amoxycillin/cotrimoxazole)
- Bronchodilator - Inhaled ipratroium bromide/salbutamol
- Anti inflammatory - Some patients may benefit from corticosteroid administration.
- Low dose 2 litres/min - Home oxygen therapy decreases pulmonary hypertension
- Surgical excision of bulla in emphysematous patients.

Treatment of Acute Exacerbation of Chrome Bronchitis
- Treatment of infection with antibiotics
- Nebulised salbutamol and ipratropium bromide
- Oxygen inhalation
- IV-corticosteroids if there is a previous response to steroids
- IV Aminophylline
- IV diuretics
- If severe exacerbation - Non invasive/ventilation support.

Dental aspects of COPD
- Perform all dental procedures under local anaesthesia and avoid IV sedation (barbiturates, morphine)
- General anaesthesia if required after proper preoperative respiratory assessment and only in hospital setting.
- There is increase chance of deep vein thrombosis postoperatively because of polycythemia.

BRONCHIAL ASTHMA

Definition
Respiratory disorder characterised by recurrent attacks of wheeze, cough, chest tightness and dyspnea due to chronic inflammation of airways and airway hyper responsiveness.

Pathogenesis
Genetic and environmental factors predispose to formation of antibodies to external allergens (atopy). These cause antigen antibody reaction on the bronchial mucosa and chronic airway inflammation.

Atopy
Condition characterised by formation of antibodies to external allergens causing extrinsic asthma. Extrinsic asthma starts in childhood and is associated with skin allergy.
Adult onset asthma: There is no atopy in these individuals and resulting asthma is intrinsic asthma.

Factors which Play Role in the Pathogenesis of Asthma

- Genetic susceptibility
- Polygenic inheritance plays a role in the genesis of asthma.

Environmental Factors

Allergens which are responsible for precipitance of asthma. House dust, mites, pet animal allergens and also fungal spores, sulphur dioxide and cigarette smokes, grass and flower of pollens.

Factors which Aggravate Asthma

Drugs: β-blockers, aspirin (NSAIDS) can induce bronchospasm.

Infections: Viral and bacterial infection can aggravate asthma.

Psychological stress: Physical, psychological stress and emotional upsets can precipitate an attack of asthma.

Pathological Features of Bronchial Asthma

- Chronic inflammatory cell infiltration over the bronchial mucosa like eosinophils and macrophages
- There will be edema of airways with mucus plugging.
- Later stages:
  - Airway wall thickening
  - Increased smooth muscle mass
  - Hypertrophy of mucus secreting glands and narrowing of airways.

Clinical Features

Symptoms

- May be persistent/episodic
- Exacerbations of asthma can occur after an attack of viral infection/exposure to allergens.
- Recurrent attacks of cough, dyspnea and wheeze.
- Starts in childhood and progresses to adulthood in extrinsic (atopic) asthma.
- Nocturnal attacks can disturb sleep (nocturnal asthma)
- Attacks of wheeze and chest tightness can occur during exercise (exercise induced asthma).

- Adult onset asthma - symptoms can persist throughout the year (not related to allergens).

Signs

- Person is dyspneic
- Hyper inflation of lung fields
- There will be bilateral rhonchi with prolonged expiration of breath sounds.

Acute severe asthma (Status asthmaticus)

- Person is severely dyspnoeic and is unable to talk in sentences
- Tachycardia and pulsus paradoxus
- Central cyanosis
- Silent chest (due to severe airflow obstruction): Rhonchi are absent
- Altered sensorium
- Late stages - bradycardia

Investigations

- Complete blood picture: Blood eosinophil count is increased.
- Chest X-ray: During an attack of bronchospasm, hyper inflated chest. There may be pneumonic consolidation/collapsed segment due to mucus plugging and in severe cases may reveal pneumothorax.
- Pulmonary function tests: There will be obstruction to the airflow - $FEV1 < 80\%$
- Peak expiratory flow rate (PEFR): PEFR will show marked variation and increase after bronchodilators (> 15% increase of PEFR after nebulised bronchodilators).
- Arterial blood gas
  - Hypoxia is usually present during severe attack of asthma.
  - Useful in monitoring the response to therapy.

Complications

- Respiratory failure
- Polycythemia
- Pneumothorax

Management

General measures

- Stop smoking
- Avoid exposure to allergens

- Avoid severe exertion
- Avoid drugs which precipitate asthma
- Take regular medication

Management of Chronic Persistent Asthma

Drugs used

- *Bronchodilators*
  - β2 agonists: Salbutamol/terbutaline tablets, inhalers, nebulisers
  - Anticholinergics: Ipratropium bromide inhalers
- *Anti-inflammatory*
  - Corticosteroids - Inhalers, budesonide, beclamethasone, fluticasone
  - Tablets and injectable steroids are available.
- *Mast cell inhibitors:* Inhaled sodium chromoglycate.
- *Methyl xanthine derivatives:* Theophylline tablets/injection.

Above drugs are used alone or in combination depending on the severity.

Step Care Therapy for Bronchial Asthma

Mild Intermittent Attack of Asthma

Less than 2 attacks of breathlessness/week and less than 2 attacks at night/month: Only inhaled β_2 agonist as required, e.g salbutamol.

Mild Persistent Attack

- More than 2 attacks/week and more than 2 attacks at night/month
- Low dose inhaled steroids, e.g. Budesonide 100 micrograms 2 times/day.
- Inhaled β_2 agonists as required.

Moderate Persistent

Daily attack of asthma and more than 1 attack at night/week

- Inhaled steroids - Low to medium doses Budesonide (400–800 micrograms/day), Budesonide microgr/day + longer acting β_2 agonists (Salmetrol).
- Inhaled β_2 agonists (if required theophylline can also be added)

Severe Persistent

Continuous attack during day time and frequent attack at night:

- Inhaled high dose steroids along with longer acting β_2 agonists and oral steroids if required and oral theophylline.

Management of Acute Severe Asthma

- High flow oxygen - 60% O_2 inhalation with monitoring of blood gas
- Nebulised β_2 - agonists salbutamol/terbutaline nebulisers repeated within 30 minutes
- IV Hydrocortisone 200 mg or inj. Methyl Prednisolone and then oral prednisolone 30–60 mg/day
- Monitor peak expiratory flow rate, arterial blood gas
- Maintain adequate hydration
- Treat respiratory infections.

Other Measures

- Nebulised ipratropium bromide
- Inj. Terbutaline 0.5 mg subcutaneously and can be repeated.
- Inj. Aminophylline 0.5 to 5 mg/kg/hour
- Look for complications like pneumothorax, collapse of part of lung due to mucus plug blocking.

If the patient deteriorates inspite of the above measures and if the patient develops altered sensorium exhaustion and respiratory arrest keep the patient on mechanical ventilator.

Once the patient has improved, patient can be put on inhaled bronchodilators with tapering of corticosteroids at the time of discharge.

Dental Aspects of Bronchial Asthma

- Carry out all dental procedures under local anaesthesia and avoid general anaesthesia as far as possible.
- Patient should take all asthmatic medications while coming to dental treatment.
- IV sedation can depress the respiration in asthmatics.
- NSAIDs, beta-blockers can precipitate an attack of asthma.
- Patients with asthma may also develop anaphylaxis to other drugs like penicillins and history of drug allergy should be enquired before the procedure.

- Thiopentone, opiates, suxamethonium, tubo-curare, should be avoided. Halothane or isoflurane are preferred anesthetics.

INFECTIONS OF THE RESPIRATORY SYSTEM

Pneumonia

- Pneumonia indicates inflammation of the lung parenchyma associated with radiological development of opacity in the lung.
- Pneumonia may involve segment or the whole lobe of the lung (lobar pneumonia).

Classification of Pneumonia

Classification by Site of Involvement

- Lobar pneumonia
- Lobular pneumonia
- Bronchopneumonia

Aetiological Classification

- Bacterial
- Viral
- Protozoal
- Fungal
- Chemical
- Radiation induced

Classification depending on the host's condition

- Community acquired
- Hospital acquired
- Aspiration pneumonia
- Pneumonia in immune compromised host

Important organisms which cause community acquired pneumonia

- *Pneumococcus*
- *Mycoplasma pneumoniae*
- *Legionella pneumophilia*
- *Staphylococcus aureus*
- *Klebsiella pneumoniae*
- *Hemophilia influenza*

Clinical Features of Lobar Pneumonia

- *Causative organism:* Pneumococcus (*Streptococcus pneumoniae*)

- *Symptoms*
  - Acute onset of fever with chills and rigors.
  - Initial dry cough with later rusty sputum.
  - Pleuritic type of chest pain
  - Associated headache, vomiting
  - Herpes labialis may be present
  - Preceding upper respiratory infection symptoms
- *Signs*
  - High grade fever
  - Tachycardia
  - Signs of consolidation in the lung: dull percussion note, tubular bronchial breathing and crepitations
  - Pleural rub and pleural effusion may be present.

Note
- Klebsiella pneumonia usually involves upper lobe and may produce red currant jelly sputum.
- Staphylococcal pneumonia can cause multiple lung abscesses.
- Mycoplasma pneumonia can cause patchy lung involvement, hemolysis, myocarditis and meningoencephalitis.
- Legionella pneumonia involves both lobes, can cause gastrointestinal tract symptoms, hyponatremia and hepatitis.

Investigations of Pneumonia

Blood Picture

- Total WBC count is increased with neutrophilia and high ESR.
- Chest X-ray (Fig. 4.10)
  - Homogenous opacity involving a lobe or segment.
  - Pleural effusion may be detectable.
- *Sputum:* Should be examined for gram stain, AFB and culture and sensitivity.
- *Blood culture and serology :* Blood culture and sensitivity and serological tests for corresponding organism.
- *Arterial blood gas:* To detect respiratory failure

Complications of Pneumonia

- Formation of lung abscess
- Pleural effusion /empyema and pyopneumothorax
- Septic syndrome

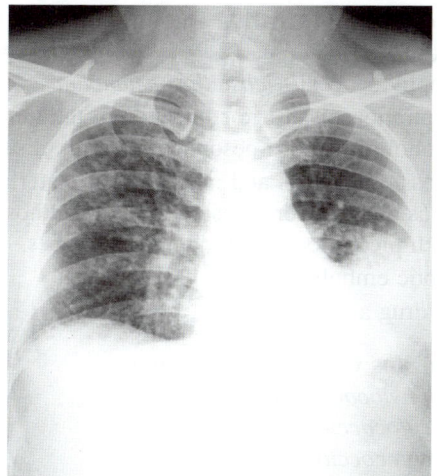 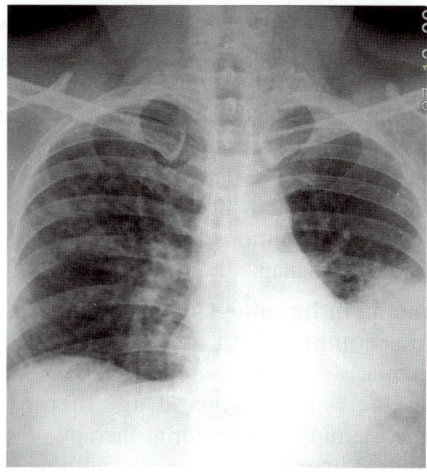

Fig. 4.10 X-ray picture of lobar pneumonia

- Respiratory failure
- Rarely pancreatitis, hepatitis, meaningo ence-phalitis and endocarditis.

Differential Diagnosis of Pneumonia

Following conditions should be differentiated from pneumonia

- Pulmonary tuberculosis
- Pulmonary infarction
- Pulmonary oedema
- Bronchogenic malignancy with secondary infection.
- Pulmonary eosinophilia and granulomatous diseases of the lung.

Management

General Measures

- Antipyretics, e.g. paracetamol
- Adequate hydration
- Analgesics for pleuritic pain
- Oxygen administration if hypoxia is present.
- Chest physiotherapy to clear the secretions

Specific Therapy

Gram Positive Organisms

For example, pneumococcus: Amoxycillin 500 mg oral/IV 8th hrly for 7–10 days.

Staphylococcal pneumonia: Flucloxacillin 500 mg QID 7–10 days

Gram Negative Organisms

Inj. Gentamicin 3 to 4 mg/kg x 7–10 days
Inj. Ceftazidime 1 to 2 gr 8th hrly 7–10 days
Mycoplasma/Legionella: Erythromycin 500 mg QID 7–10 days.

Hospital Acquired Pneumonia

- Hospital acquired (nosocomial) pneumonia suggests development of pneumonia after 48 hours of hospital admission.
- Organisms which cause pneumonia in hospital admitted patients
  - *Klebsiella pneumoniae*
  - *Escherichia coli*
  - Pseudomonas species
  - Staphylococci.

Factors Predisposing to Pneumonia in Hospital Admitted Patients

1. Dental infection, endotracheal intubation and ventilation: Organisms can directly enter the lower respiratory tact

2. Anaesthesia, corticosteroids, diabetes mellitus, post operative debility can alter the defence mechanisms of the host. Reduced cough reflex

and altered oropharyngeal flora can lead onto aspiration and pneumonia.

3. Altered sensorium, vomiting can lead on to aspiration of stomach contents into the lungs.
4. Intravenous sites, septic embolisation can cause lung abscess.

Clinical features of hospital acquired infection depends on the condition of the patient and organism and should be managed accordingly.

Pneumonia in Immune Compromised Host

Immune compromised status associated with pneumonia.

1. Immune suppressive drug therapy, e.g. corticosteroid/cytotoxic drug therapy
2. Acquired immune deficiency syndrome (AIDS)
3. Neutropenias, defective T cell response and antibody production, e.g. CLL, lymphoma, splenomegaly, plasma cell dyscrasias.
4. Diseases like diabetes mellitus and alcoholism.

Organisms which cause respiratory infection in immune compromised host

- *Bacterial:* Staphylococci, pseudomonas, klebsiella, mycobacterium tuberculosis
- *Viral:* Cytomegalovirus, herpes virus
- *Fungal:* Aspergillosis, *Candida albicans, Pneumocystis carnii.*

Clinical features, and management depend on the organisms and predisposing chest condition.

Dental Aspects of Pneumonia

- Only perform emergency dental treatment in patients with pneumonia.
- General anaesthesia is contraindicated in patients with pneumonia.

SUPPURATIVE PNEUMONIA
(LUNG ABSCESS)

Suppurative Pneumonia

Pneumonia characterised by lung parenchymal destruction by inflammatory process. There will be microabscess formation.

Lung Abscess

There will be pus collection in the lung with formation of pulmonary cavity.

Causes of Suppurative Pneumonia and Lung Abscess

1. Staphylococcal/*Klebsiella pneumoniae*
2. Aspiration of gastric contents into the lung, e.g. alcoholism, gastro-oesophageal reflux disease
3. Gross oral sepsis and inhalation of material into lungs during operations on mouth and nose, e.g. tooth pieces, oral bacteria and anaerobes.
4. Septic embolisation into the lungs
5. IV drug abusers

Organisms Causing Lung Abscess

- *Staphylococcus aureus*
- *Streptococcus pneumoniae*
- *Streptococcus pyogenes*
- *Hemophilus influenzae*
- *Klebsiella pneumoniae*

Clinical Features

- High grade fever with chills and rigors
- Fatigue and weight loss
- Large amount of sputum, yellow and may be foul smelling
- Haemoptysis
- Pleuritic pain

Signs

- Halitosis
- Clubbing
- Signs of consolidation/cavity: Dull percussion note, tubular/cavernous breathing and crepitations
- Pleural rub

Investigations

- Blood counts - Increase WBC count with neutrophilia
- Sputum-gram stain, culture sensitivity and AFB.
- Chest X-ray shows evidence of consolidation/ cavity may be with fluid level.

Complications of Lung Abscess

- Haemophysis
- Emphysema
- Metastasis
- Septicemia

Treatment

General
- General antipyretics
- Analgesics for chest pain
- Chest physiotherapy and postural drainage

Specific (Antibiotics)
- Inj. Amoxycillin 500 mg 8th hrly/day
- Inj. Gentamycin 3–4 mg/kg/body weight
- Antibiotics - Oral/I.V. should be given for 4–6 weeks depending on the culture sensitivity of the organism.
- If anaerobic infection-give metronidazole oral/IV. 500 mg 8th hrly for 7–10 days
- Removal of the precipitating cause and bronchial obstruction.
- Surgical treatment if chronic lung abscess.

Dental Aspects of Lung Abscess
Use protective devices like rubber dam while doing dental procedures to prevent aspiration of materials into the lungs. If inhalation of tooth fragment and dental instruments occur urgent chest X-ray and bronchoscopy may be required for removal of the tooth fragment/instrument.

BRONCHIECTASIS

Definition
Bronchiectasis is defined as abnormal permanent dilatation of bronchi with destruction. Usually it is associated with recurrent infection of the lower respiratory tract.

Causes

Congenital-Due to abnormal ciliary function
- Immotile ciliary syndrome
- Kartagener's syndrome
- Fibrocystic disease of the lung
- Primary hypogamma globulinemia

Acquired - In children
- After measles and whooping cough
- Foreign body inhalation
- Pulmonary tuberculosis

In Adults
- Necrotising pneumonia
- Obstruction to the bronchus
- Bronchopulmonary aspergillosis
- Tuberculosis of the lung

Pathology
Chronic inflammation of bronchial wall with hypertrophy of bronchial arteries. There will be inflammation of the surrounding lung parenchyma.

Clinical Features

Symptoms
- Chronic cough with expectoration of large amount of purulent sputum which is usually foul smelling.
- Hemoptysis
- Recurrent attacks of pneumonia, pleuritis and exacerbation of symptoms.

General Features
- Weight loss, loss of appetite and fever

Signs
- Halitosis
- Clubbing
- Bilateral coarse leathery crepitations
  May develop signs of consolidation, collapse and cavity formation in the lung.

Complications

Respiratory
- Recurrent pneumonia/lung abscess
- Hemoptysis
- Pleural effusion / empyema
- Respiratory failure

Systemic
- Cerebral abscess
- Septicemia
- Systemic amyloidosis

Investigations
- *Complete blood picture:* ESR is raised, WBC count is increased
- Hb% may be decreased
- *Sputum:* For Gram stain, AFB and culture and sensitivity.

- *Chest X-ray:* May be normal or shows cystic spaces/honey combing pattern
- *CT scan:* High solution CT scan detects bronchiectasis
- Patients with congenital bronchiectasis should undergo ciliary function assessment.

Management

General Measures
- Improvement of nutrition
- Pneumococcal and *H. Influenza* vaccination.

Specific Measures
- Postural drainage and chest physiotherapy
- Bronchodilators and mucolytic agents if required
- Antibiotics - depending on the culture sensitivity of organism for 4–6 weeks
- Treatment of complications
- Surgical treatment: If localised and recurrent complications.

PULMONARY TUBERCULOSIS

- Tuberculosis is a granulomatous disease caused by *mycobacterium tuberculosis. Mycobacterium bovis* can also cause human infections.
- Even though any tissue can be involved by tuberculosis following are the common sites of involvement
  – Lung
  – Lymph nodes
  – Skin
  – Soft tissues

Atypical Mycobacteria
(environmental mycobacteria)
- *Mycobacterium avium* complex (MBC) can cause infection in patients with HIV infection.
- These come under the category of environmental mycobacteria.
- They may cause human disease
- Atypical mycobacteria cause infection in immune compromised hosts (e.g. in patients with AIDS).

Examples of Atpical Mycobacteria
- *Mycobacterium arium intracellularae*

- *Mycobacterium ulcerans*
- *Mycobacterium kansasii*
- *Mycobacterium scrofulaceum*

  Atypical mycobacteria commonly involve lymph nodes, skin, lungs and soft tissues. Mycobacterium avium intracellularae infection is common when CD4 count is less than 50 cell/cmm.

Predisposing Factors for the Development of Tuberculosis
- HIV infection
- Diabetes mellitus
- Malnutrition
- Extremes of ages
- Post gastrectomy
- Close contact with sputum positive pulmonary TB
- Haematological malignancies

Microbiology
- *Mycobacterium tuberculosis* is an anaerobic rod shaped bacilli.
- It is an acid-fast bacilli. It cannot be decolourised by acid/alcohol once stained.
- *Mycobacterium bovis* can be transmitted by unpasteurised milk, can also cause tuberculosis.

Pathophysiology
- Primary site of infection: Usually in the lung
- Rout of spread: Inhalation of infected droplets.

Primary Complex
- Primary complex occurs after inhalation of *Mycobacterium tuberculosis*. This includes superficial focus (Ghon's focus) in the lung and hilar lymphadenopathy. Primary complex 85–90% heal spontaneously. 10 to 15% of primary complex progresses to progressive pulmonary tuberculosis. It can also spread to pleura, pericardium, GIT, genitourinary tract, bones and may progress to active tuberculosis.
- 80–95% of primary complex heal
- Healed primary complex may later progress to:
  - Post primary tuberculosis
  - May develop reinfection (especially with HIV infection).

Pathology

Pathologically tuberculosis is a form of chronic granuloma consisting of central caseation surrounded by epithelioid cells and Langerhans type of giant cells.

Clinical Features of Pulmonary TB

Primary Pulmonary TB (initial infection)

Usually occurs in childhood, may be asymptomatic or can have influenza like illness. May also develop pleural effusion, hilar lymphadenopathy, meningitis, pericarditis and erythema nodosum.

Clinical features of post primary/progressive TB

* Occurs in adults

Features

* Fever: May be at evening times
* Cough, hemoptysis
* Anorexia, weight loss

Clinical examination may be normal or may have features of consolidation, cavity, pleural effusion and pneumothorax (Fig. 4.11).

Miliary TB (Fig. 4.12)

* Due to dissemination of infection in the blood, all organs may be involved.

Features

* Fever of 2–3 weeks, weight loss, dry cough, involvement of lymph nodes, meninges, hepatosplenomegaly and severe anemia.
* Chest X-ray in miliary TB: Shows 1–2 mm lesions spread throughout both the lung fields (Fig. 4.12).

Complications of Tuberculosis

Pulmonary

* Fibrosis of lung and cavity formation
* Massive haemoptysis
* Pleural effusion.
* Bronchiectasis
* Empyema
* Pneumothorax

Extrapulmonary

* Laryngitis

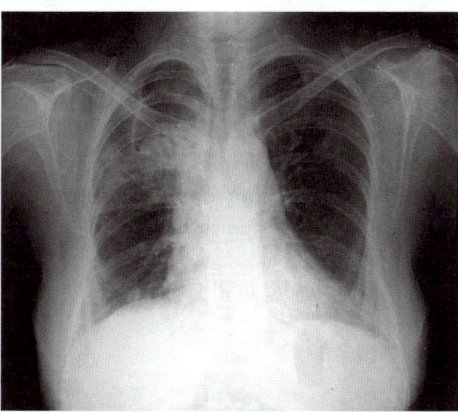
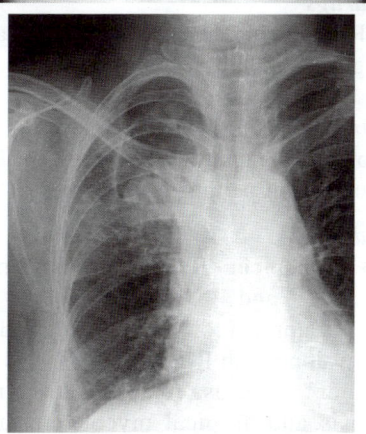

Fig. 4.11 Upper lobe cavity in the lung

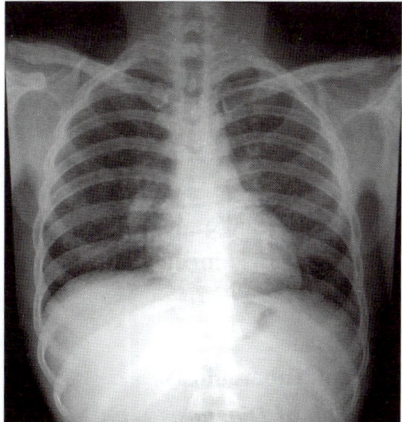

Fig. 4.12 Miliary mottlings in the lung

- Enteritis
- Meningitis
- Genitourinary tuberculosis
- Addison's disease
- Eye involvement
- Osteomyelitis

Different Types of Extrapulmonary Tuberculosis

Tuberculous lymphadenitis
- Cervical and mediastinal lymph nodes are most commonly affected.

Tuberculosis of gastrointestinal tract presents as
- Ileocaecal thickening
- Ileocaecal ulcers
- Intra-abdominal lymphadenopathy
- Peritoneal involvement with ascites

Central nervous system disease presents as
- Meningitis/tuberculoma
- Cerebrovascular accident
- Spiral cord compression TB spine

Cardiovascular involvement in tuberculosis
- Presents as pericarditis and pericardial effusion
- Constrictive pericarditis
- Tuberculous myocarditis

Genitourinary Tuberculosis
- It presents with urinary disturbances like increased frequency of urine and haematuria.
- Urine examination reveals presence of pus cells but urine culture is negative
- Female patient develops infertility due to tubo-ovarian disease/endometriosis.
- Epididymo-orchitis and prostatitis can develop in male patients.

Skeletal Tuberculosis
- Presents as vertebral involvement
- Intervertebral disc involvement
- Psoas abscess
- Arthritis

Diagnosis of Tuberculosis

Confirmation of Diagnosis
- Detection of *mycobacterium tuberculosis* (acid fast bacilli) by Ziehl Neelsen stain in the sputum/ any body fluid/specimen.

Other Supportive Investigations
- Raised ESR
- *Mantoux Test:* Using 10 Tuberculin units: positive test: Indicated by induration of >10–15 mm after 48 hrs.

Other Methods of Diagnosis
- Culturing AFB: Using Lowenstein-Jensen medium/BACTEC technique.
- By amplification of nucleic acid and using polymerase chain reaction (PCR).

Treatment

General
- Adequate nutrition
- Symptomatic therapy for fever and cough.

Specific

Chemotherapy with anti tubercular drugs

Drugs used - Ist line drugs (Table 4.2)

2nd line drugs
- Quinolones - Ofloxacin/ciprofloxacin
- Macrolides - Azithromycin/clarithromycin
- Ethionamide
- Cycloserine
- Paraamino salicylic acid (PAS)

Drug Regimes

Using 4 drugs
- INH+Rifampicin+Ethambutol + Pyrizinamide/inj S.M.1g for 2 months
  and
- C- Rifampicin + INH-For 4 months
- Pyridoxine 20 mg/day should be given along with INH to prevent peripheral neuropathy.

Using 3 drugs
- INH + Rifampicin + Ethambutol for 2 months
  and
- INH + Rifampicin for 7 months + pyridoxine 20 mg/ day along with INH.

Treatment failures, relapses, drug resistant tuberculosis and atypical mycobacteria require different treatment regimes.

Table 4.2 First line drugs

Name of the drug	Dose/kg body wt	Side effects
Isoniazid (INH)	5mg/kg body weight	Hepatitis Peripheral neuropathy Psychosis
Rifampicin	10 mg / kg	Orange discoloration of body fluids Flu like syndromes Hepatitis Thrombocytopenia
Pyrizinamide	25–35 mg\kg	Hepatitis Hyperuricemia
Ethambutol	15–25 mg/kg	Optic neuritis
Streptomycin (S M)	0.75–1g/day	Nephrotoxicity Labyrinthine toxicity

Corticosteroid is required for tuberculosis of pericardium, pleura, meninges, genitourinary tract, adrenals and tuberculous toxaemia.

Dental Aspects of Tuberculosis
- Anti tuberculosis drugs with oral side effects
  - Rifampicin - Orange discolouration of oral secretions.
  - Streptomycin - Circum oral paraesthesia
- Tuberculosis can affect the oral cavity and person can develop oral ulcers.

Dental Treatment
- Dental staff who are infected with pulmonary tuberculosis (AFB +ve) should take precautions while treating patients as they can transmit the infection to the patients.
- Patients with sputum AFB +ve can transmit the infection to dental staff.
- General anesthesia is contraindicated in patients with active pulmonary tuberculosis.
- Streptomycin can cause blockage of neuromuscular junction in patients undergoing general anaesthesia.

Different Anti-TB drug regimes in special circumstances
1. Drug resistance to INH or intolerance to INH alone: Combination of Rifampicin + Pyrizinamide + Ethambutol for 6 months.

2. If there is resistance to both INH and rifampicin: Injection of streptomycin + combination of pyrizinamide + Ethambutol + Quinalone for 18 to 24 months (Inj. Streptomycin can be discontinued after 2 months).
3. If there is resistance to all first line drugs: Inj. Amikacin/kanamycin + combination of ethionamide, cycloserine, ciprofloxacin and para-amino salicylic acid (3 out of 4 drugs) for 24 months.
   - Inj. Amikacin/kanamycin can be stopped after 2 months
   - Quinalones: Ciprofloxacin/ofloxacin/gatiflo-xacin
   - Ethionamide: 15 m/kg. body wt.
   - Cycloserine: 750 mg 1-0-1

Retreatment Regime
- Total 8 months of therapy
- For initial 3 months: inj. Streptomycin + INH + Rifampicin + Pyrizinamide + Ethambutol
- For later 5 months: INH + Rifampicin + Ethambutol.

Drugs	Dosage
Ethionamide	15–20 mg/kg body wt.
Cycloserine	15–20 mg/kg body wt.
Ciprofloxacin	750 mg 1-0-1/day
Gatifloxacin	400 mg/day
Amikacin	15 mg/kg body weight

BRONCHOGENIC CARCINOMA

Aetiological factors responsible for development of bronchogenic carcinoma

Smoking

- Chronic heavy cigarette smoking (2 packs a day for 20 years) increases the risk of bronchogenic carcinoma by 60 to 70 times.
- Passive exposure to cigarette smoke increases the risk of bronchogenic carcinoma by 1.5 times.
- Exposure to radiation, atmospheric pollution (tobacco smoke), industrial exposure to asbestos and chronic lung disease like COPD also increases the risk of bronchogenic carcinoma.

Different Histological Types of Bronchogenic Carcinoma

- Squamous cell carcinoma
- Adenocarcinoma
- Small cell carcinoma
- Large cell carcinoma

Clinical Features

Symptoms

- Intractable cough: Expectoration may result from secondary lung infection.
- Hemoptysis
  - May be massive and fatal. Occasionally only blood streaked sputum may be present.
- Breathlessness
  - Due to the growth pressing over the bronchus or intra bronchial growth with collapse of the lung.
  - Due to massive pleural effusion.
  - Due to pressure over the trachea by the enlarged lymph nodes in the mediastinum.
- Chest pain
  - Due to involvement of intercostal nerves or brachial plexus by the tumour
  - Due to pleural involvement by the tumour causing pleuritic pain.
  Other symptoms due to compression effect by the tumour
  - Pressure over the oesophagus - Dysphagia

- Pressure effect on the cervical sympathetic trunk causing Horner's syndrome.
- Tumour in the apex of the lung causes compression on the lower part of the brachial plexus causing pain in the upper limb with involvement of C8, T1 nerve roots (Pancoast's tumour).
- Patient can have symptoms due to hormone like substances released by the tumour (paraneoplastic syndrome) like hypercalcemia, gynaecomastia, increased ADH secretion (SIADH) and increased ACTH secretion and neurological syndrome. Bronchogenic carcinoma can metastasize to brain, liver, kidney and bone, etc.

Other nonspecific symptoms of bronchogenic carcinoma

- Fever, weight loss and loss of appetite can be due to bronchogenic carcinoma.

Signs

Clinical examination may be normal. Following signs can be due to bronchogenic carcinoma

- Clubbing and pulmonary osteoarthropathy
- Cervical lymphadenopathy
- Signs of pleural effusion
- Signs of pulmonary collapse.
- Signs of consolidation or mass lesion in the lung (Fig. 4.13).
- Signs of superior venae caval obstruction
- Signs due to metastasis and paraneoplastic syndrome.

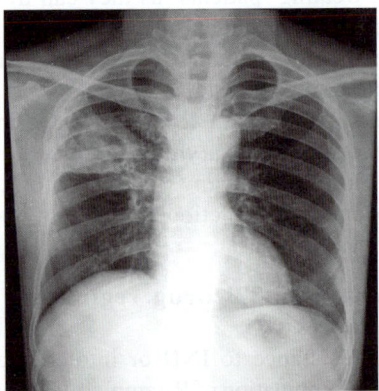

Fig. 4.13 Malignancy of the lung

Investigations
- Sputum cytology showing malignant cells.
- Chest X-ray/CT scan chest
  - May show evidence of mediastinal mass, mass in the lung and pleural involvement.
- Supraclavicular lymph node biopsy for evidence of malignant cells.
- Bronchoscopy
  - May show evidence of obstruction of the bronchus by the growth.
  - Bronchial washings may be positive for malignancy.
- CT guided fine needle aspiration cytology (FNAC) or biopsy of the intrathoracic lesion can be positive for malignancy.
- Investigations should also be done for metastatic lesions in the liver, brain and bone, etc.

Treatment
- Malignancy if localised: surgical resection can be done.
- Radiotherapy for palliative treatment, can decrease the pressure symptoms.
- In patients with inoperable lesion chemotherapy can be combined with radiation.

Dental Aspects
Bronchogenic carcinoma can have secondaries in the oral cavity or jaw. General anaesthesia is not advisable in patients with severe lung involvement due to bronchogenic carcinoma.

PLEURAL EFFUSION

This term is used to describe the presence of fluid in the pleural cavity (Fig. 4.14).

Transudative Pleural Effusion
- Fluid accumulates in the pleural cavity either due to increased hydrostatic pressure or decreased osmotic pressure, e.g. CCF, nephrotic syndrome, cirrhosis of liver

Exudative Pleural Effusion
- Fluid accumulates in the pleural cavity due to the inflammation of pleural layers.
  For example, pneumonia, pulmonary TB, etc.

Common Causes of Pleural Effusion
- Tuberculosis
- Pneumonia
- Malignancy bronchogesic/secondaries
- Connective tissue diseases
- CCF
- Cirrhosis of liver
- Nephrotic syndrome.

Clinical Features

Symptoms
- Fever
- Pleuritic chest pain
- Dry cough
- Breathlessness
- Symptoms of underlying disease like tuberculosis, malignancy, etc.

Signs
- Mediastinal shift to the opposite side
- Decreased movements of chest wall
- Stony dull note on percussion
- Breath sound intensity is decreased

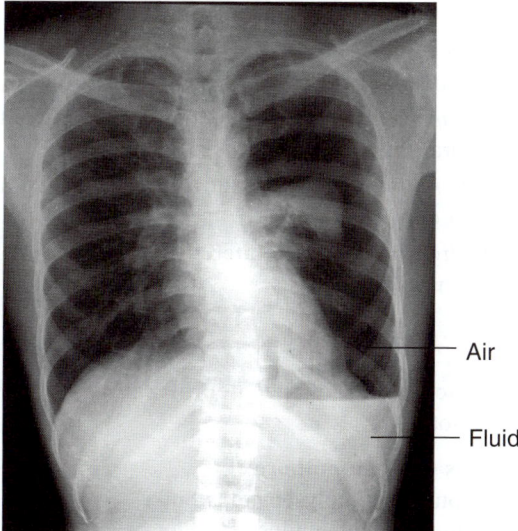

Fig. 4.14 X-ray showing air and fluid in the pleural cavity (hydropneumothorax)

Investigations
- WBC count and ESR may be increased
- Mantoux test is positive in TB effusions.
- *Sputum:* Gram stain, AFB and culture and sensitivity
- Chest X-ray demonstrates dense homogenous opacity with shift of mediastinum to opposite side
- Pleural fluid analysis to find out the cause of the disease

Characteristics of Pleural Fluid Analysis

Exudative Effusions
- *Pleural fluid:* serum protein ratio > 0.5
- *Pleural fluid:* serum LDH ratio > 0.6
- Increase in the fluid cell count > 250 cell/cm either neutrophils/lymphocytes/malignant cell.

Transudative Effusions
- *Pleural fluid:* serum protein ratio < 0.5
- *Pleural fluid:* serum LDH ratio < 0.6
- Pleural fluid cell count not increased

Chest CT scan, antinuclear antibodies, pleural biopsy and cervical lymph node biopsy for the aetiological diagnosis of pleural effusion.

Treatment
- If the patient is breathless aspiration of the pleural fluid
- Treatment of the cause of pleural effusion
- *Parapneumonic effusion:* complete tapping of the pleural fluid and antibiotics.
- *Tuberculous effusion:* Anti tuberculous therapy with corticosteroids
- *Malignant effusion:* Intercostal drainage with chemical pleurodesis

PNEUMOTHORAX

Presence of air in the pleural cavity is called pneumothorax.

Causes of Pneumothorax
- Rupture of emplysematous bulla
- Pulmonary tuberculosis
- Lung abscess
- COPD
- Bronchogenic carcinoma
- Chest trauma

Different Types of Pneumothorax

Closed Type (Fig. 4.15a)
- Communication between pleural space and the lung closes after the air has escaped into the pleural cavity.

Open Type (Fig. 4.15b)
- Communication between pleura and lung persists and air and pus collects in the pleural cavity (pyopneumothorax)

Tension Type (Fig. 4.15c)
- Air enters into the pleural cavity during inspiration and escape of air from the pleural cavity is prevented due to a valve like mechanism. Large amount of air accumulates and interferes with inspiration and cardiovascular function.

Clinical Features of Pneumothorax
- Sudden onset of chest pain and dyspnoea.
- Symptoms of underlying lung disease may be present.

Signs
- Patient is breathless especially in tension pneumothorax
- Mediastinum is shifted to the opposite side
- Chest movement is reduced on the affected side.
- Hyper resonant note on percussion on the affected side.
- Absence of breath sound on the affected side.
- Tension pneumothorax may be associated with tachycardia, hypotension and cyanosis.

Investigation
- Complete blood picture and ESR
- Sputum AFB and culture sensitivity
- Chest X-ray reveals presence of air in the pleural cavity
- CT scan of chest reveals presence of air in the pleural cavity.

Treatment
- Treatment of the cause

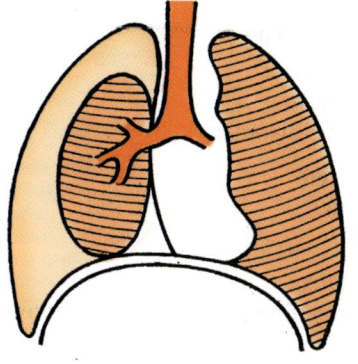 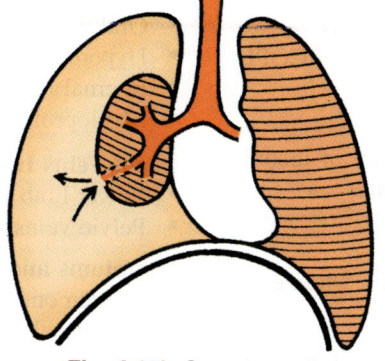 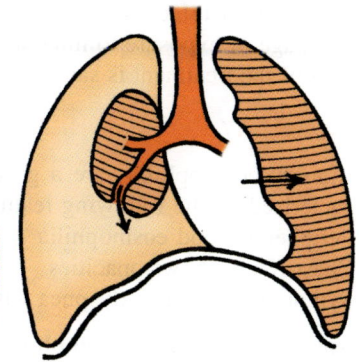

Fig. 4.15a Closed pneumothorax

Fig. 4.15b Open type of pneumothorax

Fig. 4.15c Tension pneumothorax

- Closed pneumothorax heals spontaneously
- Open pneumothorax requires surgical management and treatment of infection
- Tension pneumothorax under water seal drainage and treatment of the cause.
- Recurrent pneumothorax requires obliteration of pleural cavity by administration of irritants in to the pleural cavity called pleurodesis.

PNEUMOCONIOSIS

- Pneumoconiosis is a group of disorders characterised by the development of diffuse pulmonary fibrosis due to chronic exposure to inorganic dusts.
- Chronic exposure to inorganic dusts causes inflammatory and fibrotic response in the lung causing pulmonary damage.
- Chronic exposure to dusts of iron, beryllium and tin oxide can also cause lung damage.
- Exposure to toxic gases like chlorine ammonia, nitrogen dioxide can also cause acute lung injury.

Coal Workers Pneumoconiosis
- Develops after exposure to coal dust.

Simple Coal Worker's Pneumoconiosis
- There will be development of nodularity in the lung. Disease stops if the person avoids exposure to dust.

Progressive Massive Fibrosis
- There will be development of lung nodules with cavitation. Person will have cough, sputum, dyspnoea and signs of COPD. Person can develop progressive massive fibrosis. Tuberculosis may complicate the disease.

Silicosis
- Silicosis develops after chronic exposure to silica dust. Silica is a most fibrogenic particle. Person with silicosis develops symptoms and signs of COPD. Tuberculosis can complicate the underlying disease.

Asbestosis
- Asbestosis develops due to chronic exposure to asbestos. Person may develop pleural plaques, pleural effusion, mesothelioma of pleura and even bronchogenic carcinoma.
- All types of pneumoconiosis can be prevented by early avoidance of exposure to mineral dusts. Table 4.3 lists some important types of pneumoconiosis.

Treatment of Pneumoconiosis
- Symptomatic treatment for cough and dyspnoea

Table 4.3 Important types of pneumoconiosis

Types of dust	Corresponding disorder
Asbestos	Asbestosis
Coal dust	Coal worker's pneumoconiosis
Silica	Silicosis

- Treatment of infection
- Stoppage of exposure to mineral dusts
- Rest of the treatment is same as that of COPD

PULMONARY EOSINOPHILIA

Pulmonary eosinophilia are a group of disorders characterised by the following features.
1. Peripheral blood eosinophilia
2. Chest X-ray shows opacities
3. Symptoms of cough, dyspnea with wheeze

Cause of Pulmonary Eosinophilia
- Worm infestations, e.g. ascariasis, filariasis
- Fungal infection, e.g. bronchopulmonary aspergillosis
- Drug induced, e.g. nitrofurantoin, sulfasalazine, Paraamino salicylic acid
- Pulmonary eosinophilia associated with poly-arteritis nodosa and Churg Strauss disease.
- Cryptogenic eosinophilic pneumonia and hyper eosinophilic syndrome.

Treatment
- Remove the cause, i.e. stoppage of drugs.
- Treatment of worms and fungal infections.
- Corticosteroids.

Tropical Pulmonary Eosinophilia

- Occurs in patients infected with lymphatic filariasis.
- Person is usually from endemic area of filariasis
- Patient presents with recent onset of cough, wheeze (nocturnal) with fever and lymph-adenopathy.
- Absolute neutrophil count is more than 2,500 cells/ cmm.
- Serum IgE cells are raised with positive antifilarial antibodies.
- Patient responds to treatment with diethyl-carbamazine.

DEEP VEIN THROMBOSIS

Predisposing Factors
- Elderly age
- Bed ridden state

- Postoperative states
- Oral contraceptive intake
- Hypercoagulable states
- Internal malignancy
- Myeloproliferative disorder

Usual Veins Involved
- Lower limb veins
- Pelvic veins

Symptoms and Signs
- Sudden onset of calf pain and swelling of lower limb-usually unilateral.
- There may be history of fever
- Calf will be tender to touch
- On dorsiflexion of foot, patient will complain of calf pain (Homan's sign).
- Deep vein thrombosis can result in pulmonary embolism and sudden death.

Investigations
- Venous Doppler of the lower limb can detect the thrombus and venous occlusion.
- Detailed laboratory evaluation is required to detect the cause of venous thrombosis.

Treatment
- Immediate anticoagulation with intravenous heparin followed by oral anticoagulation with warfarin.
- Oral anticoagulation may have to be continued for minimum period of 6 months depending on the cause.
- Treatment of the cause.

Pulmonary Embolism

- Most of the causes of pulmonary embolism results from deep vein thrombosis in the lower limb and pelvis.
- Predisposing factors: As mentioned under deep vein thrombosis.

Acute Massive Pulmonary Embolism

Features

Symptoms
- Sudden onset of chest pain

- Breathlessness
- Syncope

Signs
- Tachycardia
- Hypotension
- Right ventricular failure
- Sudden death

Investigations

Chest CT scan and CT angiogram are the investigation of choice in a patient of pulmonary embolism.

Other investigations which are helpful in diagnosing pulmonary embolism

- *ECG:* Shows tachycardia and right ventricular dominance (T1 inversion in lead V1 and V2).
- *Chest X-ray:* May be normal or may show an opacity.
- *Venous Doppler of the lower limb:* May demonstrate deep vein thrombosis (DVT).
- *Ventilation perfusion scanning of lung:* Abnormal in pulmonary embolism
- *Echocardiogram:* Demonstrate right ventricular dysfunction
- *Arterial blood gas analysis:* Demonstrated hypoxia and decrease PCO_2.
- Positive plasma D - Dimer assay.

Treatment

- Immediate administration of oxygen
- IV Heparin or low molecular weight heparin and followed by oral anticoagulation with warfarin. Duration depends on the aetiology (minimum 3–6 months).
- *Other forms of therapy:* Thrombolysis and thrombectomy
- Treatment of risk factors for pulmonary embolism in deep vein thrombosis (see Chapter Cardiology II).

Dental Aspects

- Elderly, post operative patients are at greatest risk of pulmonary embolism.
- Prophylactic anticoagulation may be required in high risk patients.
- Early mobilisation and leg exercises are essential in preventing pulmonary embolism in post operative patients.

SARCOIDOSIS

- Sarcoidosis is a multisystem disease due to formation of chromic granulomas.

Aetiology

- Not definitely known
- May be due to impaired cell mediated immune response.

Pathology

- Sarcoidosis is characterised by formation of epithelioid cells and non caseating granulomas.

Structures Involved

- Pulmonary involvement seen in 90% of cases.
- Lymph nodes
- Parotid glands
- Skin, eye, liver and spleen
- Hypercalcemia and bone involvement.
- Renal calculi

Clinical Features

- *Constitutional symptoms:* Fever, weight loss.
- *Respiratory:* Hilar adenopathy, pulmonary infiltration causes cough and dyspnoea.
- *Eye:* Acute uveitis, glaucoma and cataract.
- Lymph nodes, liver and spleen: Generalised lymphadenopathy, hepato splenomegaly.
- *Bones and joints:* Joint pain, hypercalcemia.
- *Renal:* Renal calculi formation
- *Skin:* Erythema nodosum
- *Neurological:* Cranial/peripheral neuropathy.

Investigations

- Raised ESR and decreased lymphocytes.
- Negative skin test for tuberculosis
- Positive skin test for sarcoidosis-Kveim test.
- Tissue biopsy: Non caseating granuloma.
- Raised levels of serum calcium and angiotensin converting enzyme levels.

Management

- *Minor symptoms:* Symptomatic therapy with NSAIDS.

- Systemic involvement: Corticosteroids—Short course and maintenance therapy.
- Immunosuppressive therapy with methotrexate.

Dental Aspects of Sarcoidosis
- Any oral tissues can be involved in Sarcoidosis.
- Most commonly lacrimal and parotid glands can be involved. (Heerfordt's syndrome - parotid enlargement with uveitis).
- Gingival hypertrophy can occur during the course of the disease.
- Biopsy of the oral tissues demonstrate sarcoid like granulomas.

Upper Respiratory Tract Infections (URTI)

- Viral infection is the most common cause of upper respiratory tract infection.
- These infections readily spread through respiratory route and difficult to prevent.

Main Clinical Patterns of Upper Respiratory Infection
- Common cold syndrome (coryza)
- Sinusitis
- Pharyngitis and tonsillitis
- Laryngotracheitis.
  Secondary streptococcal infection occurs usually after viral infection of the upper respiratory tract.

Common Cold Syndrome
Etiological agents
- Viruses (Table 4.4)

Features
- Nasal discharge
- Nasal obstruction
- Throat irritation
- Throat pain

Systemic Features
- Fever and bodyache
  Secondary bacterial infection due to streptococci can cause sinusitis. Occasionally complications like pharyngeal/tympanic oedema or otitis media can occur. Common cold may be a preceding illness due to measles/influenza.

Treatment of Common Cold

Symptomatic Treatment
- Antihistaminics
- Nasal decongestants
- Paracetamol for fever and bodyache
- Antibiotics if secondary bacterial infection.

Sinusitis
Infection of the paranasal sinuses occurs usually secondary to viral upper respiratory tract infection.

Clinical Features

Frontal Sinusitis
- Fever, frontal headache and tenderness over the frontal sinus.

Ethmoidal Sinusitis
- Headache and tenderness over the ethmoid sinuses.

Maxillary Sinusitis
- Pain in the cheek/upper teeth which increases by tilting the head or lying down.

Table 4.4 Common cases of upper respiratory tract infection	
Disorder associated	*Organisms*
Common cold	Rhinoviruses Para influenza viruses ECHO viruses Coxsackie viruses Respiratory syncytial viruses
Pharyngitis and tonsillitis	Influenza viruses Adeno viruses Epstein-Barr viruses

- Nasal obstruction with mucopurulent nasal discharge.
- Tenderness over the maxillary sinus.

Patients with frontal and maxillary sinusitis will have haziness in the X-ray with fluid level.

Treatment of Sinusitis
- 1% ephedrine nasal drops
- Karvol steam inhalation
- Antibiotics - Co-Trimoxazole/Erythromycin

Pharyngitis / Tonsillitis

Etiological Agent
- Viruses (Table 4.4)
- Organisms like *Streptococcus pyogenes*, *Mycoplasma pneumoniae* and *H. influnenzae* can cause pharyngitistonsillitis.

Features
- Irritation in the throat
- Pain on swallowing
- Fever
- Congestion of pharynx and tonsils

Treatment
- Symptomatic for fever and throat pain, e.g. Paracetamol
- Antibiotics for bacterial infection, e.g. amoxycillin/azithromycin

Complications of Tonsillitis/Pharyngitis
- Can result in peritonsillar abscess
- Streptococcal infection can result in scarlet fever, acute glomerulonephritis and rheumatic fever.

Laryngotracheitis
- Laryngo tracheitis can occur due to viruses as mentioned above and can be complicated by

secondary bacterial infection (Streptococcus\ *H. influenzae*).

Features
- Hoarseness of voice, loss of voice, persistent cough and stridor (noisy respiration due to partial laryngeal obstruction).

Treatment
- NSAIDS
- Nasal decongestants
- Steam inhalation
- Oxygen inhalation, antibiotics (β-lactum: Amoxycillin 500 mg 1-1-1 × 7 days, Azithmomycin 500mg/day × 3 days) and tracheostomy if required.

Halitosis (bad breath)

Causes
1. Disorders of the oral cavity
   - Infection
   - Fermented food
   - Dry mouth
   - Drugs: Alcohol
   - Abuse of solvents
   - Smoking
2. Disorders of the nasal cavity and sinuses
   - Nasal infection
   - Atrophic rhinitis
   - Maxillary antral infection
3. Systemic diseases
   - Bronchiectasis
   - Fetor hepaticus in liver disease
   - Fruity odour of diabetic ketoacidosis
   - Ammoniacal smell of uremia
   - Gastrointestinal disease

5a Gastrointestinal Tract I

History and Approach to a Patient of Gastrointestinal Disease

Symptoms and History of Present Illness

- Pain abdomen
- Nausea and vomiting
- Heart burn, flatulence and water brash
- Haemetemesis and malena
- Distension of abdomen
- Dysphagia
- Constipation and diarrhoea
- Altered bowel habit
- Jaundice, itching and high coloured urine
- Fever
- Weight loss

Miscellaneous Symptoms

- Pain in the oral cavity
- Dry mouth and altered taste
- Halitosis
- Hiccups

PAIN ABDOMEN

It is a significant symptom of gastrointestinal disease.

Pain abdomen is invariably organic in origin.

Different Mechanisms Contributing for Pain Abdomen

1. *Visceral pain:* Pain may be due to distension, inflammation or perforation of viscera.
   - Pain is conducted by sympathetic supply from T5 to L2 segments.
   - Unpaired intra-abdominal organs can cause midline pain.
2. *Parietal peritoneal pain:* Due to irritation or inflammation of parietal peritoneum.
   - Pain is felt in the distribution of somatic supply of the peritoneum.
3. *Excessive smooth muscle contraction*
   - Specific pain and usually colicky in nature and well localised, e.g. biliary or intestinal colic.

Check list in a Patient of Abdominal Pain

- Onset
- Site
- Type of pain
- Aggravating factors
- Relieving factors
- Referred/radiation of pain
- Other associated symptoms

Onset and Duration of Pain

The causes of acute onset of pain in abdomen are biliary, ureteric or intestinal colic, torsion of testis, ovarian, caecal and sigmoid colonic pathology.

Characteristics of different types of pain abdomen depending on the onset

- *Hollow viscous perforation:* Person was asymptomatic before and sudden onset.
- *Aortic aneurysm rupture:* Acute/sudden onset of severe pain.
- *Occlusion of mesenteric artery:* Pain progresses rapidly and becomes diffuse all over the abdomen.
- *Acute appendicitis:* Pain progress is slow and in a steady manner
- *Acute cholecystitis/Acute diverticulitis:* Pain persists for hours to days

- *Chronic pancreatitis:* Pain will be persisting for few months to years
- *Peptic ulcer:* There will be recurrent exacerbation of pain

Note: Suspect massive GI bleed acute pancreatitis, aortic aneurysm rupture or rupture of ectopic pregnancy (in a female) in all patients with abdominal pain and shock.

Different types of pain abdomen depending on the site of pain

- *Epigastric pain:* For example, peptic ulcer
- Umbilical: Small intestinal disease
- *Right hypochondrium:* Diseases of the liver and gall bladder, hepatic flexure of colon.
- *Left hypochondrium:* Diseases of the spleen, pancreas and splenic flexure of colon.
- *Right iliac pain:* Disease of the appendix, caecum, terminal ileum, mesentery, right urinary tract and uterine adnexa.
- *Left iliac fossa:* Diseases of the sigmoid colon, diverticulitis, left urinary tract and left uterine adnexa.
- *Hypogastric region:* Usually urinary bladder in origin.

Type of Pain

- *Burning type of pain:* Peptic ulcer disease.
- *Colicky type of pain:* Intermittent, spasmodic pain - pain of hollow viscous. For example Ureteric colic, biliary colic.
- *Diffuse abdominal pain:* Peritonitis, intestinal obstruction, and gaseous distension of abdomen.
- *Dull aching pain:* Enlargement of solid viscera like liver and spleen. [Rapid stretch of liver capsule (Glisson's) and splenic capsule causes pain].
- *Nocturnal pain:* Usually organic, e.g. pain of duodenal ulcer.

Aggravating Factors

1. Food aggravating pain (gastric ulcer)
   - Biliary colic
   - Occasionally pancreatitis
   - Allergy to food
2. Pain on physical activity and jolting
   - Biliary/ureteric calculus

3. Pain on reclining forwards
   - Hiatus hernia
4. Pain after roughage intake
   - Inflammatory bowel disease
5. Pain increases during menstruation
   - Spasmodic dysmenorrhoea
   - Endometriosis
   - Pelvic inflammatory disease
6. Hunger pain (may be nocturnal)
   - Duodenal ulcer.
7. Drug induced pain (NSAIDS, corticosteroids)
   - Peptic ulcer disease
8. Abdominal pain, which increases after passing stool, may suggest local colonic disease.

Posture and Abdominal Pain

- Abdominal pain predominantly on reclining may be due to hiatus hernia.
- Abdominal pain occurring on jolting may suggest biliary or ureteric colic.
- Patients of acute peritonitis are usually immobile in the bed.
- Pain of chronic pancreatitis decreases on knee elbow position.

Relieving Factors

- Food relieves pain in a patient of duodenal ulcer.
- Pain responding only to antispasmodics suggests colicky pain.
- Sitting up and stooping forward relieves pain in a patient of pancreatitis.
- Abdominal pain, which is relieved by passing flatus and stool, may be seen in patients with irritable bowel syndrome.

Referred Pain

Pain is felt in the area of somatic supply (cutaneous area) which converges on the same segment of the spinal cord to which the visceral pain is conveyed.

For example, pain from the liver abscess, tumor invading the diaphragm and sub diaphragmatic abscess may be referred to shoulders.

Radiation of Pain

Pain radiates from the original site of pain to a distant site. Examples of pain radiation:

- Pain of penetrating peptic ulcer, from epigastrium to back
- Pain of pancreatic disease, from center of the abdomen to back
- Pain of rectum and sigmoid colon, radiates posteriorly to the sacral area

Importance of Associated Symptoms with Abdominal Pain
- Onset of abdominal pain in a patient with previous history of constipation may suggest the possibility of carcinoma colon or diverticular disease.
- Suspect aortic aneurysm rupture in a patient of severe hypertension with abdominal pain and shock.
- Suspect mesenteric ischaemia in a patient of abdominal pain with CCF, atrial fibrillation and peripheral vascular disease.
- Preceding history of dyspepsia (belching, bloating, nausea, anorexia and vomiting) with sudden onset of abdominal pain may suggest peptic ulcer perforation.
- Follicular rupture usually causes pain abdomen in the middle of menstrual cycles.

Metabolic causes of Pain Abdomen
- Hypercalcemia
- Porphyria
- Diabetic ketoacidosis
- Haemochromatosis

Nongastrointestinal Causes of Abdominal Pain
- Diaphragmatic pleurisy
- Sickle cell disease
- Myocardial infarction
- Dissecting aneurysm
- Herpes zoster
- Collagen vascular disease

Characteristic Features of Common Types of Abdominal Pain

Peptic Ulcer
- Episodic attacks of pain
- Nocturnal or hunger pain relieved with food/ antacids

- Pain may be severe- burning/colicky type
- May radiate posteriorly to the back

Biliary Colic
- Severe spasmodic pain associated with vomiting
- Pain is felt in the right hypochondrium/ epigastrium
- Pain may be of longer duration for hours
- Pain refers to right scapula/ shoulder tip

Ureteric Colic
- Pain starts in the loin spreads to groin and genitalia, spasmodic and severe restlessness, vomiting, haematuria and dysuria may be associated with pain.

Appendicitis
- Colicky/ severe pain
- Associated with fever and vomiting
- Initial visceral pain - vague pain around the umbilicus
- Involvement of parietal peritoneum - pain will be felt in the right iliac fossa.
- Rupture of appendix - generalised abdominal pain due to peritonitis.
  "Consider appendicitis in all cases of acute right iliac pain."

Pancreatitis
- Acute onset severe pain - epigastrium/hypochondrium.
- Pain may increase after food/alcohol.
- Pain decreases with sitting up and stooping forward.
- Pain may persist for hours, associated with vomiting, jaundice and shock.

Nausea and Vomiting

Nausea
Feeling or discomfort that occurs before vomiting. Nausea may be associated with symptoms like sweating, faintness and salivation.

Vomiting
Forceful expulsion of contents of gastrointestinal tract through the oral cavity.

Regurgitation

Contents of stomach enter the oral cavity through reflux.

Not associated with forceful act of vomiting.

Approach to a Patient of Nausea and Vomiting

All acute abdominal conditions are associated with vomiting

For example, acute gastritis, pancreatitis, cholecystitis and acute hepatitis.

Vomiting associated with Pain Abdomen

For example, peptic ulcer disease, carcinoma stomach, ureteric colic, pancreatitis, intestinal obstruction, biliary obstruction and cholecystitis

Vomiting without Pain Abdomen

For example, pregnancy, alcoholism, pyloric obstruction, psychogenic, renal failure.

Projectile Vomiting

There is no preceding nausea before vomiting. Raised intracranial tension is a common cause of projectile vomiting.

Note: Oesophageal and gastric obstruction and achalasia cardia may not have nausea before vomiting.

Self-induced Vomiting

Patients themselves may induce vomiting for pain relief in peptic ulcer disease.

In conditions like bulimia nervosa also person himself may induce vomiting.

Causes of Severe Vomiting

• Duodenal ulcer

• Food hypersensitivity
• Meniere's disease
• Migrainous head ache

Conditions Associated with Early Morning Vomiting

• Chronic alcoholism
• Incipient uremia
• Psychogenic vomiting
• Pregnancy

Relationship between the time of onset of vomiting and consumption of food

• Peptic ulcer disease and psychogenic vomiting
  – May vomit immediately after food
• Pyloric/ duodenal obstruction
  – Vomiting may occur later in the day
  – Recurrent vomiting few hours after food
  – Vomitus may contain food eaten the previous day.

Note
• Patients with carcinoma stomach can have foul smelling vomitus.
• Pyloric obstruction will not have bile stained vomitus.
• Rarely vomitus may contain pus (swallowed) or parasites like round worms.

Table 5.1 lists contents of vomitus in GI disorders.

Nongastrointestinal Causes of Vomiting

Vomiting is invariably the manifestation of Gastrointestinal tract. But following conditions are the examples of nongastrointestinal causes of vomiting

Table 5.1 Contents of vomitus

Gastrointestinal disorders	*Contents of vomitus*
Upper gastrointestinal bleed	Blood in the vomitus
Vomiting of gastric cause	Pungent odour/ penetrating smell
Achalasia	No taste or smell to the vomitus
Pyloric obstruction	Large amount, may be foul smelling (due to fermentation
of	Oesophageal regurgitation ingested food).
Gastrocolic fistula	Vomitus can have faecal odour and can contain faecal matter.
Distal ileal obstruction	
Colonic obstruction	
Reflux of duodenal contents into stomach	Vomitus contains bile (yellowish green) and can have bitter taste.

- *Metabolic:* Hypercalcaemia, hypoadrenalism, diabetic ketoacidosis and renal failure.
- *Neurological:* Increased intracranial tension, labyrinthine disease, migraine, severe pain, febrile states.
- *Drug induced:* NSAIDS, digoxin, morphine, alcohol
- *Psychogenic:* Bulimia and anorexia nervosa

Psychogenic Vomiting
- Symptoms of depression are usually associated with psychogenic vomiting.
- Vomiting is usually in the early morning and late evening hours.
- No organic cause can be found out.

HEART BURN, INDIGESTION AND FLATULENCE

Heart Burn (Pyrosis)

Person feels burning type of sensation behind the sternum. Food intake, lying down immediately after food and forward bending increases the retrosternal burning.

Antacids and H_2 blockers relieve heartburn. Reflux of acid, pepsin or bile into the oesophagus causes heartburn.

Note: Heartburn can also be a manifestation of duodenal ulcer. Occasionally cardiac pain may present like heartburn.

Causes of Heart Burn
- Reflux oesophagitis
- Hiatus hernia
- Reflux of acid can occur due to relaxation of lower oesophageal sphincter or increased intra-abdominal pressure.

Water Brash
- Condition associated with reflux increase of salivation and mouth fills with excess saliva.
- Water brash is usually associated with reflux oesophagitis and duodenal ulcer.

Dyspepsia
Benign disorder

Characteristics
- Symptoms of peptic ulcer disease
- Endoscopy fails to detect an ulcer

Different Types of Dyspeptic Disorders
- Reflux type of symptoms: For example, retrosternal burning
- Peptic ulcer like symptoms: Pain and vomiting. Food or antacids relieve pain.
- Symptoms of disturbed motility: Early fullness, recurrent belching.
- Peptic ulcer disease and occasionally IHD can cause symptoms of dyspepsia.

Flatulence

This refers to the condition associated with increased belching and passing excess flatus through rectum.

Flatulence may be associated with audible bowel sounds (borborygmi) due to movement of fluid and gas due to altered intestinal motility.

Excess flatus production can occur due to:
- Aerophagia (swallowing of air)
- Malabsorption
- Lactase deficiency
  Intestinal obstruction can result in total absence of passing flatus

Note: Normally flatus is produced by fermentation of carbohydrates by colonic bacteria due to poor absorption.

HAEMETEMESIS

Indicates presence of blood in the vomitus.

Common Causes of Haemetemesis
- Oesophageal variceal bleed
- Erosive gastritis
- Mallory-Weiss syndrome
- Peptic ulcer disease
- Stomach/oesophageal malignancy.

Approach to a patient of Upper Gastrointestinal Bleed
- Vomiting of bright red vomitus indicates bleeding at the pharyngeal or oesophageal level.
- Coffee ground vomitus: Suggests bleeding into

the stomach. Color of the vomitus is characteristically brownish and may contain coffee ground sediment.

- Colour is due to the conversion of haemoglobin to acid haematin by gastric acid.
- Previous history of chronic pain abdomen and dyspepsia with upper gastrointestinal bleed is common with peptic ulcer disease.
- History of retching and violent vomiting especially after alcohol indicates Mallory- Weiss tear.
- Consumption of NSAIDs and steroids prior to hemetemesis is common with erosive gastritis.
- Presence of chronic liver disease with hemetemesis is usually indicative of variceal bleed.
- Elderly person with weight loss and haemetemesis may be suggestive of gastrointestinal malignancy.

Lower Gastrointestinal Bleed

Causes

- Acute bacterial or amoebic dysentery.
- Lower gastrointestinal malignancy (40 years of age, recent change of bowel habit).
- Diverticulosis
  Characteristics
  – Abdominal discomfort
  – Constipation and altered bowel habit.
- Ulcerative colitis and Crohn's disease and ischaemic colitis
  Characteristics
  – Lower abdominal pain
  – Diarrhoea
  – Rectal bleeding
- Acute mesenteric infarction
  Characteristics
  – Abdominal rigidity
  – Altered bowel habit
  – Lower gastrointestinal bleed

MALENA

Term is given to the passing of black tarry stools.

- Suggests upper gastrointestinal bleed above the attachment of ligament of Treitz.
- Minimal of 60 ml of bleeding is required for the appearance of malena.

- Tarry colour is due to the action of lower bowel secretions on the blood.
- Malena stool is usually sticky (intake of iron and bismuth salts will produce tarry stool but will not be sticky).
- Stool color may remain black for several days even after the stoppage of bleed.

Haematochezia

Indicates passing frank blood per rectum.

Common Causes

- Colitis
- Bleeding piles
- Fissure in ano
- Malignancy rectal/colon
- Inflammatory bowel disease

Rare Causes

- Diverticulosis
- Polyposis of colon
- Ischaemia of bowel
- Massive upper gastrointestinal bleed with rapid intestinal-transit.

Bleeding from the Anal Canal and Rectum

Characteristics

- Bleeding piles
  – Massive bleeding with splashing of blood
  – Bleeding continues even after passing the stool
- Anal canal bleed
  – Can only soil the toilet paper. Usually bright red and separate from the fecal matter.
- Anal fissure bleed
  – Severe pain is associated with bleeding while passing the stool
- Infection/Inflammation of colon
  – Loose stools associated with blood and mucus and tenesmus.

ABDOMINAL DISTENSION

Five common causes of abdominal distension.

- F   Fluid accumulation
- F   Fat accumulation

- F   Faecal matter (e.g. intestinal obstruction, chronic constipation)
- F   Flatus (e.g. intestinal obstruction)
- F   Foetus.

Check list for Abdominal Distension
- Onset and duration
- Pain abdomen
- Vomiting
- Constipation
- Puffiness of face
- Pedal oedema
- Urine output
- Acute and rapid distension of abdomen along with pain may be due to peritonitis.
- Distension of abdomen associated with vomiting, abdominal pain and absolute constipation suggests presence of intestinal obstruction.
- Gradually progressive distension may also due to accumulation of fluid.
- Combination of puffiness of face, swelling of feet and abdominal distension occurs in conditions like cirrhosis of liver, nephrotic syndrome and congestive cardiac failure.
- In cirrhotic patients: Abdominal distension is predominant compared to pedal oedema due to the combined effect of hypoalbuminemia and portal hypertension.

KEY POINTS 5.1

- Constipation, distension of abdomen and the child not soiling the clothes with faecal matter may suggest Hirschsprung's disease.
- Acute development of tense ascites is usually due to intra-abdominal malignancy, infectious peritonitis, hepatic or portal vein obstruction.
- Painless abdominal distension in women may be indicative of pregnancy or ovarian cyst.
- Abdominal distention in an elderly may occasionally be due to pseudo obstruction as a result of autonomic neuropathy or use of anticholinergics.
- Massive enlargement of liver/spleen or any abdominal viscera can cause non uniform distension of abdomen.

DIARRHOEA

Definition
Frequent passage of unformed stools with stool quantity more than 200 gm/day.

Causes
- Acute (less than 2 weeks)
  - Infective- viral, bacterial, amoebic dysentery
  - Drug allergy
- Chronic (more than 4 weeks)
  - Tuberculosis of intestine
  - Colonic neoplasm
  - Malabsorption syndrome
  - Parasitic infestation
  - Inflammatory bowel disease
  - Endocrinal - thyrotoxicosis, Addison's disease,
  - Irritable bowel syndrome
  - Zollinger - Ellison syndrome

Approach to a Patient of Diarrhoea
- *Infective or inflammatory disease:* Diarrhoea associated with fever and abdominal pain.

KEY POINTS 5.2

- Diarrhea associated with weight loss and diarrhoea that is nocturnal is usually organic.
- Enquire the history of consumption of laxatives, antacids and long term antibiotics as they themselves can cause diarrhoea.
- Diarrhea after consumption of milk or milk products suggests either primary or secondary lactase deficiency.
- Constipation and rectal impaction can cause overflow resulting in spurious diarrhoea.
- Small intestinal diarrhea is usually characterised by large volume with less frequency.
- Large bowel diarrhoea is characterised by small volume and more frequency.
- Presence of tenesmus suggest rectal pathology and presence of blood mixed with stool suggests ulcerative lesion in the colon.
- Consider tuberculosis, HIV infection and thyrotoxicosis in a patient with diarrhoea associated with significant weight loss.

- *Inflammatory bowel disease:* Diarrhoea associated with arthritis, skin rash and ocular symptoms.
- *Malabsorption syndrome:* Presence of pale bulky greasy stool (steatorrhoea). Foul smelling stools, excessive flatulence, difficult to flush the pan.
- *Intestinal mucosal disease:* Presence of abdominal bloating with flatulence and diarrhea.
- *Ulcerative lesion in the colon:* Blood and mucus with stool
- *Irritable bowel syndrome:* Diarrhoea alternating with constipation with large quantities of mucus.
- *Food poisoning:* History of diarrhoea in several members of close community.

CONSTIPATION

The term is used if the stool frequency is less than 3 times/week (term is highly individualised and depends on the bowel habit of each individual).

Causes
- Lesions causing pain on defecation, e.g. proctitis, fissure in ano.
- Endocrine disorders: Hypercalcemia and hypothyroidism.
- Intestinal obstruction: Carcinoma, stricture
- Hirschsprung's disease
- Lesions involving sacral nerve roots: Cauda equina syndrome
- Drugs: Aluminium hydroxide, opiates
- Decreased fibre intake
- Lack of physical activity
- Psychogenic factors like depression

Dyschezia

Difficulty in emptying rectum with requirement of excess straining at stool, a form of rectal constipation.

Due to the loss of tone of rectal musculature requiring greater amount of stool collection to initiate the act.

ALTERED BOWEL HABIT

Irritable bowel syndrome is a common cause of alternate diarrhoea and constipation (especially below the age of 50 years).

Recent changes in the bowel habit in an elderly person, consider and rule out malignant disease of the bowel.

Tenesmus

A sensation of incomplete rectal emptying or frequent desire to pass stool.

Common Causes of Tenesmus
- Colonic infection
- Irritable bowel syndrome
- Carcinoma rectum
- Prolapse of the rectum

JAUNDICE

Yellowish discolouration of skin, sclera and mucosa due to excess circulating bilirubin.

Check list for Jaundice
- Duration
- Color of urine
- Fever
- Obstructive symptoms
- Pain abdomen
- Appetite and weight loss
- Altered bowel habits
- Bleeding tendencies
- Abdominal pain

A. Duration
1. Acute causes of jaundice
   - Acute hepatitis
   - Acute cholecystitis
   - Acute haemolysis
2. Gradually progressive jaundice
   - Chronic parenchymal liver disease
   - Chronic hepatitis
3. Causes of progressive jaundice due to obstruction to the bile flow:
   - Gall stones
   - Carcinoma head of pancreas
   - Carcinoma ampulla of vater

B. Colour of Urine

1. Deep yellow (high coloured) urine with jaundice
   - Due to the presence of conjugated bilirubin in the urine, e.g. parenchymal liver disease and extra hepatic biliary obstruction.
2. Presence of jaundice with normal urine colour
   - Due to increase of unconjugated bilirubin in circulation which cannot be excreted in the urine (acholuric jaundice). For example, hemolytic jaundice.

Symptoms of Obstructive Jaundice

High coloured urine, itching and clay coloured stool.

Colour of Stool

Clay coloured stool in a patient of jaundice suggests obstruction to the biliary flow (due to the absence of stercobilinogen in the stool).

Itching

Suggests obstructive jaundice with increase level of bile salts.

FEVER

Jaundice Associated with Fever

For example, acute hepatitis of any cause, acute cholecystitis, sepsis syndrome, acute malaria.

Jaundice with Bony Pain and Bleeding Tendencies

Defective absorption of vitamin D and vitamin K occurs in patients with obstructive jaundice.

KEY POINTS 5.3

- Painless progressive jaundice may be due to carcinoma head of pancreas.
- Fluctuating jaundice may be due to gall stone disease.
- Recurrent attack of jaundice since child hood may be due to hemolytic disease or familial hyper bilirubinemias.

Defective vitamin D metabolism causes bony pain and defective vitamin K metabolism causes bleeding tendencies.

Note: All causes of hepatocellular jaundice and primary biliary cirrhosis can cause intra hepatic cholestasis and obstructive jaundice.

Jaundice with Abdominal Pain

- Dull aching abdominal pain is associated with hepatomegaly and parenchymal liver disease.
- Colicky pain in the right hypochondrium suggests obstructive biliary tract disease.
- Epigastric pain radiating to the back suggests pancreatic disease.

Gastrointestinal Disorders Associated with Fever

(All infective and inflammatory disorders of gastrointestinal tract)

For example, acute hepatitis, appendicitis, acute peritonitis, pyelonephritis, tuberculosis abdomen, inflammatory bowel disease and malignancies like abdominal lymphoma, pancreatic carcinoma and renal cell carcinoma.

MISCELLANEOUS SYMPTOMS OF GASTROINTESTINAL DISEASE
(Symptoms of oral disease)

Pain in the Oral Cavity

Causes
- Nutritional deficiency
  - Glossitis due to B complex and iron deficiency
- Mechanical causes
  - Ill fitting denture
  - Carcinoma
- Infections
  - Oral thrush
  - Herpes simplex infection
  - Vincent's angina
- Dermatological

– Ulcers due to lichen planus and due to pemphigus
- Drug therapy
  – Ulcers due to drug allergy
  – Steven-Johnson syndrome
- Collagen disease
  – Mouth ulcers
- Idiopathic
  – Apthous ulcers

BAD BREATH (HALITOSIS)

Bad breath is usually due to putrefaction of food in the oral cavity.

Putrefaction of food occurs as a result of overgrowth of organisms in the oral cavity, gum or tonsil.

Conditions Associated with Bad Breath
- Disease of the oral cavity
- Carcinoma stomach
- Bronchiectasis/ lung abscess
- Intestinal obstruction
- Diabetic ketoacidosis - Acetone odour
- Uraemia - Ammoniacal odour
- Hepatic encephalopathy - Musty odour

HICCUPS

Hiccups occurs as a result of diaphragm and intercostal contraction resulting in sudden inspiration which is terminated by closure of glottis.

Some of the Causes of Hiccups
- Dilatation of stomach
- Ischaemic heart disease
- Oesophageal irritation
- Hyponatremia
- Diaphragmatic irritation
- Alcoholism

Cough
Cough may rarely be a manifestation of alimentary disease like gastroesophageal reflux disease and hiatus hernia.

SPECIFIC SYMPTOMATOLOGY OF LIVER DISEASE

- Fatigability
- Anorexia
- Weight loss

These Occur in All Forms of Acute and Chronic Liver Disease
1. Patients with cirrhosis can have weight gain due to fluid retention.
2. Disordered taste and smell: Jaundiced persons (usually with viral hepatitis) cannot tolerate cigarette smell.
3. Nausea and vomiting: Occurs in parenchymal and obstructive liver disease.
4. Abdominal distension and pain
   - Abdominal pain- Parenchymal and biliary tract disease (see abdominal pain).
   - Abdominal distension and pedal edema: Occurs in (see abdominal distension) cirrhotic with ascites. Abdominal distension can also occur due to enlarged liver and spleen.
5. Jaundice (see jaundice)
6. Bowel function and stool
   - Constipation precipitates encephalopathy in cirrhotics
   - Clay coloured stool suggests cholestasis.
   - Steatorrhoea occurs in chronic biliary obstruction.
   - Black tarry stool can occur as a result of upper gastrointestinal bleeding due to oesophageal varices.
7. Oliguria and nocturia
   - Oliguria can occur in cirrhotics and hepatic outflow obstruction.
   - Nocturia due to increased renal blood flow in recumbent position.

Pruritis of Hepatobiliary Disease
- Common in patients with cholestasis
- Pruritis may be mild to severe, more on hands and feet.
- Increases after hot bath and troublesome at night.
- Alcoholic liver disease is a rarer cause of pruritis.

- Pruritis is supposed to be due to increasing concentration of circulating bile salts, irritating the nerve endings.

Fever with Rigors and Skin Eruption
- Viral hepatitis especially hepatitis B is associated with fever and rash.
- Fever with rigors occurs in conditions like cholecystitis, liver abscess and cholangitis.

Encephalopathy Symptoms
1. *Inverse sleep rhythm:* Somnolence during the day with lack of sleep at night.
2. Change in mental functions with neuropsychiatric manifestations.
3. Altered consciousness
4. Memory impairment and decreased intelligence

Impotence and Sexual Dysfunction
- Common in patients with chronic parenchymal disease like cirrhosis.
- Impotence is more common in alcoholic cirrhotics than non alcoholics.
- Sexual desire significantly decreases in cirrhotics
- Menstrual irregularities occur in female patients with liver disease.

Bleeding Tendency, Night Blindness and Bony Pain

Defective absorption of fat soluble vitamins like K, A and D in patients with hepatobiliary disease result in bleeding tendency, night blindness and bony pain.

Bleeding tendency may also be due to defective prothrombin synthesis in parenchymal liver disease.

Symptoms of Systemic Disease

Enquire always symptoms of other systemic disease, which can secondarily involve the liver.

Past History
- Previous history of fever with jaundice may be present in patients of chronic liver disease due to hepatitis B and C.
- Recurrent history of jaundice occurs in patients with chronic hepatitis, gall stone disease and hepatic decompensation.
- Previous history of pain abdomen, dyspeptic symptoms are common in patients with peptic ulcer complications like perforation and haemorrhage.
- Previous history of transfusions, vaccinations, injections and needle sharing is significant in patients with acute hepatitis B and C and in chronic liver disease of viral aetiology.
- High risk behaviours like intravenous drug abuse and multiple sexual partners is important in patients with parenchymal liver diseases like hepatitis B and C and HIV infection.
- Previous history of surgery is significant in patients with biliary stricture, retained gall stones and damage to portal vein.
- History of staying in endemic areas of schistosomiasis should be enquired in patients with portal hypertension.

History of Taking Drugs

Drugs Causing Hepatic Abnormalities
- INH, rifampicin, pyrazinamide, methyldopa - hepatitis.
- Sex hormones - Cholestatic jaundice, adeno-matous changes
- Anabolic steroids - Hepatocellular carcinoma
- Paracetamol > 10 gm (single dose) can cause hepatic necrosis.
- Long duration of methotrexate therapy can cause cirrhotic changes in the liver.

Family History

GIT Disorders with Familial Tendency
- Peptic ulcer
- Gluten sensitive enteropathy
- Inflammatory bowel disease
- Familial polyposis coli
- Gastrointestinal malignancy

Liver Disorders with Familial Tendency
- Wilson's disease
- Congenital hyperbilirubinemia

- Alpha-1 antitrypsin deficiency

History of parental consanguinity is important in patients with Wilson's disease, galactosemia and hereditary fructose intolerance.

Several family members can be affected with viral hepatitis and it is ideal to vaccinate other partner of a hepatitis B patient.

Personal History

Loss of Appetite
Appetite loss occurs in all disorders of hepatobiliary and gastrointestinal tract.

Loss of weight
- Occurs in acute and chronic liver disease.
- Chronic disorders of gastrointestinal tract like malignancy, malabsorption, tuberculosis, HIV induced gastrointestinal disorders are associated with significant weight loss.
- Patients of chronic duodenal ulcer can gain weight due to excessive eating to relieve hunger pain. Weight gain can also occur due to fluid retention in cirrhotics.

Smoking
Details of amount and duration of smoking should be enquired.

Smoking can contribute to the development of peptic ulcer disease and reflux esophagitis. Smoking can also delay the healing of peptic ulcer.

Patients with acute viral hepatitis may not tolerate the smell of cigarette smoke.

Alcohol
Amount and duration of alcohol consumed is important in causing liver disease.

Consumption of 60–80 gm of alcohol/day for about 10 years may be necessary in males for the development of cirrhosis of liver. (Females tolerate alcohol less than males - about 30 gm/day for 10 years is adequate to develop cirrhosis).

Hepatic abnormalities caused by alcohol
- Fatty liver
- Acute hepatitis

- Chronic hepatitis
- Cirrhosis of liver
- Hepatocellular carcinoma

Gastrointestinal disorders caused by alcohol
- Pancreatitis
- Peptic ulcer disease
- Reflux oesophagitis

Occupational History

- Occupations related to alcohol are more predisposed for the development of alcoholic liver disease.
- Laborers coming in contact with contaminated water can develop leptospirosis.
- Medical and paramedical personal have additional risk of contacting hepatitis B and C.
- History of travel to endemic areas of viral hepatitis should be enquired in patients with jaundice.
- Occupations associated with stress and irregular eating patterns are more likely to be associated with peptic ulcer disease.

Personal History

Weight Loss
Chronic disorders of gastrointestinal tract like malignancy, malabsorption, tuberculosis, HIV induced gastrointestinal disorders are associated with significant weight loss.

Weight Gain
Can occur in patients with chronic duodenal ulcer due to excess eating to relieve hunger pain.
Weight gain can also occur due to fluid retention in cirrhotics.

Sleep
Reversal of sleep rhythm occurs in patients with early hepatic encephalopathy.

Hunger pain disturbing sleep can occur in patients with chronic duodenal ulcer.

Urine and stool (see history of present illness)

High-risk behavior (see history of present illness)

Menstrual history

Patients with chronic parenchymal liver disease will have decreased menstrual flow or amenorrhea.

EXAMINATION OF THE GASTROINTESTINAL TRACT

Scheme of Examination

General Physical Examination
- Build
- Nourishment
- Vital signs
  - Pulse
  - Blood pressure
  - Respiratory rate
  - Temperature
- Pallor, clubbing, edema,
- Icterus, cyanosis, lymphadenopathy

Examination of Oral Cavity

EXAMINATION OF THE ABDOMEN

Inspection
- Shape of the abdomen
- Pulsations
- Scar mark
- Flanks
- Veins
- Hernial orifices
- Umbilicus
- Peristalsis
- Genitalia
- Movement of different parts
- Visible mass

Palpation
- *Superficial:* Tenderness, temperature, guarding/rigidity.
- *Deep palpation:* Liver, spleen, kidney or any other mass.

Percussion
- Liver and splenic dullness, free fluid

Auscultation
- Bowel sounds, bruit, venous hum

EXAMINATION OF OTHER SYSTEMS

Examination of the Gastrointestinal Tract

Build and Nourishment

Loss of muscle bulk and subcutaneous fat occurs with chronic liver disease and chronic gastrointestinal disorders.

Rarely anabolic steroid abuse can cause unduly large muscles.

Pallor

Significant anemia, develops in following gastrointestinal disorders.
- Gastrointestinal bleeding
- Malabsorption syndrome

Chronic liver disease can result in anemia due to the following reasons
- Bleeding due to oesophageal varices
- Portal hypertension with splenomegaly causing hypersplenism
- Bleeding tendencies due to defective prothrombin synthesis.
- Anemia of chronic disease

Icterus
- Icterus appears when serum bilirubin level reaches above 3 mg/dl.
- Icterus appears early in the sclera than in other parts of the body.

Causes (see general physical examination)

Clubbing

Gastrointestinal and hepatic causes of clubbing
- Cirrhosis especially in biliary cirrhosis
- Hepatocellular carcinoma

- Ulcerative colitis and Crohn's disease
- Malabsorption syndrome.

Cyanosis

Portal hypertension can cause pulmonary AV shunting, O_2 desaturation and hypoxia and cyanosis.

Lymphadenopathy

Causes of significant lymphadenopathy associated with gastrointestinal disease

- Left supraclavicular node-Virchow's node (Troissier's sign)
- Node enlarges due to metastasis from gastro-intestinal and testicular malignancy spreading through the thoracic duct.
- Viral infections, lymphoma and leukemias associated with generalised lymphadenopathy can also involve gastrointestinal tract and para-aortic nodes.

Pedal Oedema

- Cirrhosis of liver is associated with swelling of feet.
- Patients of hepatic out flow and inferior venacaval obstruction can also have pedal oedema.

Examination of Face and Eyes in Relation to Gastrointestinal Tract

- *Exopothalmos:* Thyrotoxicsis can be associated with diarrhea and weight loss.
- *Jaundice:* Suggestive of hepatobiliary disease.
- Subconjunctival hemorrhage: Leptospirosis is associated with subconjunctival hemorrhage and liver involvement.
- *Keiser-Fleischer ring:* Brownish green ring appears due to deposition of copper on the descemet membrane of the cornea found in patients with Wilson's disease.
- *Xanthelasma:* Yellowish deposit near the eyelids, associated with chronic cholestasis.

Nails

Nails become white (leuconychia), bilateral nails will show transverse white lines parallel to lunula, e.g. cirrhosis

Skin

- Needle tracks may be visible with IV drug abusers.
- Skin excoriations are seen in patients with severe itching due to primary biliary cirrhosis and sclerosing cholangitis. Skin pigmentation may be a feature of haemochromatosis, primary biliary cirrhosis or chronic cholestasis.

> *Note*
> - Vitiligo can occur due to autoimmune hepatitis/ primary biliary cirrhosis.
> - Chronic cholestasis, primary biliary cirrhosis and liver disease associated with haemochromatosis can be associated with skin pigmentation.

SIGNS OF LIVER CELL FAILURE

Icterus

Parenchymal and obstructive liver diseases are associated with icterus.

Parotid Swelling

- Parotid swellings are commonly associated with alcoholic liver disease.
- Parotid enlargements are usually not painful
- Parotid swelling may be related to alcohol itself or due to malnutrition.

Spider Naevi

Characteristics

- Central arteriole with radiating small vessels resembling spider legs which blanch on pressure.
- Pin head to 2 cm size
- Giant spiders seen to pulsate and may bleed.

Distribution of Spider Naevi

- Upper part of the body in the territory of superior venacava.

Causes of Spider Naevi

- Cirrhosis of liver
- Thyrotoxicosis
- Pregnancy
- Rheumatoid arthritis

- Estrogen therapy
- Alcoholic hepatitis

> *Note*
> - Occasionally normal persons can have spiders (usually less than 5 in number).
> - Increasing the size of previous spider or appearance of new spider is abnormal.
> - Upper part of the body is more prone to skin trauma making prone to develop spider naevi.

Differential Diagnosis of Spider Naevi
- Campbell de Morgan spots
- Hereditary telengiectasia

Palmar Erythema

- Redness of thenar and hypothenar eminences, sole of feet, pulp of fingers can also become erythematous.
- Hands are usually warm, bright red, blanches on pressure with rapid return of color.

Causes
- Cirrhosis of liver
- Pregnancy
- Thyrotoxicosis
- Chronic rheumatoid arthritis

Gynaecomastia

Palpable enlargement of glandular tissue beneath the areola. Areola may become enlarged and pigmented.

Gynaecomastia may be tender (for further details see endocrinology).

Common Causes of Gynaecomastia
- Cirrhosis of liver
- Spironolactone therapy
- Testicular disease

Testicular Atrophy

Testis becomes soft and small.

Normal testicular size in adult males is around 4.6 cm (15–20ml /vol) measured by pralid orchidometer. Testicular size less than 3 cm usually suggests testicular atrophy. Testicular atrophy is more commonly related to alcoholic liver disease and alcohol induced pituitary abnormality.

Dupuytren's Contracture

Common in patients with alcoholic liver disease. Characterised by flexion deformities of fingers due to thickening and shortening of palmar fascia. Occurs as a result of free radical damage to the connective tissues caused by alcohol. Mainly related to alcohol rather than cirrhosis itself.

Breast Atrophy in Females

Female patients with cirrhosis develop atrophy of gonads and ovulatory failure. They may develop breast atrophy and infertility. Menstrual cycles become altered with oligomenorrhea or amenorrhea. All these are closely related to alcoholic liver disease.

Loss of Axillary and Pubic Hair

Cirrhotic men will shave less and will have loss of axillary and pubic hairs.

Bleeding Tendencies

Petechiae and echymoses can occur due to:
- Hypoprothrombinaemia
- Liver disease
- Decreased platelets as a result of hypersplenism due to portal hypertension.

Pedal Oedema

Patients of cirrhosis of liver will have pedal edema due to decrease of albumin synthesis.

Hepatic Encephalopathy

Characteristic Features
- Altered conscious level
- *Personality changes* (loss of family concern and irritability)
- Handwriting becomes impaired
- *Intellectual deterioration* (deterioration of intellectual function)

- *Constructional apraxia* - inability to reproduce simple diagrams with blocks or matches.
- Flapping tremors
- *Other features* - hypothermia, fetor hepaticus.

Flapping Tremors (Asterixis)

Failure to actively maintain posture results in flapping tremors.

Significance of Flapping Tremor
- Indicates hepatic encephalopathy
- Flapping tremors are due to difficulty in maintaining posture. These are not seen on voluntary movement and are absent at rest.
- Sustained posture is more likely to result in flapping tremor and is usually bilateral.

Elicitation
- Ask the patient to outstretch the arms and keep the wrist hyperextended while supporting the forearm and maintain this position for about 15 sec.

Observation
- Lateral movement of fingers
- Flexion and extension movement of wrist and metacarpophalangeal joints.

Pathogenesis
Defective posture maintenance is due to defective relay of joint sense and other informations to brain stem reticular formation concerned with posture maintenance.
Other causes of flapping tremor are CCF, uraemia, CO_2 narcosis.

Mechanisms Causing Spider Naevi and Palmar Erythema
- Due to oestrogen induced vasodilatation and altered ratio of oestrogen/free testosterone
- Pathogenesis behind endocrine abnormalities in cirrhosis
- Alcohol induced liver damage
- Decompensated liver disease with abnormal hormone metabolism
- Alcohol induced pituitary dysfunction
- Spironolactone induced anti androgen effect.

EXAMINATION OF THE GASTRO INTESTINAL TRACT

Examination of the Oral Cavity

Buccal Mucosa
Observe for mouth ulcers

Causes of Mouth Ulcers
- Aphthous ulcers
- Inflammatory bowel disease
- Herpes simplex stomatitis
- Malignancy
- Herpes zoster
- Collagen vascular disease
- See also under causes of pain in the oral cavity

Characteristics of Lesions in the Oral Cavity

Infective Disorders
Oral thrush (moniliasis) (Figs 5.1 a to d)

See also oral lesions

It is caused by *Candida albicans*. Lesions will have sheets of curdy white patches difficult to remove and leave behind a raw surface after removal.

Conditions associated with oral thrush
- Immunosuppressive and corticosteroids therapy
- Long term antibiotic therapy
- Diabetes mellitus
- Acquired immunodeficiency syndrome

Causes of White Lesions in the Oral Cavity apart from Oral Thrush
- Lichen planus
- Leukoplakia
- Ulcers of other causes

Streptococcal Tonsillitis

Exudates appear as yellow punctate lesions over the tonsil.

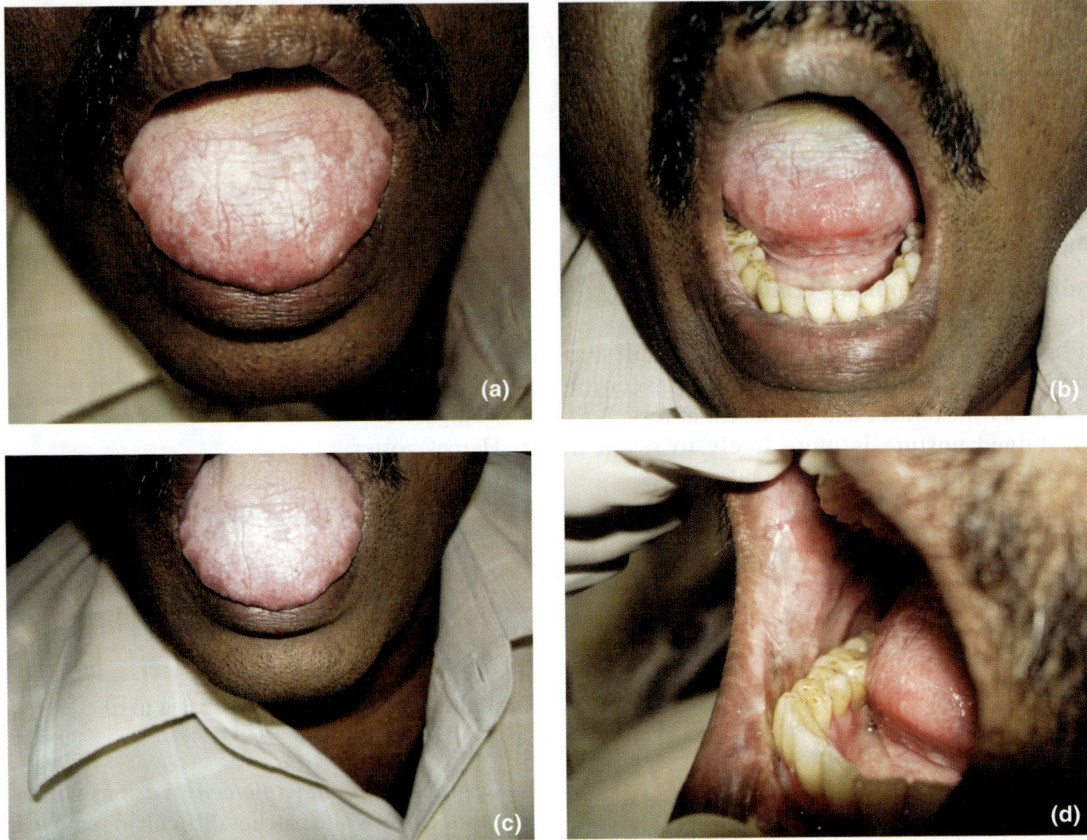

Figs 5.1a to d Oral candidiasis

Infectious Mononucleosis

- Redness of pharynx
- Fauces and palate are edematous
- Tonsils are enlarged and covered with white exudate

Diphtheria

Characterised by white or greenish colored membrane formation. Membrane spreads from tonsil to pharynx.

Herpes Zoster

Vesicles over the oral mucosa

Measles

Characterised by the presence of Koplik's spots.

Koplik's Spots
- Bluish white spots surrounded by an area of redness.
- Usually seen opposite the molar teeth.

Chickenpox
Vesicles can appear in the oral mucosa.

Pigmentation of Oral Cavity

Causes
- Congenital

- Addison's disease
- Malabsorption syndrome
- Haemochromatosis
- Peuz-Jegher's syndrome (associated with multiple polyposis of intestine)
- Racial hyperpigmentation.

Miscellaneous Lesions in the Oral Cavity
- Cleft palate
- Telengiectasia
- Haemorrhages
- Pallor, cyanosis and jaundice
- Abnormal palate and uvula movement in 10th nerve palsy.

Gross oral sepsis can lead onto endocarditis, lung abscess and can aggravate dyspepsia and gastritis.

Examination of the Teeth

Teeth Abnormalities
- Check for number and condition of the teeth
- Discoloration
- Decaying (caries)
- Abnormal configuration and artificial denture

Cause of discoloration of teeth [see Gastrointestinal tract II]

Hutchinson's teeth (See infectious disease)

Hypoplastic teeth (poorly developed)
- Occurs in patients with hypoparathyroidism.
- Delayed teeth eruption occurs due to hypocalcaemia in infancy.

Examination of Gum

Gingivitis
- Deep red congestion of gums, which bleed easily on touch.

Pyorrhea
- Teeth are loose, covered with a greenish yellow exudate.
- Pus can be squeezed from the gum margins.

Acute Herpetic Gingivostomatitis

It is caused by herpes simplex virus associated with greenish gray slough with halitosis.

Vincent's Angina
It refers to ulceration and sloughing of gingiva caused by infection due to spirochetes and fusiform bacilli.

Lead Poisoning
Blue line at gum may due to deposition of lead sulfide in gum tissues.

Scurvy
Gums are soft, spongy swollen and bleed easily.

Hypertrophy of Gums

Causes
- Pregnancy
- Long term phenytoin treatment.
- Scurvy
- Acute myeloid leukemia (gums are hypertrophied and bleed easily)

Tongue

Check for Following Abnormalities
- Atrophy of papillae
- Tremors
- Ulcers and white lesions
- Atrophy of musculature
- Enlargement of tongue

Atrophy of Papillae
- Pale and bald tongue - iron deficiency
- Pink and bald - B-complex deficiency
- Magenta colored - Riboflavin deficiency
- Beefy red - Niacin deficiency

Tremors of the Tongue
- Thyrotoxicosis
- Parkinsonism
- Anxiety states

Ulcers Over the Tongue
All causes of ulcers in the oral cavity

Atrophy of Tongue Musculature
LMN type of 12th nerve palsy

Enlargement of Tongue
Causes
- Acromegaly
- Myxedema
- Amyloidosis
- Down's syndrome (may be fissured)

Miscellaneous lesion in the tongue and curdy white patches over the tongue suggests oral candidiasis.

Hairy leukoplakia (see Gastrointestinal tract II)

Central Cyanosis
Bluish discoloration of the tip of the tongue.

Ventral Surface of the Tongue
Hemorrhages, neoplastic ulcers, leukoplakia and jaundice can be made out.

EXAMINATION OF THE ABDOMEN

General Principles

1. Proper positioning of the patient is essential for examination of the abdomen. Patient should be completely resting supine with the arms on sides.
2. Examiner stands on the right side of the patient.
3. Expose the abdomen preferably from xiphisternum to inguinal region. Cover the genitalia except during the examination of genitalia.

For the purpose of description abdomen is divided into 9 different regions as shown in the Figure 5.2.
- *Vertical line 1 and 2:* Line drawn upwards from mid-inguinal region to mid-clavicular region
- *Horizontal line I:* Connects the lowest part of 10th costal cartilage on both sides.
- *Horizontal line II:* Connects the highest points of iliac crest on both sides.

Inspection of the Abdomen

Distension of Abdomen
- Uniform distention caused by 5 Fs (discussed above).
- Ascites is the most important cause of uniform distension of abdomen.

- Flanks become full in patients with uniform distention of abdomen.
- *Localised distention:* Caused by massive enlargement of intra abdominal viscera.
- *Epigastric fullness:* Occurs in patients with distension of stomach due to pyloric obstruction.
- Fullness of suprapubic region occurs due to
  - Uterine enlargement
  - Distended urinary bladder
  - Ovarian tumors

Scaphoid Abdomen

Causes
- Severe starvation
- Disorders like TB/ malignancy

Umbilicus
Normal position of the umbilicus is at the center of the abdomen. It may be inverted and retracted.

Bulging of the umbilicus occurs due to umbilical hernia which can be confirmed by impulse on coughing.

Umbilicus is transversely stretched in patients with massive ascites.

Discharge from the Umbilicus
Serous and sero-purulent discharge occurs due to infection of the umbilicus and patent urachus.

Displacement of umbilicus can occur in upper and lower abdominal mass lesions.

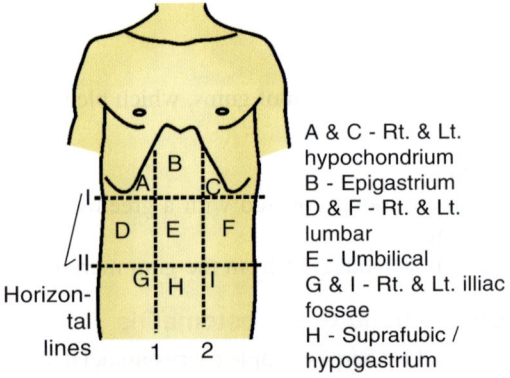

A & C - Rt. & Lt. hypochondrium
B - Epigastrium
D & F - Rt. & Lt. lumbar
E - Umbilical
G & I - Rt. & Lt. illiac fossae
H - Suprafubic / hypogastrium

Horizontal lines

Fig. 5.2 Different parts of the abdomen

Skin Striae

White, colorless lines over the abdomen occur in patients with gross distention of the abdomen. Enormous stretching of the skin causes rupture of elastic fibers causing white striae.

Examples
- Pregnancy
- Massive ascites
- Excessive weight gain

Purple striae occurs in patients with cushing's syndrome.

Campbell De Morgan spots: Small angiomas occur in elderly patients.

Scars

Previous surgery or laparoscopy (immediately below the umbilicus) can cause multiple scars over the abdomen.

Discoloration of Skin

Cullen's Sign
Bluish discoloration around the umbilicus suggests bleeding into the peritoneal cavity.

For example, rupture of ectopic pregnancy and acute pancreatitis

Turner's Sign
Bluish discoloration (ecchymosis) of flanks due to hemoglobin undergoing tissue catabolism.

For example, acute pancreatitis

Sister Joseph Nodule

Metastatic nodule in the umbilical area indicates intra peritoneal tumor with metastasis

Note: Branding marks of different size and shape indicate pain and distress in that part of the abdomen.

Movement of the Different Parts of the Abdomen
- Normally all parts of the abdomen move equally with respiration.
- In males abdomen moves outwards during inspiration.

- Localised or generalised peritonitis or intra abdominal disease causes decrease movement of that region of the abdomen.
- Tense ascites can also cause decrease movement of the abdomen.

Visible Pulsations

Visible epigastric pulsation may be due to
- Abdominal aorta in thin individuals
- Right ventricular hypertrophy

Pulsatile liver causes predominantly right hypochondrial pulsation.

Aortic aneurysm produces expansile pulsation. Mass overlying the aorta can have transmitted pulsations through the mass. (Pulsation will decrease on knee elbow position as the mass falls away from the aorta).

Divarication of Rectus Abdominis
Persons with chronic intra abdominal pressure increase will have wide separation of recti muscles in the midline (may be due to weakness of muscles).

When the person is asked to sit upright from supine position without support, linea alba bulges between the two recti.

For example, common in multiparous individuals, can also occur in patients with long standing massive ascites.

Visible Veins

Normally there may be thin small veins below the costal margin.
- Dilated tortuous veins are more of pathological significance.
- Visibility of veins is made out better in standing position.

Demonstration of Direction of Flow in a Collateral Vein
- Select a part of the collateral vein of about 3–4 cm which is free of branches.
- Press the two fingers over the middle part of this vein and empty the vein by drawing apart the two

fingers without releasing the finger pressure being applied.
- Lift one of the fingers at a time and note the direction of filling up of the emptied vein.

Caput Medusa (Fig. 5.3 b)

Characteristics
- Veins radiating away from the umbilicus
- Flow is away from the umbilicus
- Caput medusa suggests intrahepatic portal hypertension.
- Portal vein drains through collateral vessels along the falciparum ligament.
- In extrahepatic portal hypertension, umbilical veins are not prominent.

Inferior Venacaval Obstruction (Fig. 5.3c)
- Dilated anastamotic channels predominantly seen over the flanks and back.
- Blood flow is from below upwards.
- Anastamoses occur between superficial epigastric and superficial circumflex iliac veins below and lateral thoracic veins above.

Hepatic Outflow Obstruction
Patient may have prominent back veins draining from below upwards.

Visible Mass
- Visible mass appears as an area of localised fullness of the abdomen.
- Massively enlarged liver and spleen can produce visible mass in the hypochondrium.

Visible Peristalsis
- Visible peristalsis may be a normal feature in a very thin elderly person with lax abdominal muscles.
- Vigorous tapping or flickering the skin of the abdomen can augment peristalsis.

Pyloric Obstruction
- Massively enlarged stomach can cause epigastric fullness.
- Ask the patient to drink water and observe for peristaltic waves moving from left to right hypochondrium.
- *Succussion splash over the abdomen:* A splashing sound is heard when the patient is shaken in cases of pyloric obstruction.

Small Intestinal Obstruction
Abdomen is usually distended. Peristalsis appears as writhing movement in the center of the abdomen or may appear as a ladder pattern.

Colonic Obstruction
- In transverse colonic obstruction, waveform appears moving from right to left in the upper abdomen.
- In ascending and descending colonic obstruction- wave form appears to be moving up and down or appears as an alternatively appearing or disappearing mass.

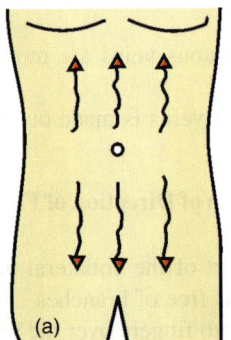 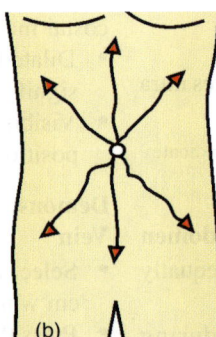 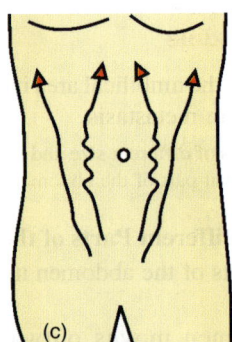

(a) (b) (c)

Fig. 5.3a to c Abdominus venous flow patterns (a) Normal (b) Portal hypertension (c) IVC obstruction

Hernial Orifices

Hernial orifices should be carefully inspected especially on standing and on coughing for cough impulse.

- Umbilical hernia appears as a bulge through the umbilicus.
- Epigastric hernia: Extraperitoneal fat bulging through the defect in the linea alba producing a small epigastric swelling.
- Incisional hernia: Herniation occurs due to defective healing of the incision wound after the surgery
- Femoral and inguinal hernia: Herniation through the femoral and inguinal hernial orifices.

Inspect the groin in a male for any abnormality of penis, scrotum, position of the testis and testicular swelling.

Palpation

Methods of Palpation

Different Methods of Abdominal Palpation
- Superficial palpation
- Deep palpation
- Bimanual palpation
- Ballotment
- Dipping method

Superficial Palpation

Gentle and light palpation is required predominantly with the flat of the hand and observe for tenderness, guarding and rigidity.

Area of Tenderness

Indicative of inflammatory lesions of underlying viscera and surrounding peritoneum.

Generalised tenderness over the abdomen occurs in patients with generalised peritonitis.

Rebound Tenderness

- Initial routine palpation does not result in pain.
- Slow and deep palpation over the abdomen and then sudden release of pressure by withdrawing the hand. Patient experiences pain. This indicates peritoneal inflammation.
- Pain on release of hand is due to sudden movement of intra abdominal inflamed structure or viscera.

Note
- Pressure in the left iliac fossa may cause pain in the right iliac fossa in cases of appendicitis.
- Gaseous distension of intestinal coils may give rise to temporary abdominal tenderness.

Guarding and Rigidity

Indicate resistance of the muscle for palpation.

Guarding

State of voluntary contraction of the abdominal muscles by the patient (patient expects a painful palpation).

Rigidity

State of reflex involuntary spasm of the muscles of the whole of the abdominal wall.

Rigidity is indicative of generalised peritonitis and abdominal wall does not move with respiration. Whole abdominal wall becomes hard and board like (board like rigidity).

Edema of the Abdominal Wall

Abdominal wall edema is demonstrated by applying finger pressure or pinching a fold of skin over the abdominal wall producing a depression (pitting). Abdominal wall edema occurs in patients with anasarca.

KEY POINTS 5.4

- Patient's position
  - Patient is lying down comfortably on his back.
  - Head is raised slightly and arms are kept to the side.
  - Knees are semiflexed (for relaxing the abdomen)
  - Cover the genitalia until they are examined.
- Examiner sits by the side of the patient and keeps the palpating hand parallel to the abdomen.
- Patient should breath more deeply than normal with mouth open.
- Use flat of the hand and mould it to the abdominal wall and exert pressure by the finger tips and avoid sudden poking of the abdomen.
- Avoid palpating the tender area unless required.

Deep Palpation

Each area of the abdomen should be palpated starting from remote area of tenderness and observe for palpability of underlying mass or viscera.

Structures which may be felt normally on Palpation

1. Lower border of the liver on deep respiration.
2. Lower pole of right kidney.
   • Felt in thin and lax abdominal wall on deep inspiration.
3. Abdominal aorta: Palpable in thin individuals.

In thin individuals with lax abdominal wall occasionally pelvic colon, caecum and transverse colon may become palpable.

An intra abdominal mass may become less prominent if the person is asked to raise the head from supine position without support, whereas mass arising from the abdominal wall becomes more prominent.

PALPATION OF LIVER

Palpation in the Right Hypochondrium (Fig. 5.4)
• Examiner sits on the side of the patient.
• Flat of one hand or both hands are kept side by side lateral to the rectus abdominus below the costal margin and the patient is asked to take deep breath.
• It is preferable to move the hand upwards from much below the costal margin to avoid missing a greatly enlarged liver
• Firm upward and inward pressure is given with the hand with the fingers directed towards the costal margin.
• Border of the liver is felt by the tips of the fingers.
• Define the border of the liver from the right hypochondrium to the epigastrium.
• Liver normally moves about 1–3 cm downwards on inspiration.

Palpation from the Right Iliac Fossa (Fig. 5.5)
• Keep the right hand in the right iliac fossa with its border parallel to the costal margin.
• Move the hand upwards until the edge of the liver is felt by the border of the hand.

Note the following features whenever the Liver is Palpable

1. Extent of enlargement from the costal margin in the mid-clavicular and mid-sternal line
2. Edge or border
3. Surface
4. Consistency
5. Tenderness

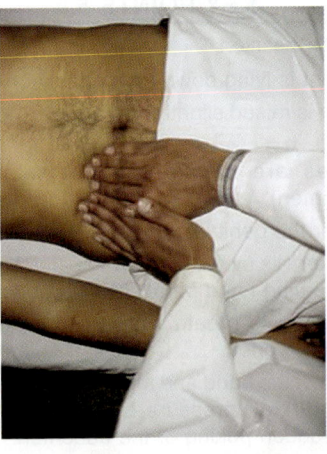

Fig. 5.4 Palpation of liver from right hypochondrium

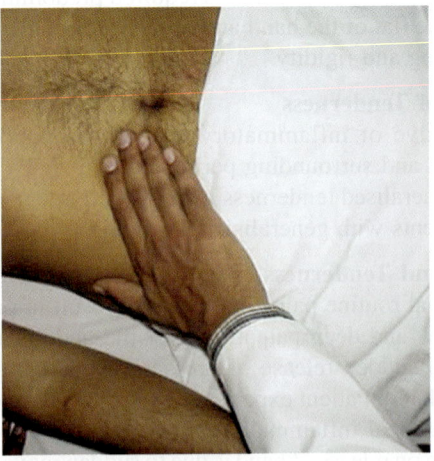

Fig. 5.5 Palpation of liver from right iliac fossa

6. Movement with inspiration
7. Pulsation

Features Favoring a Hepatic Mass
- Presence in the right hypochondrium
- Movement with respiration
- Getting above the mass is not possible
- Finger can not be insinuated between the costal margin and the mass

Left Lobe of Liver

Left lobe of the liver may be palpable in the epigastrium between the xiphoid process and umbilicus. Left lobe is continuous with the right lobe in the hypochondrium.

Reidel's Lobe

Tongue like projection of a part of the liver, which is felt superficially in the mid-clavicular line occasionally may become palpable at the level of the umbilicus.

Reidel's lobe moves freely with respiration and may be mistaken for a mobile kidney or a gall bladder.

Features of Normal Liver
Sharp and regular border, soft in consistency, smooth surface, moves with respiration.

Hepatomegaly

Indicates enlargement of liver with increase in the liver span.

In conditions like pleural effusion and emphysema, liver may be pushed down, becoming palpable without enlargement (normal liver span).

Causes of Hepatomegaly
- Acute
  - Viral hepatitis
  - Enteric fever
  - Acute malaria
- Chronic
  - Cirrhosis of liver
  - Fatty liver
  - Lymphoma and leukemias

Tender and Enlarged Liver

Causes
- Congestive cardiac failure
- Amoebic liver abscess (may cause pre-dominant upward enlargement)
- Viral hepatitis
- Pyogenic liver abscess

Abnormalities of Palpable Liver
- Round border liver: For example, congestive cardiac failure
- Firm liver: All causes of chronic liver disease, e.g. cirrhosis
- Nodular liver
  1. Macronodular cirrhosis (e.g. post necrotic cirrhosis)
  2. Malignancy of liver
  3. Hepar lobatum-congenital syphilis
- Hard liver (Table 5.2)
  1. Primary hepatocellular carcinoma
  2. Secondaries in the liver

Pulsatile Liver

Causes
Tricuspid stenosis, tricuspid regurgitation and aortic regurgitation.

Palpation of Pulsatile Liver
Place two fingers over the surface of the liver well separated. Observe for further separation of two fingers with each pulsation suggesting pulsatile liver.

Table 5.2 Difference between hepatocellular carcinoma and secondaries in the liver

Hepatocellular carcinoma	*Secondaries in the liver*
Hard enlarged liver	Hard single or multiple nodules
Bruit over the liver	Bruit is absent
	Umbilication over the nodule (Central softening due to degeneration of cells)

Causes of massive liver enlargement (>10 cm below the costal margin)

Common causes

- Tricuspid regurgitation and CCF
- Malignancy of liver
- Hepatic amoebiasis
- Hepatic outflow obstruction

Rarer causes

- Myelofibrosis
- Chronic myeloid leukemia
- Lymphoma

Causes of painless hepatomegaly

- Cirrhosis of liver
- Hematological disorders (leukemia, lymphoma, etc).
- Fatty liver
- Biliary obstruction
- Chronic malaria
- Amyloidosis
- Infiltrative and storage disorders

GALL BLADDER

- Normally not palpable.
- Enlarged gall bladder is felt as a round smooth swelling
- Gall bladder swelling usually moves with respiration.
- Enlarged gall bladder is felt at the angle formed by the lateral border of the rectus abdominus and the right costal margin.

Enlarged Gall Bladder without Jaundice

Cystic duct obstruction can cause enlarged gall bladder due to mucocele or empyema without causing jaundice.

Causes of Palpable Gall Bladder

1. Carcinoma of head of pancreas - patient is deeply jaundiced
2. Mucocele of gall bladder - patient is not jaundiced.
3. Carcinoma of gall bladder - felt as a hard irregular swelling.

Murphy's Sign

- In patients with acute cholecystitis (usually secondary to gall stone) tenderness is felt below the right costal margin, midway between the xiphisternum and the flank.
- In patients of acute cholecystitis, if the fingers are kept over the above said area and the patient is asked to take deep breath. Inspiration suddenly gets arrested due to sudden occurrence of pain (Murphy's sign).

Palpation of Spleen

- Normally spleen is not palpable.
- Spleen should enlarge by 2–3 times to become palpable.
- Direction of enlargement of spleen is in the long axis of spleen towards the right iliac fossa.

Method of Palpation of Spleen (Fig. 5.6)

- Examiner sits or stands on the right side of the patient.
- Flat of the right hand is placed in the right iliac fossa with the fingers pointing towards the left costal margin.
- Flat of the left hand is placed over the lower left rib cage posterolaterally and continuous pressure is applied medially and downwards.
- Right hand is moved upwards after each inspiration until spleen is felt. (pressing the finger upwards and inwards may be helpful).
- Entire left costal margin is to be palpated starting from lateral to medial aspect.
- Spleen is felt as a round border swelling with direction of enlargement towards the right iliac fossa.

Method of Palpation for just Palpable Spleen

- Turn and keep the patient on the right lateral side (Fig. 5.7).
- Apply inward pressure from the left hand, which is applied over the posterolateral aspect of left lower rib cage.
- Left hip and knee may be flexed at right angle.
- Tip of the spleen can be palpated with the right hand below the left costal margin.

Hooking Method

Examiner can stand on either side of the patient, Place the left hand of the patient under his lower chest. Fingers of the examining hand are curled under the left costal margin starting from most lateral aspect. Patient is asked to take deep inspiration. Just palpable spleen can be felt with this method.

Massively enlarged spleen may also be palpated by bimanual method.

Features Favoring Splenic Mass

- Present in the left hypochondrium
- Enlarges towards the right iliac fossa
- Notch can be felt
- Dull to percuss
- Getting above the mass is not possible

Features of Splenomegaly

Size: Measure the dimension of splenomegaly from the costal margin.

Consistency

- Normally soft
- Acute enlargement of spleen causes soft splenomegaly.
- Chronic enlargement of spleen causes firm splenomegaly.

Edge: Is usually regular occasionally one or two notches may be felt.

Tenderness: Tender splenomegaly can occur in the following conditions

- Enteric fever
- Infective endocarditis
- Rupture and infarction of spleen

Massive splenomegaly: Spleen is palpable more than 8 cm below the costal margin.

Bimanual Method of Palpation (Fig. 5.8)

- Left hand is placed in the region of loin and the right hand is placed anteriorly in the lumbar region.
- Patient is asked to take deep breaths.
- Two hands are brought together gently.
- Mass will be palpable touching the two hands, e.g. kidney mass, massive splenomegaly.

Different Mechanisms Involved in Splenomegaly

1. Congestive splenomegaly, e.g. CCF, portal hypertension, hepatic outflow obstruction)
2. Reticuloendothelial system hyperplasia, (e.g. hemolytic anemias)
3. Hyperplasia due to immunological disorders (e.g. collagen vascular disease, infective endocarditis)
4. Infiltrative disorders, (e.g. storage disorders, lymphoma)

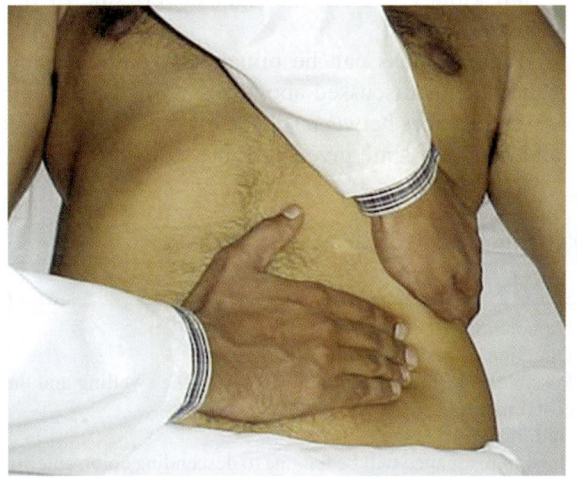

Fig. 5.6 Palpation of spleen

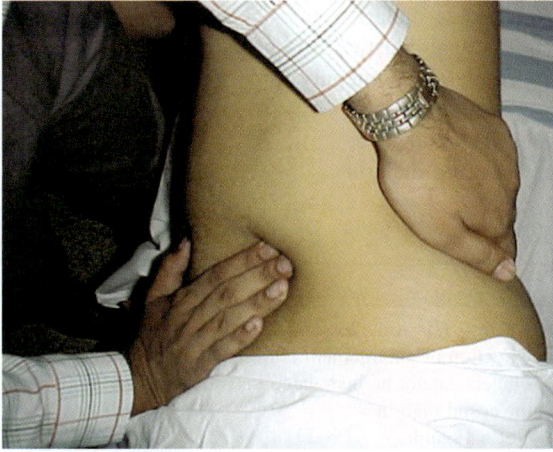

Fig. 5.7 Palpation of spleen - Patient in the right lateral position (lateral view)

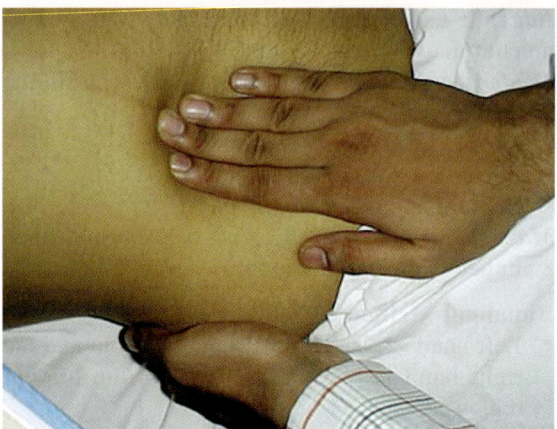

Fig. 5.8 Bimanual palpation of the kidney

Ballotment
Keep one hand in the area of loin and place the other hand over the abdominal wall anteriorly over the mass. Move the mass forwards and backwards between the two hands.

Renal mass is ballotable and bimanually palpable.

Causes of Splenomegaly

- Mild splenomegaly
  - Infective endocarditis
  - Typhoid fever
  - Acute malaria
  - Megaloblastic/iron deficiency anemia
- Acute splenomegaly
  - Infective
  - Typhoid fever
  - Acute malaria

- Massive splenomegaly
  - Chronic malaria
  - Chronic myeloid leukemia
  - Lymphomas
  - Myelofibrosis
  - Kala azar
- Chronic splenomegaly
  - Portal hypertension
  - Chronic malaria
  - Chronic myeloid leukemia

Causes of Hepatosplenomegaly

Acute
- Acute viral hepatitis
- Typhoid fever
- Acute malaria

Chronic
- Cirrhosis of liver
- Lymphomas
- Chronic leukemias

Palpation of Kidney

Occasionally lower pole of the right kidney may be palpable in thin asthenic individuals.
- Left kidney is usually not palpable.
- Right kidney is palpated from the right side and left kidney is from the right or left side of the patient.

Kidney mass can be bimanually palpable and ballotable as discussed above.

Differences between splenic mass and renal mass and renal mass are given in Table 5.3.

Table 5.3 Difference between splenic mass and renal mass

Spleen	*Kidney*
Notch is felt in the lower medial border	No notch is felt
Direction of enlargement is in the spino-umbilical line	Direction of engagement is downwards
Fingers cannot be insinuated between the swelling and the costal margin	Possible to insinuate the fingers between the swelling and the costal margin
Not ballotable	Ballotable
Mass is dull to percuss	Band of resonance will be felt due to descending colon anterior to the mass.

Unilateral Kidney Enlargement

Causes

- Tumors of the kidney
- Hydronephrosis
- Hypertrophy of one kidney due to atrophy/ agenesis of the other kidney

Bilateral Kidney Enlargement

Causes

- Polycystic kidney - Usually bilateral, irregular mass and deeply situated.
- Amyloidosis of the kidney

AORTA

Aorta is not readily palpable except in thin individuals.

Palpation of Aortic Pulsation

- Dip the tips of fingers deeply into the abdomen
- Aortic pulsation is usually felt little above and to the left of umbilicus.
- Width of aortic pulsation can be made out if the same technique as mentioned above is repeated a few cms to the right of previous site of palpation.

Transmitted pulsation: There is no separation of two fingers which are kept parallally over the area of pulsation.

Expansile pulsation: There is separation of two fingers which are kept parallally over the area of pulsation.

Paraaortic Nodes

- Feel for the aortic pulsation as mentioned above.
- Palpate along the left border of aortic pulsation.
- Nodes are palpable when they are significantly enlarged.
- Paraaortic nodes become palpable when they become significantly enlarged. They are usually found along the left border of aorta in the umbilical region and felt as round firm masses.

Causes

- Tuberculosis
- Lymphoma
- Intra abdominal malignancy
- Germ cell tumors

URINARY BLADDER

Normally urinary bladder is not palpable.

Features of Urinary Bladder Swelling

- History of retention of urine.
- Mass is present in the hypogastrium with regular margin
- Mass is firm in consistency and usually oval in shape
- Upper border can be readily made out but lower border cannot be made out.

Differentiate bladder swelling in a female from enlarged uterus and ovarian cyst

COLON

Descending colon may be palpable occasionally in normal persons as a firm tube in the left iliac fossa and also caecum may become palpable occasionally.

Hernial Orifices

- Check for Inguinal hernia at superficial inguinal ring.
- It is ideal to ask the patient to stand and look for the cough impulse.
- Invaginate the finger into the external abdominal ring through the scrotum and ask the patient to cough, early herniation can be made out.
- Look also for the cough impulse in the epigastrium and umbilical region.

Dipping Method of Palpation

- Dipping method is used for palpation is patients with massive ascites.
- Keep one hand or both the hands (left hand over the right hand) over the area to be palpated.
- Give sudden dipping movements to the finger tips which will displace a quantum of fluid temporarily.
- Displacement of fluid allows the edge of the viscera to come in contact with the finger tips.

PERCUSSION

Percussion is an important aspect of abdominal examination.

Percussion is helpful in detecting following intra abdominal abnormalities.

KEY POINTS 5.5

- It is beneficial to carryout light percussion over the abdomen.
- Tympanitic note will be heard while percussing over gas containing viscera.
- Dull note is produced by solid viscera enlargement, fluid collection and solid mass.

1. Ascites
2. Gaseous distention
3. Solid tumor/cyst
4. Enlarged intra abdominal organs

Detection of Ascites

1. Puddle Sign
Detects as little as 120 ml of ascitic fluid within the abdomen.

Elicitation
- Keep the patient in the knee elbow position and maintain it for several minutes.
- Percuss around the umbilicus - presence of fluid will result in dull note.

Note: Normally there will be tympanitic note around the umbilicus.

2. Horse Shoe Shaped Dullness (Fig. 5.9)
Helpful in detection of moderate to massive ascites.
Fluid usually occupies the area of flanks and hypogastric region.

Method of detection
- Percuss from the umbilical region towards each flank on both sides of the abdomen.
- Percuss also the suprapubic region.
- In presence of ascites - Both flanks and suprapubic areas are dull to percuss due to the collection of fluid.

3. Shifting Dullness (Figs 5.10 and 5.11)
Shifting dullness indicates free fluid in the abdomen (may detect ascites > 1000 ml).

Method of elicitation
- Ask the patient to lie down flat on his back.

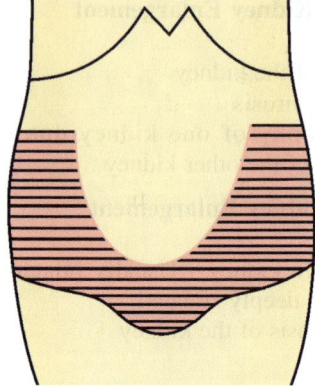

Fig. 5.9 Ascites representing horseshoe-shaped dullness

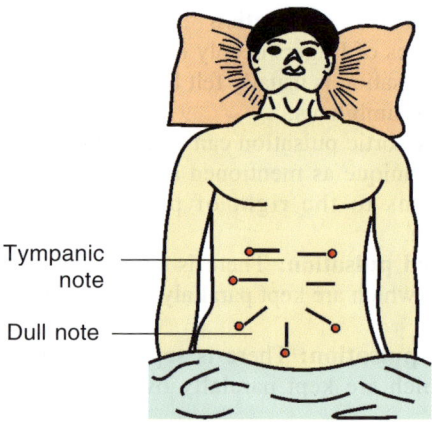

Tympanic note
Dull note

Fig. 5.10 Demonstration of shifting dullness

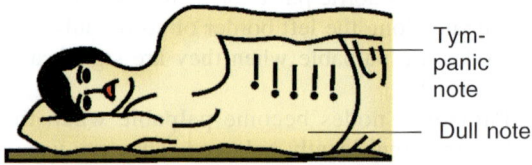

Tym-panic note
Dull note

Fig. 5.11 Shift of dullness to dependent site

- Examiner percusses from center of the abdomen (around the umbilicus) towards one flank till dull note is obtained (normally only lateral abdominal musculature produces dull note).

- Keep the finger in the area of dull note and turn the patient to the opposite side.
- Percuss the area of previous dull note and observe for the change of note.
- In the presence of ascites previous area of dull note changes to resonant note due to shift of fluid and floating up of intestinal coils.
- Percuss back towards the midline. Observe for dull note which was previously resonant.
- Repeat the above procedure on the other side of the abdomen.

In the following circumstances ascites can be present without shifting dullness
- Massive ascites
- Adhesions of coils of intestine preventing the fluid to shift.

4. Fluid Thrill (Fig. 5.12)
Fluid thrill usually signifies presence of massive ascites.

Technique of detection
- Ask the patient to lie flat on his back.
- Ask a bystander to keep the ulnar border of his hand in the center of patient's abdomen along the linea alba to prevent the transmission of vibrations through the abdominal wall fat.

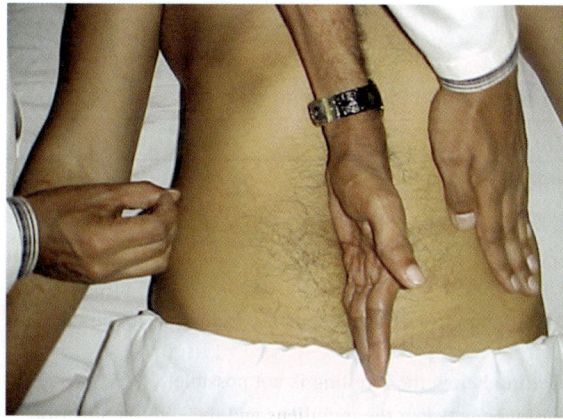

Fig. 5.12 Elicitation of fluid thrill

- Give a tap from one hand to one of the flanks while keeping the flat of the other hand over the opposite flank.
- Appreciate the thrill by the palpating hand when he tap is delivered.

Causes of Fluid Thrill other than Ascites
- Large ovarian cyst (Table 5.4)
- Large hydronephrosis
- Large hydatid cyst

Percussion of Liver

Upper Border
- Start percussing from the right 2nd intercostal space in the mid-clavicular line till dullness. Heavy percussion is beneficial.
- Normally upper border of liver dullness is at the level of 5th intercostal space.
- Liver dullness will extend down till the lower border.

Lower Border
- Percuss from the right iliac fossa upwards towards the costal margin till dullness with light percussion.

Liver Span
Vertical distance measured between upper most and lower most part of liver dullness.
   Normal liver span: Males 10–12 cm, females 8–11 cm.

Causes of Decrease of Liver Dullness
Acute
- Fulminant hepatic failure (massive liver cell necrosis)
- Air under the diaphragm, perforated hollow viscera in the abdomen.

Chronic
- Shrunken liver-cirrhosis
- In conditions like emphysema, right pneumothorax, liver dullness may decrease.
- In a condition called Chilaiditi syndrome (interposition of colon between the liver and diaphragm) liver dullness decreases.

Causes of Ascites

- Transudate
  - Cirrhosis of liver
  - Nephrotic syndrome
  - CCF
- Exudate
  - Pyogenic peritonitis
  - TB peritonitis
  - Peritoneal malignancy

Points Favoring Ascites

- Umbilicus is transversely stretched
- Flanks are dull to percuss
- Detection of shifting dullness
- Presence of fluid thrill.

Note: Ultrasound can detect as little as 100 ml of ascitic fluid.

Patients with ascites can have pleural effusion (predominantly right sided) due to the following mechanisms:

1. Movements of fluid through the diaphragm:
   - Through trans-diaphragmatic lymphatic channels.
   - Anatomic defects in the diaphragm.
2. Disorders associated with decrease serum albumin and decrease osmotic pressure with fluid leakage.
3. Lymph leakage from thoracic duct channels which are over burdened by ascitic fluid reabsorption.

Splenic Dullness

Significance of splenic dullness

1. Splenic dullness detection helps in the diagnosis of splenomegaly before becoming palpable.
2. Alerts the examiner, the site where the spleen may be palpable.
3. Presence of increase in the area of splenic dullness over the left flank may suggest splenic enlargement in suspected cases of splenomegaly.
4. Splenic dulness increases in patients with traumatic rupture and subscapular hematoma of spleen.

Method of Detection of Splenic Dullness

- Keep the patient in the right lateral position.
- Start percussing from the lower part of left lung resonance in the posterior axillary line.
- Percuss towards the left costal margin.
- Splenomegaly: Area of dullness of more than 8 cms.

Note: Splenic dullness extends from 10th rib posteriorly from mid-axillary line to the anterior chest.

Auscultation

Normal Bowel Sounds

- Auscultate in one area constantly for minimum of one minute (may be at the right of umbilicus).
- Peristaltic sounds may appear every 5 secs or every 10 secs in a normal individual.

Table 5.4 Differentiating features between ascites and large ovarian cyst

Ascites (Fig. 5.13)	Large ovarian cyst (Fig. 5.14)
Umbilicus is :	**Umbilicus is :**
Transversely stretched	Pushed upwards and may be vertical
Dullness: Flanks are dull	Dullness: Flanks are resonant
Upper border of dullness will have concavity upwards	Upper border of dullness will have convexity upwards
Distance between the umbilicus and anterior superior iliac spine on either side is equal	Maximum girth of the abdomen is below the umbilicus
	Getting below the swelling is not possible
	Distance between the umbilicus and the anterior superior iliac spine on either side is unequal

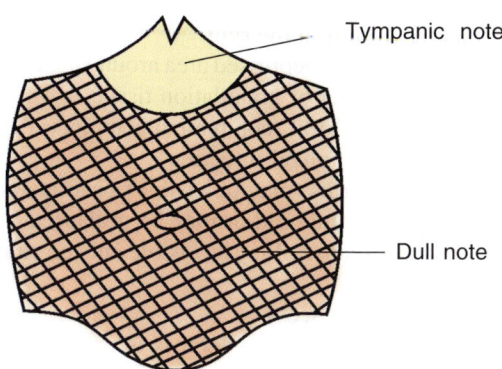

Fig. 5.13 Massive ascites

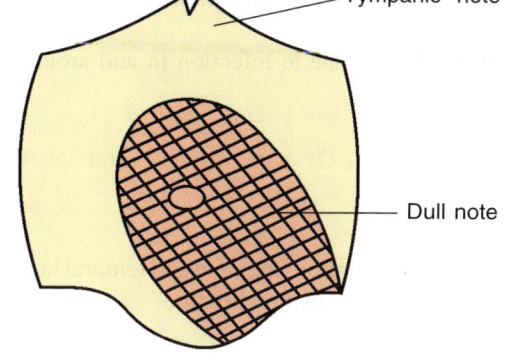

Fig. 5.14 Large ovarian cyst

- Minimum of 3–5 minutes of auscultation is required to confirm that peristaltic sounds are absent.

Increased Intensity of Bowel Sounds

Causes
- Massive bleeding into the gastrointestinal tract with rapid intestinal transit of blood.
- Malabsorption syndrome
- Early and acute intestinal obstruction
- Carcinoid syndrome

Intestinal Obstruction

- Bowel sounds become greatly exaggerated (Borborygmi) and sounds may have high pitched twinkling quality.
- Absence of peristalsis sounds
  - Late stages of intestinal obstruction
  - Peritonitis
  - Drugs - anticholinergics

Succussion Splash

- Place the hands over the lower ribs and shake the patient quickly from side to side.
- A splashing sound is palpable or auscultated over the abdomen.
- Normally succussion splash may be present up to 2 hours after a main meal.
- Succussion splash heard 4 hours after meal suggests delayed gastric emptying.

Causes of succussion splash over the abdomen
For example, pyloric obstruction, paralytic ileus and autonomic neuropathy.

Vascular Sounds

- ***Arterial bruits:*** Sounds produced due to the turbulence of blood flow occurring through narrowed or compressed blood vessel during systole.
- ***Aortic bruit:*** Auscultated just above and to the left of umbilicus.
- ***Renal bruit:*** Can be auscultated on either side of umbilicus. May also over the renal areas posteriorly.
- ***Liver bruit:*** Heard in cases of alcoholic hepatitis, hepatoma, hepatic artery aneurysm.
- ***Venous hum:*** Usually heard in patients with portal hypertension.
  Site
  - Between xiphisternum and umbilicus and increases on inspiration.
  - Due to the turbulence in the well developed collateral circulation (like opening of umbilical vein).

Friction Sound (rubs)

Conditions associated with hepatic rub
- Perihepatitis
- Hepatocellular carcinoma
- After liver biopsy (transiently)

Conditions associated with splenic rub

- Splenic infarction
- Peri splenitis due to infection in and around the spleen.

EXAMINATION OF INGUINAL REGION AND GENITALIA

Males

- Look for herniation (Inguinal and femoral herniae)
- Swelling in the inguinal region

Causes

- Inguinal lymphnodes
- Hydrocele
- Varicocoele
- Orchitis
- Epidydymitis
- Testicular mass

EXAMINATION OF ANAL CANAL AND RECTUM

Pre requisites

- Proper explanation of the procedure to the patient.
- Adequate lighting facilities should be available.

Note: Per rectal examination can cause discomfort to the patient but usually not painful.

Positioning of the patient

- Left lateral
- Buttocks at the edge of the examining couch.
- Perineum should be clearly visible (knees are flexed upwards with heels away from the perineum)

Finger used

Index finger of the examining hand (adequately lubricate the gloved fingers).

External Examination of the Anal Canal

Check for the following abnormalities

- Ulcerations, e.g. TB, syphilis, etc.
- Pilonidal sinus
  - Located in the natal cleft (mid line posteriorly)
  - Hairs may be surrounding the sinus

- Anal fissure - Separate the anal ring-look for a tear or a split in the ring.
- Anal fistula - Depressed area around the anus with surround area of granulation tissue.
- Warts, e.g. Viral (condyloma acuminata)
- Infection - Fungal infection
- Thread worms (may be visible) - causes pruritis
- Piles - Thrombosed or may be prolapsed
- Rectal prolapse - May be visible only on straining.
- Abscess
  - Perianal abscess
  - Ischaeorectal - Tenderness is present between the anus and the ischeal abscess tuberosity.

Indications

General medical indications

- Fever of unknown origin
- Evaluation of bony pain and back ache
- Evaluation of blood loss and iron deficiency
- Evaluation of weight loss

Gastrointestinal disorders

- Evaluation of pain abdomen
- Evaluation of altered bowel habit
- All acute abdominal conditions

Urogenital disorders

- Prostatic disorders
- Obstructive uropathy
- Urinary disturbance
- Genital infections

Per Rectal Examination

- Position of the patient and prerequisites -same as for inspection of anal canal and rectum
- Introduce the index finger of the examining hand into the anal canal and rectum. Turn the finger all around and palpate all parts of the rectum.

Feel for the following structures while finger is in the anal canal

- Anal sphincter tone and tone of muscles.
- Ano rectal junction - Felt as a thick band of muscle
- Irregularity and ulceration in the anal canal

Following conditions produce severe pain and tenderness on per rectal examination
- Anal fissure
- Ulcers
- Thrombosed hemorrhoids

Feel for the following structures while the finger is in the rectum
- Ulcers, growth, feel for the narrowing (strictures) and polyps.
- Feel the lateral sides of the pelvis and check for the tenderness.
- Lateral wall tenderness may be suggestive of peritonitis.

P/R examination in a male
Check for
- Seminal vesicles
- Prostate gland
- Recto vesicle pouch

Seminal Vesicles
- Lie above the prostate - running upwards from its margins.
- Can be felt only if it is full.

Thickening of Seminal vesicles: May be suggestive of tuberculosis

Prostate
- Felt as firm swelling with smooth and regular surface.

- Malignancy of the prostate is felt as hard and irregular mass.

Prostatic massage: Smears are useful in diagnosis of prostatitis and malignancy of prostate.

Prostatic tenderness: Suggestive of prostatitis.

Rectovesical Pouch
- Tender swelling lying above the prostate suggests the presence of pelvic abscess.
- Hard nodules in the rectovesicle pouch suggest the presence of malignant deposits.

Note: Normally seminal vesicle and rectovesicle pouch are not palpable.

P/R Examination in a Female
Normal person: Cervix and retroverted uterus can be felt on the anterior wall of the rectum.

Tenderness on the lateral wall: It may be suggestive of salpingitis.

Abnormalities detectable in the retrouterine pouch (pouch of douglas)
- Uterine fibroid
- Malignant deposit
- Abscess in the pelvis
- Ovarian cyst

Withdraw the finger after per rectal examination and check the finger for
- Color of stool
- Presence of blood and mucus

Causes of Granulomatous Lesions in the Oral Cavity

- Tuberculosis
- Foreign bodies
- Leprosy
- Brucellosis
- Sarcoidosis
- Beryllium poisoning

DRY MOUTH (XEROSTOMIA)

Causes

1. Disorders of salivary gland - Sjögren's syndrome, sarcoidosis, mumps, salivary calculi
2. General medical disorders - Volume depletion, diarrhoea and vomiting, diabetes mellitus and diabetes insipidus
3. Irradiation of major salivary glands
4. Drug induced - Anticholinergics, tricyclic anti depressants
5. Psychogenic
6. Mouth breathing

HYPERSALIVATION (SIALORRHOEA)

Drooling of Saliva is Common in

- Infants
- Mentally retarded
- Facial palsy
- Neuromuscular incoordination of facial musculature.

True Hypersalivation

Causes

- Foreign body in the oral cavity

- Inflammatory lesions and ulcers in the oral cavity
- Rabies
- Anticholinesterase administration
- Heavy metal consumption
- Defective swallowing
- Parkinsonism
- Oesophageal obstruction
- Psychogenic

Several cases of hypersalivation can be treated with parotid duct transplanted into the pharynx, so that saliva directly enters into the pharynx. Similarly submandibular duct can also be implanted into the pharynx.

Swelling of the Salivary Glands

Causes

Infective/ Inflammatory disorders

- Bacterial infection of the salivary gland - sialadenitis.
- Viral parotitis, e.g. mumps
- Obstruction to the salivary duct
- Sarcoidosis
- Sjogren's syndrome

Metabolic/Endocrine disorders

- Diabetes mellitus
- Alcoholic liver disease
- Protein calorie malnutrition
- Acromegaly

Tumors of the salivary gland

- For example, mixed parotid tumor

Drug induced

- Iodides, phenylbutazone

Pigmentation of Oral Cavity

Causes

Endocrine/metabolic
- Addison's disease
- Ectopic ACTH syndrome
- Nelson's syndrome
- Hemochromatosis
- Malabsorption syndrome

Drug induced: Cytotoxic drugs
- For example, busulphan, antimalarials
- Metals: Lead, mercury, bismuth and silver

Neoplastic
- Melanosis secondary to metastatic carcinoma.
- Congenital-Peutz-Jegher's syndrome
- Racial hyperpigmentation.

Causes of Discoloration of Teeth

Local causes
- Trauma
- Caries tooth
- Resorption of teeth
- Poor oral hygiene
- Smoking

Drug induced
- Tetracycline therapy in childhood (Fig. 5.16)
- Iron therapy

General medical disorders
- Fluorosis

- Kernicterus
- Porphyria

Angular Stomatitis
Characterised by inflammation of angle of mouth.

Causes
- Oral candidiasis
- Staphylococcal infection
- Iron deficiency anemia
- B_{12} deficiency
- Denture-induced stomatitis

Hairy Leukoplakia
- Raised white areas of thickening on the lateral border of the tongue. Hairy surface is due to keratin projections.
- Hairy leukoplakia is supposed to be caused by Epstein Barr virus.
- It is a premalignant condition.
- It may be develop into squamous cell carcinoma.

DYSPHAGIA

Term indicates difficulty in swallowing.
Felt as a sensation of food sticking in the throat or chest while swallowing.

Causes of Dysphagia
1. Painful lesions of mouth, throat and oesophagus, e.g. ulcers, peritonsillar abscess.
2. Mechanical causes

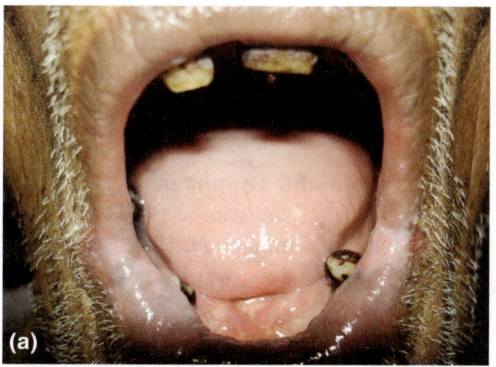
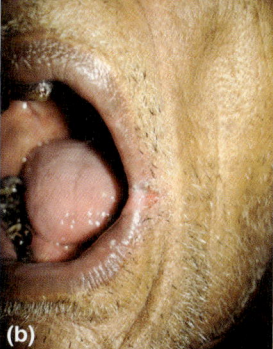

Fig. 5.15a and b (a) Glossitis (b) Stomatitis

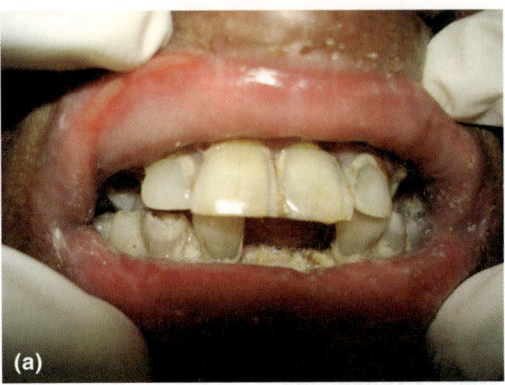 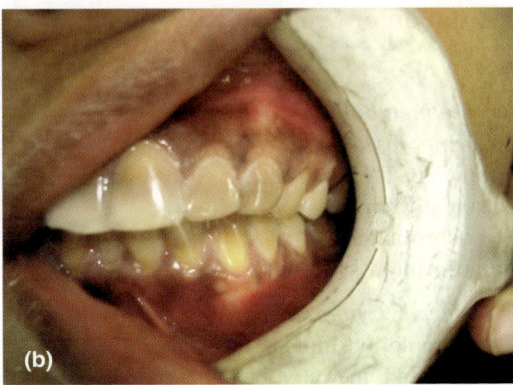

Figs 5.16a and b Tetracycline-induced stained teeth

- Neoplasm of oral cavity, pharynx and oesophagus
- Extrinsic compression of oesophagus
- Stricture of oesophagus
- Oesophageal webs:
  For example, post cricoid web in iron deficiency anemia.
3. Neuromuscular disorders
   - Bulbar and pseudobulbar palsy
   - Myasthenia gravis
   - Achalasia cardia
4. Miscellaneous
   - Globus hystericus

Approach to a Patient of Dysphagia

Following details are important in a patient of dysphagia.
1. Duration of dysphagia
2. Level at which dysphagia occurs (sensation of food sticking)
3. Intermittent/progressive
4. Associated with pain or painless
5. Type of dysphagia (for solids/liquids)
6. Associated symptoms of reflux

Types of Dysphagia

- Symptoms of dysphagia occurring immediately (1–2 sec) after food usually suggests pathology in the oral cavity or pharynx.
- Patients with difficulty in swallowing initially for liquids than solids associated with coughing suggests neurological cause for dysphagia.
- Dysphagia initially for solids and later both for solids and liquids suggests mechanical cause for dysphagia.
- In patients with long standing oesophageal obstruction food may be regurgitated long after it was taken.
- Achalasia cardia may cause initially intermittent dysphagia.

Level of Dysphagia

1. Dysphagia occurring at the level of cricoid cartilage may be due to growth, narrowing of oesophagus or even pharyngeal pouch.
2. Obstruction anywhere along the course of oesophagus may cause sensation of dysphagia at suprasternal notch.
3. Dysphagia occurring at the lower part of the oesophagus is usually due to disease of the lower oesophagus like growth, achalasia cardia or oesophagitis due to reflux disease.

Pain and Dysphagia

Severe pain can be felt at the site of narrowing due to food impaction. Regurgitation of food or passing of food downwards can relieve the pain.

Causes of Painful Dysphagia

For example, infective/inflammatory disorders of oral cavity, reflux oesophagitis.

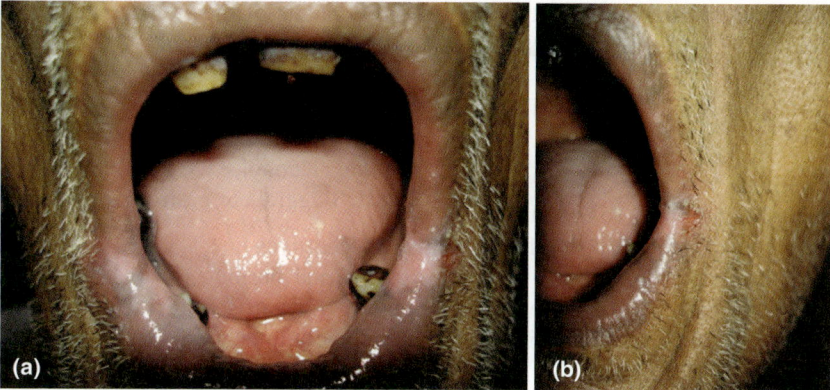

Figs 5.17a and b Angular chelitis

- Oesophageal pain may be due to muscle contraction above the level of obstruction to the oesophagus.
- Oesophageal pain may be retrosternal and may radiate to the neck and interscapular area.
- Lower oesophageal burning type of pain may be due to reflux oesophagitis.
- Occasionally painless dysphagia can be due to tumor invasion causing denervation.

Oropharyngeal Dysphagia
Symptoms of drooling of saliva, hoarseness of voice and dysarthria are common in patients with oropharyngeal dysphagia. There may be difficulty in initiating the act of swallowing and symptoms of nasal regurgitation and aspiration into the trachea are usually present.

Oesophageal Dysphagia
Person may complain of sticking of food at the level of obstruction. Person may have difficulty in swallowing of solids initially and then for liquids indicating mechanical obstruction.

Associated symptoms along with Dysphagia
- Malignant disorders with dysphagia cause severe weight loss.
- Lesion in the distal oesophagus may cause hiccups.
- Localised wheeze over the chest with dysphagia may indicate mediastinal mass.

- Esophageal obstruction, reflux oesophagitis and oesophageal spasm cause retrosternal chest pain.
- History of corrosive intake and radiation in a patient of dysphagia suggests oesophageal stricture.
- Painful swallowing indicates oesophagitis and can occur due to herpes simplex, NSAID intake, cytomegalovirus and candidiasis.
- Nasal regurgitation and aspiration into the lungs may be due to tracheo-oesophageal fistula/ pharyngeal paralysis.

Examination of a Patient of Dysphagia
- Look for swelling in the neck for thyroid enlargement and lymphadenopathy.
- Examine the oral cavity for evidence of pathological lesions.
- Look for evidence of 9th and 10th cranial nerve palsy and other neurological disorders.
- Rule out collagen vascular disease/ seleroderma which can cause dysphagia.
- Examine the respiratory system for evidence of aspiration pneumonia.
- Search for evidence of malignancy like lympha-denopathy and secondaries in the lung and liver.

Globus Hystericus
- Not a true form of dysphagia
- Person feels as though there is a foreign body or lump sticking in the throat.

- Person has no difficulty in swallowing or eating.
- There will be associated history of suppressed emotional feeling .
- Crying or emotional outbursts can relieve dysphagia.

Investigations of Dysphagia
- *Upper gastrointestinal endoscopy:* To detect the exact site and nature of obstruction. Biopsy of the lesion can also be performed.
- *Barium swallow:* Can detect the site of obstruction type of obstruction and motility disorder of oesophagus.
- *Oesophageal manometry:* Detects the oesophageal motility disorder.
- *Videofluroscopy of orophageal swallowing:* For oral causes of dysphagia.

Treatment
- Treatment of the cause

Dental aspects of Dysphagia
- Oral ulcers, viral infections in the oral cavity and tonsillitis commonly cause dysphagia.
- Carcinomatous ulcers of the tongue can occasionally cause dysphagia.
- Parapharyngeal abscess and Ludwing's angina can interfere with swallowing.
- Dry mouth and lower cranial nerve palsies should also be considered in patients with dysphagia.

REFLUX OESOPHAGITIS

- Gastro-oesophageal reflux develops due to the reflux of gastric contents into the oesophagus.
- Prolonged contact of lower part of oesophagus with gastric contents results in oesophagitis.

Factors Responsible for the Development of Reflux Oesophagitis
- Function of lower oesophageal sphincter becomes abnormal.
- Reflux oesophagitis is more common in patients with hiatus hernia.
- Defective peristaltic activity of oesophagus causes delayed oesophageal clearance.

- Acid contents of the stomach cause irritation of lower part of oesophagus.
- Increased intra-abdominal pressure and delayed gastric emptying can precipitate reflux oesophagitis.
- Smoking, alcohol, excess coffee consumption and NSAIDS aggravate gastrooesophageal reflux.

Clinical Features
- Retrosternal burning (heart burn) increasing on bending forwards especially after lying down immediately after food.
- Excess salivation (water brash)
- Oesophageal spasm can cause retrosternal chest pain.
- Nocturnal cough due to aspiration of oesophageal contents into the larynx.

Complications
- Benign oesophageal stricture
- Blood loss and anemia
- *Barrette's oesophagus:* Due to chronic oesophagitis normal squamous epithelium of lower part of oesophagus is replaced by columnar epithelium (premalignant condition). This is called Barrett's oesophagus.

Investigations
Upper gastrointestinal endoscopy, barium swallow oesophagus and oesophageal motility studies can demonstrate reflux oesophagitis.

Management
- Life style management
  - Loosing weight
  - Stoppage of smoking
  - Avoidance of alcohol
  - Avoid excess coffee consumption and NSAID intake.
  - Head end elevation while sleeping.
- H_2 receptor blockers
      T. Ranitidine-150 mg 1-0-1 × 4–6 weeks
                            or
- *Proton pump inhibitors:* T-Omeprazole 20 mg/day 4–6 weeks and if required for longer duration.

- Drug therapy may be required till symptoms subside/lifelong.
- *Barrette's oesophagus:* Surgical correction is required
- *Persistant oesophagitis:* Fundoplication surgical technique may be performed.

ORAL ULCERS

Causes of Oral Ulcers

Local Causes
- Burns
- Trauma
- Irritation by chemicals
- Recurrent aphthous ulcers
- Malignant ulcers

Systemic Causes

Blood disorders
- Deficiency anemias
- Leucopenia
- Leukemias

Gastrointestinal tract disorders
- Inflammatory bowel disease
- Malabsorption syndrome

Collagen diseases
- SLE
- Behcet's syndrome

Dermatological
- Lichen planus
- Pemphigus
- Erythema multiforme

Infections
- Viral infections
- Tuberculosis
- Syphilis

Drug induced
- Steven-Johnson syndrome due to cytotoxic drugs/antibiotics.

Miscellaneous
- Malignant ulcers
- Kaposi's sarcoma in HIV patients.

APHTHOUS ULCERS

Minor Aphthous Ulcers (Fig. 5.18a)
Characteristics
- Predominantly affects younger population (children and adolescents)
- Usually associated with positive family history.
- Recurrences and remissions are common.
- Invariably round or oval in shape and painful.
- Usually 2–4 mm in diameter, single or multiple with erythematous border and majority heal within 10 to 14 days.
- Minor aphthous ulcers are self limiting and ceases before middle age.
- *Sites:* Oral and labial mucosa, floor of the mouth, soft palate, lateral and ventral aspect of tongue.

Major Aphthous Ulcers (Fig. 5.18b)
Ulcers are of several centimeters, persists for years and heal with scarring.

HERPETIFORM APHTHOUS ULCERS
Multiple ulcerations with wide spread erythema.

Aetioloy of Aphthous Ulcers
- Exact cause not known
- Following factors are associated with aphthous ulceration:
  – There is a familial association
  – May appear during luteal phase of menstruation
  – Associated with stress and trauma.

Disorders associated with Recurrent Aphthous Ulcers
1. *Nutritional deficiency:* Iron, folic acid and vitamin B_{12}
2. *Inflammatory bowel disease:* Crohn's disease, ulcerative colitis
3. Behcet's syndrome
4 Cyclical neutropenia

Management
- Rule out primary disorders like deficiencies, stress, inflammatory bowel disease, blood

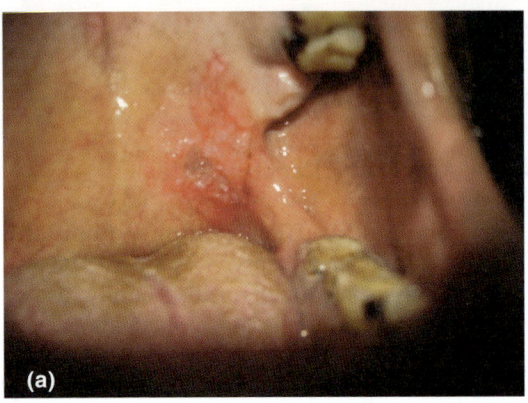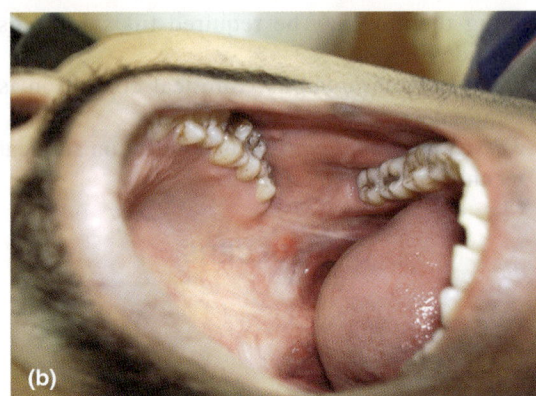

Fig. 5.18a and b (a) Major Apthous (b) Minor Apthous ulcers

dyscrasias before labelling as idiopathic aphthous ulcer.
* Rarely biopsy of the ulcer is required.
* May subside spontaneously.

Treatment

Mouth wash
* Chorhexidine gluconate (0.2%) keeps good oral hygiene and may decrease ulceration.

Symptomatic relief
* Lignocaine gel or solutions

Mouth washes
* Some patients respond to tetracycline or tetracycline with nystatin or amphotericin mouth washes.

Topical steroids
* Application of triamcinalone acetonide paste to the ulcer.
* Hydrocortisone hemisuccinate pellets (2.5 mg) dissolved in mouth, 4 times daily.
* *Oral corticosteroids:* Recurrent severe aphthous ulcers require oral tablets of prednisolone.

PEPTIC ULCER

Definition
* Peptic ulcer is defined as an ulcer in the lower part of oesophagus, stomach, duodenum, in the jejunum after surgical anastomoses to the stomach or rarely in the ileum adjacent to a Meckel's diverticulum.
* Peptic ulcer develops in or close to the acid secreting area.
* Peptic ulcer in the stomach is called gastric ulcer
* Peptic ulcer in the duodenum (proximal duodenum) is called duodenal ulcer
* Patients of gastric ulcer - Acid secretion normal
* Patients of duodenal ulcer - Hypersecretion of acid is present

Aetiology and Pathogenesis of Peptic Ulceration

Conditions promoting formation of peptic ulceration
* Stress
* Smoking
* *Genetic factors:* There is increased association between blood group 'O' and peptic ulcer. Peptic ulcers are common in first degree relatives of patients.
* Alcohol consumption
* *Drugs:* NSAIDS, corticosteroids.

Conditions Associated with Raised Gastrin Levels which can Manifest as Peptic Ulcer
Examples:
* Hyper-parathryroidism: Induces hypercalcemia inducing gastrin release.

- Zollinger Ellison syndrome: Gastrin producing tumor.
- Chronic renal failure: Poor gastrin metabolism.
- Infection with Helicobacter pylori: Helicobacter pylori infection can cause gastric ulcer, duodenal ulcer. It also has significant role in the development of gastric mucosal lymphoma and adenocarcinoma of the stomach.

Pathology

Gastric ulcers
- Benign gastric ulcers are found distal to the pyloric antrum
- Gastric ulcer can present as malignancy

Duodenal ulcers
- Occurs in the first part of the duodenum
- Ulcers are 1–6 cms in diameter and well demarcated with surrounding fibrosis.
- Duodenal ulcers rarely become malignant.

Features

Gastric ulcer
- Presents with epigastric pain
- Food may aggravate pain
- Vomiting may be associated

Duodenal ulcer
- Epigastric pain: Characteristic hunger pain (e.g. at 2 a.m.).
- Pain is relieved with antacids /food.
- Symptoms of epigastric fullness, nausea may also be present.

Peptic ulcer may present first time with complication like
- Hemorrhage
- Perforation of ulcer
- Pyloric obstruction
- Occasionally peptic ulcer can manifest as anemia due to chronic blood loss,

Investigations
- Upper gastrointestinal endoscopy can directly visualise the ulcer
- Biopsy of the ulcer
- Barium meal X-ray can demonstrate the ulcer

- Gastric acid studies and serum gastrin level may show abnormality.

Management
- Stop smoking
- Stop alcohol consumption

Drug Therapy of Peptic Ulcer
- H_2 receptor antagonists
  - Ranitidine 150 mg 1-0-1 or 300 mg/day
- Proton pump inhibitors
  - Omeprazole 20–40 mg/day or
  - Pantoprazole 40 mg/day
- Colloidal bismuth 125 mg 6th hrly
- Misoprostol 200 mg 6th hrly
- Sucralfate 2 g 12th hrly
- Antacids: Antacids are salts of calcium, magnesium and aluminium (dose: 30 ml 4 to 5 times a day)
  - Not used as first line of treatment of peptic ulcer
  - Used only as relief of dyspeptic symptoms

Treatment of Helicobacter pylori if required
T. Omeprazole 20 mg 1-0-l × (7 days)

\+

T.Clarithromycin 500 mg 1-0-l × (7 days)

\+

T. Metronidazole 400 mg 1-1-1 × (7 days)

Duration of Therapy
Usual duration of therapy for peptic ulcer is 4 to 6 weeks. Some patients require maintenance therapy for a longer duration.

Complications of Peptic Ulcer
- Sudden intra abdominal hemorrhage
- Perforation of ulcer
- Pyloric obstruction
- Chronic blood loss
- Chronic gastric ulcers can become malignant
- All gastric ulcers - chronic should be biopsied

UPPER GASTROINTESTINAL BLEED

Bleeding from the upper gastrointestinal tract may be an acute emergency or may result in chronic blood loss.

Causes of Upper Gastrointestinal Bleeding

1. Erosive gastritis (NSAIDS/Alcohol-induced)
2. Oesophagitis
3. Peptic ulcer
4. Oesophageal varices
5. Mallory-Weiss tear
6. Malignancy of stomach/oesophagus

Approach to a Patient of Upper Gastrointestinal Bleed

- Enquire the history of taking non steroidal anti inflammatory drugs or alcohol.
- Enquire the history suggestive of liver disease for evidence of portal hypertension and oesophageal variceal bleed.
- There will be history of hemetemesis (vomiting of blood), may be bright red or black (coffee ground)
- History of syncope may be present due to hypotension
- History of fatiguability, loss of appetite may be associated with carcinoma stomach.
- Presence of malena - Passing black tarry stool indicates upper GI bleed.
- Chronic blood loss causes anemia causing easy fatiguability.
- History of bleeding from multiple extra gastrointestinal sites indicate bleeding disorder as a cause for upper GI bleed.
- Clinical examination may reveal low volume pulse, pallor, hypotension in patients with severe blood loss.
- Signs of coexisting diseases like cirrhosis of liver, portal hypertension, peptic ulcer,
- Carcinoma stomach, bleeding disorders may be present or upper abdominal mass/ multiple bleeding spots respectively.

Investigations

1. Hb%, packed cell volume to detect severity of blood loss
2. Bleeding time, prothrombin time and platelet count to detect bleeding and clotting abnormality.
3. Renal, liver function tests for renal, hepatic dysfunction causing bleed.

4. Upper GI endoscopy to defect the site and cause of bleed.
5. Ultrasound abdomen for evidence of liver disease and abdominal malignancy.

Management

- Monitoring of pulse, blood pressure and respiration
- Correction of blood loss with intravenous fluid and blood transfusion.
- Stoppage of NSAIDS
- Injectable proton pump inhibitors.
- IV Somatostatin or Octreotide
- Treatment of the cause

MALABSORPTION SYNDROME

Malabsorption syndrome consists of group of disorders which result in defective absorption of nutrients.

Causes and Classification of Malabsorption Syndromes

1. Disorders associated with impaired digestion:
   - Chronic pancreatitis and chronic diseases of pancreas including carcinoma
   - Postgastrectomy
   - Gastrinoma
2. Disorders associated with impaired micelle formation
   - Parenchymal and cholestatic liver disease.
   - Small intestinal bacterial over growth.
   - Ileal resection, Crohn's disease
   - Drugs like neomycin.
3. Impaired mucosal absorption
   - Tropical sprue
   - Coeliac disease
   - Crohn's disease
   - Amylodosis
   - Whipple's disease
   - Lymphoma
   - Vit B_{12} and Folate deficiency
   - Genetic disorders like disaccharidase deficiency.
4. Impaired nutrient delivery to/from intestine:
   - Lymphatic obstruction, e.g lymphoma
   - CCF
   - Vasculitis

5. Endocrine and metabolic disorders
   – Hyperthyroidism
   – Diabetes mellitus
   – Carcinoid syndrome.

Clinical Features of Malabsorption
Symptoms
- *Diarrhea:* May be watery and voluminous.
- *Steatorrhea:* Pale bulky, foul smelling stool floating on the toilet (due to fat malabsorption)
- Abdominal distention and crampy abdominal pain.
- Weight loss
- Lethargy and depression

Signs
- Due to nutritional deficiency
   – Iron and folic acid and vit. B_{12} deficiency results in anemia, glossitis and angular stomatitis
   – Vitamin A deficiency results in night blindness
   – Vitamin C and K deficiency causes purpura, bruising and bleeding gum and poor wound healing
   – Hypocalcemia and hypomagnesemia causing tetany.
- Clubbing
- Peripheral neuropathy (due to vit. B_{12} deficiency)
- Edema (due to hypoalbuminemia)
- Muscle wasting (protein deficiency)
- Bone pain, osteomalacia and proximal myopathy (due to vit. D deficiency)
- Clinical features of primary diseases like hyperthyroidism, celiac disease, etc.

Investigations
1. Evaluation of anemia-serum iron, folic acid and vit. B_{12} level.
2. Serum albumin, calcium and magnesium level are decreased
3. Prolonged prothrombin time
4. Renal and liver function tests for abnormalities
5. Barium studies to know the intestinal pathology
6. Pancreatic function tests
7. Duodenal and jejunal biopsy
8. Ultrasound/CT scan abdomen for lesions like lymphoma
9. 14C-triolein breath tests for protein malabsorption

Treatment
- Supplementation of vitamins
- Supplementation of minerals
- Supplementation of calories and proteins
- Treatment of the cause

Coeliac Disease (Gluten sensitive enteropathy)
- Coeliac disease occurs due to toxic reaction of small intestinal mucosa due to the consumption of protein called gluten present in wheat, barely and oats.
- Inflammation of the intestinal mucosa occurs due to immunological response to the intake of gluten. Gliadin component of gluten leads to the formation of antigliadin antibodies leading on to immunological destruction of intestinal mucosa.
- Coeliac disease is genetically determined and can be associated with other immunologically mediated disorders.

Clinical Features
- May start at any age
- There will be destruction of villi of small intestine with inflammatory reaction.
- Diarrhoea, steatorrhea and abdominal pain develops after consumption of gluten.
- Growth retardation in children.
- Symptoms and signs of nutritional deficiencies.
- Symptoms of dyspepsia, bloating sensation in the abdomen and oral ulceration is usually present

Investigations
- Evaluation of nutritional deficiencies.
- Duodenal and jejunal biopsy to demonstrate villous atrophy.
- Detection of antigliadin and antiendomysial antibodies

Management
- Avoid gluten containing diet.
- Correction of nutritional deficiencies.
- Rarely they may develop lymphoma or gastrointestinal malignancy.

- If refractory—Corticosteroids/immune suppression is beneficial.

Dental Aspects
- Coeliac disease is usually associated with recurrent aphthous ulcers, angular stomatitis and burning mouth.
- In early age it interferes with growth and can cause enamel dysfunction.

Tropical Sprue

Persons from, in and around tropics are having malabsorption and is associated with small intestinal structural and functional abnormalities.

Disease is associated with partial villous atrophy of the small intestine.

Aetiology
- May occur after gastrointestinal infection
- Bacterial overgrowth due to *Klebsiella*, *E.coli* and *Enterobacter* are usually associated with tropical sprue. Folic acid deficiency may also be responsible for the features of tropical sprue.

Clinical features
- Diarrhea and abdominal distention
- Weight loss, loss of appetite and fatigue.
- Recurrent exacerbation and remission of symptoms
- Features of megaloblastic anemia due to folic acid deficiency.
- Occurrence of glossitis and stomatitis.

Management
- Tetracycline 250 mg 1-1-1-1 × 4wks.
- Folic acid 5 mg/day

Dermatitis Herpetiformis

- Chronic skin disease related to coeliac disease.
- There will be severely itching papulovesicular eruptions (blisters) over the extensor surfaces of back and limbs.
- Characterised by IgA deposition at dermo-epidermal junction.
- Jejunal biopsy demonstrates partial villous atrophy.

- Disorder usually responds to gluten free diet and occasionally requires dapsone therapy.

Dental Aspects
- Oral lesions like erythematous, vesicular and purpuric lesions can occur.
- Oral lesions respond to dapsone or sulfapyridine
- Dermatitis herpetiformis can rarely be associated with intestinal cancer.

DISEASES OF THE LIVER

Diseases of the liver can have following general effects on the body function
1. Impaired drug detoxification
2. Occurence of bleeding tendencies
3. Transmission of viral hepatitis to the treating doctor.

Figure 5.19 shows hepatobiliary and pancreatic system.

Metabolism of Bilirubin

Physiology of Bilirubin Metabolism

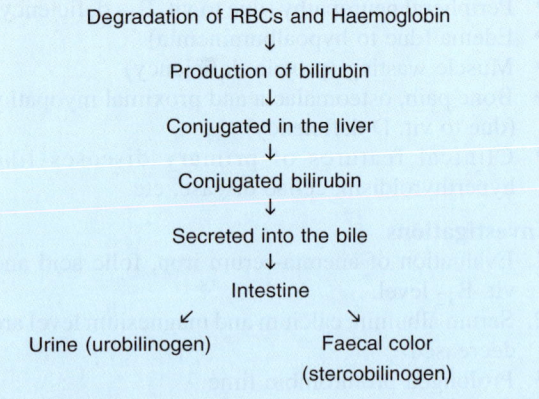

Degradation of RBCs and Haemoglobin
↓
Production of bilirubin
↓
Conjugated in the liver
↓
Conjugated bilirubin
↓
Secreted into the bile
↓
Intestine
↙   ↘
Urine (urobilinogen)   Faecal color
                    (stercobilinogen)

Abnormalities of Bilirubin Metabolism

Unconjugated Bilirubin (indirect) Increase
Causes
- Due to enzyme defect in the liver, e.g. Gilbert's syndrome

- Hemolytic anemias
- Ineffective erythropoesis

Conjugated Bilirubin (direct) Increase

Causes
- Biliary obstruction, e.g. biliary calculus
- Parenchymal liver disease, e.g. viral hepatitis
   Unconjugated or conjugated bilirubin increase leads to increase concentration of bilirubin in plasma results in the appearance of jaundice.

Classification and Causes of Jaundice
See general physical examination

Obstructive jaundice

- In obstructive jaundice, there is obstruction to the flow of bile from the gall bladder to the intestine. Obstruction may be inside the liver (intrahepatic) or outside the liver (extrahepatic). Bilirubin is not reaching the intestine. Faeces is not colored and stool becomes clay colored.
- There is increased level of conjugated bilirubin in the circulation. Conjugated bilirubin is water soluble and will be excreted in the urine and urine becomes high colored. In patients with obstructive jaundice concentration of bile salt increases in the circulation causing itching.

Note
- Unconjugated bilirubin is not water soluble and will not be excreted in urine. Urine is not colored (acholuric jaundice).

Impaired Drug Metabolism in Liver Disease
- Analgesics, sedative hypnotics and general anaesthetics - action is potentiated in liver disease and they can precipitate hepatic encephalopathy.
- Sedative hypnotics and NSAIDS should be avoided in patients with liver disease.

Plasma Proteins and Coagulation Factors in Liver Disease
- Serum albumin synthesis is decreased in the presence of chronic liver disease.
- There will be impaired absorption of vitamin K in patients with obstructive jaundice and formation of prothrombin is affected. In patients with

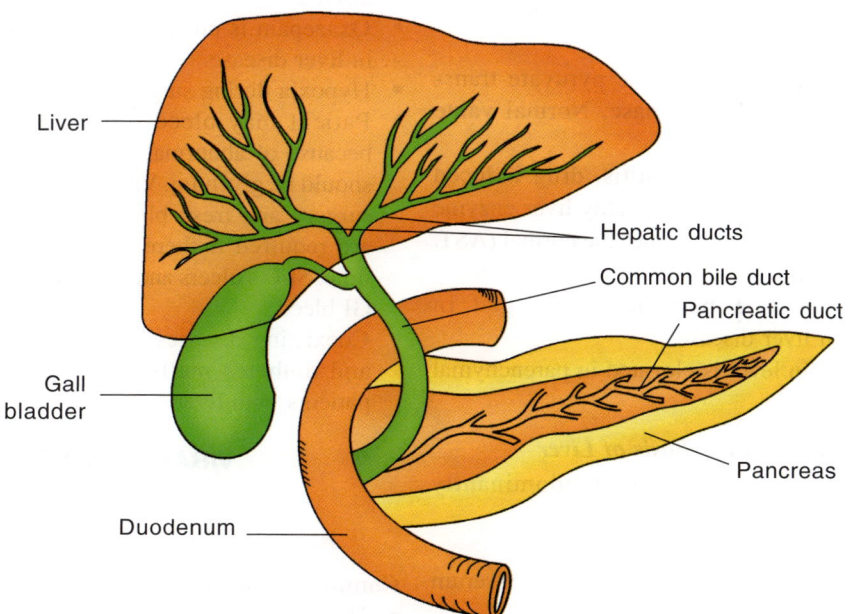

Liver

Hepatic ducts

Common bile duct

Pancreatic duct

Gall bladder

Pancreas

Duodenum

Fig. 5.19 Hepatobiliary and pancreatic system

parenchymal liver disease prothrombin synthesis is affected with prolongation of prothrombin time causing tendency for bleeding.

Portal Hypertension
- Portal vein is formed by the joining of splenic vein and superior mesenteric vein draining blood from the intestine to the liver.
- Cirrhosis of liver will cause impaired portal venous blood flow causing increased portal vein pressure resulting portal hypertension (intra hepatic). Obstruction to the portal blood flow can occur outside the liver (extra hepatic portal hypertension).
- Portal hypertension results in formation of oesophageal varices which can bleed resulting in massive hemetemesis.
- Portal hypertension can also cause hemorrhoids.

Liner Function Test (LFT) Abnormalities in Liver Disease

Parenchymal liver disease
- *SGOT (AST):* Serum glutamic oxaloacetic transaminase - alanine transaminase. Normal value 0–40 IU/L
- *SGPT(ALT):* Serum glutamic pyruvate transaminase-aspartate transaminase. Normal value 0–40 IU/L
- In patients with viral hepatitis, drug induced hepatitis and ischemic hepatopathy liver enzyme increases by more than 10 times the normal (AST, ALT > 10 times).
- Prothrombin time becomes prolonged in parenchymal liver disease.
- Direct bilirubin level is elevated in parenchymal liver disease.

LFT Abnormalities in Cirrhosis of Liver
- Bilirubin level is increased (predominantly conjugated)
- Minimal increase of AST and AST
- Decrease of serum albumin and increase of serum globulin (reversal of A:G ratio)
- Prothrombin time becomes prolonged

LFT Abnormalities in Obstructive Jaundice
- Direct bilirubin is increased.
- Significant increase in the level of alkaline phosphatase
- SGOT, SGPT and serum albumin levels are usually not affected.
- Alcoholic hepatitis AST (SGOT) is elevated more than ALT (SGPT) in the ratio of 2:1.

Dental Aspects of Parenchymal Liver Disease

Following drugs should be avoided in patients with liver disease
- NSAIDS
- Sedative hypnotics
- Anticoagulants
- Tetracycline
- Erythromycin
- Chlorpromazine
- Opiates and suxamethonium

Surgery in Patients with Liver Disease
- General anesthesia is not well tolerated in liver disease
- Oxazepam is preferred to other benzodiazepines in liver disease.
- Hypoxia during surgery should be avoided
- Patient may bleed profusely during surgery because of abnormal prothrombin time. Patient should be given Inj. Vit K 10 mg for 3 days before surgery and fresh blood or fresh frozen plasma are required if there is prolonged prothrombin time. Stress ulcers and varies can also cause upper GI bleed.
- Coexisting diseases like alcoholism, hepatitis B and diabetes mellitus require proper care in patients with liver disease.

VIRAL HEPATITIS

Causes of Viral Hepatitis

Common Causes (Hepatotrophic viruses)
- Hepatitis A
- Hepatitis B

- Hepatitis C
- Hepatitis D
- Hepatitis E

Rarer Causes

- Cytomegalovirus virus
- Coxsackie virus
- Yellow fever virus
- Epstein-Barr virus
- Herpes Simplex virus

Hepatitis A and E are transmitted through faeco - oral route.

Hepatitis B, C and D are transmitted through parenteral route. For example, Injections, needle sharing, sexual route and blood or blood product transfusion.

Hepatitis B (Serum hepatitis)

Aetiological agent

Hepatitis B virus- DNA virus

Route of Transmission

Parenteral

- Injections, needles
- Sexual (especially male homosexuals)
- Blood/blood product transfusion
- Perinatal

Incubation Period

30 to 180 days (60 to 90 days)

Clinical Features

Prodromal (pre icteric phase) up to 1 week

- Fever
- Nausea, vomiting
- Severe loss of appetite
- Bodyache
- Rash, arthralgia
- Muscle pain
- Jaundice

Icteric phase

- Appearance of jaundice at the end of 1 week
- High colored urine
- Clay colored stools

- Itching
- Enlarged tender liver
- High colored urine, clay colored stools, itching are due to intrahepatic cholestasis
- Most of the patients of viral hepatitis recover within in 2–4 weeks.

Investigations

- Serum bilirubin is increased (direct > indirect)
- Serum AST and ALT increased (> 10 times)
- Prothrombin time may be prolonged
- Urine contains bile salts and bile pigments
- Ultrasound abdomen reveals enlarged liver.

Serological Markers of Hepatitis B Infection

Hepatitis B surface antigen (Australia antigen - HBsAg)

- Transiently found in acute hepatitis B
- Persists in chronic infection
- Persists in hepatitis B carriers
- HBsAg appears 1–20 days after acute hepatitis B and disappears usually after 6 weeks.

Anti HBs Antibody

- Develops after about 6 weeks of appearance of jaundice (then HBsAg disappears).
- Persists for many years.
- Presence of anti HBs Antibody and absence of HBsAg suggests complete recovery and immunity
- Hepatitis B vaccine elicits anti HBs antibody response.

Hepatitis B Core Antibody (Anti HBcAb)

- IgM anti HBcAb develops and persists for about 3 months, indicates recent viral hepatitis B.
- IgG anti HBcAb indicates past viral hepatitis B infection. This antibody is absent in patients with hepatitis B vaccination.

Hepatitis Be Antigen (HBeAg)

- Presence of HBcAg indicates active disease and high infectivity. If it remains for more than 4 weeks there is more likely chance of liver disease.

Anti hepatitis Be Antibody (Anti HBeAb)

- Presence of anti HBeAg indicates complete recovery and loss of infectivity.

Complication of Viral Hepatitis B
- Chronic hepatitis, cirrhosis of liver
- Hepatocellular carcinoma
- Polyarteritis nodosa (30% can have HBsAg positive)
- Nephrotic syndrome
- HBsAg carrier state

HBsAg Carrier State
- Usually develops in patients with anicteric (without jaundice) hepatitis.
- HBsAg carriers may remain asymptomatic or can progress to chronic liver disease.
- HBsAg carrier state can persists up to 20 years.

High Risk Groups for Hepatitis B Transmission
- Persons receiving recurrent blood transfusion/ blood products, e.g. haemophiliacs.
- Homosexuals, IV drug abusers
- Immune suppressed individuals
- Medical, dental, paramedical and lab workers
- Tattooing and needle sharing.

Management of Hepatitis B
- Absolute bed rest
- High carbohydrate diet
- Avoid hepatotoxic drugs and alcohol
- For itching - antihistamines
- Anti viral drugs like vidarabine

Dental Management of Hepatitis B

Source of Hepatitis B in Dental Surgeons
1. Patient's saliva contains hepatitis B virus and may be a source of infection.
2. Blood, plasma and serum of the patients are infective 0.0000001 ml of HBsAg positive serum can transmit hepatitis B.
3. Needle stick injuries and human bites can transmit hepatitis B

Post-exposure Prophylaxis
If the person is not vaccinated against hepatitis B, sustains exposure to hepatitis B, person can be administered hepatitis B immunoglobulin and Hepatitis B vaccination for both active and passive immunization.

Risk of Infection in Dental Personnel
- Dental persons especially oral surgeons and periodontologists are at increased risk of contacting hepatitis B.
- Use of double gloves while treating high risk patients is beneficial.
- Hepatitis B vaccination for all dental staff will reduce the risk.

Risk of Transmission of Hepatitis B Infection to Patients
- Dentists who are HBsAg positive should wear double gloves, protective clothing while treating patients.
- Dentists who are having acute hepatitis should recover fully before treating patients.
- All persons who are HBsAg positive should be tested for HBeAg and if found positive for HBeAg, should not treat immunologically compromised patients and should take proper treatment.

Hepatitis B Vaccination
- Hepatitis B vaccination is recommended for all dental staff.
- Dose: 1 ml of vaccine IM at interval of 0, 1 and 6 months (to deltoid).
- No immediate side effect.
- Booster dose if required-after testing for anti HBsAb after 5 years.

Dental Management of a Patient with Jaundice and Viral Hepatitis
- If the person is jaundiced and if there is abnormal LFT, avoid operative procedure and consult a physician regarding management of dental treatment.
- If there is past history of jaundice try to establish the cause of jaundice and rule out hepatitis B, C or D.
- If the person is HBsAg positive, carefully do the procedure-wearing double gloves, mask and gown. Needle pricks should be avoided and needles must be disposed in non penetrable disposable containers. Syringes, masks, gloves are disposed off into a labeled plastic bag. If there is

spillage of blood disinfection can be carried out with 2% glutaraldehyde (cidex).

Acute Hepatitis A

Aetiological agent: Hepatitis A RNA virus
- Spread: faeco oral route, food borne
- Incubation period: 2–6 weeks

Clinical Features
- Clinical features are same as for hepatitis B. Rash and arthralgia are rare.
- Gives long standing immunity.
- Active and passive immunity can be obtained from vaccine and immunoglobulins respectively.
- Infection can be transmitted from oral surgeons to patients.
- Persons are infective till the appearance of jaundice.

Hepatitis C

Aetiological Agent: Hepatitis C RNA virus
- Transmission: Usually through blood transfusion/ IV drug abusers.
- Incubation period: 15 to 160 days.

Clinical Features
- Clinical features are same as that for hepatitis B.
- More likely to cause chronic liver disease and liver cancer.

Precautions
- Same as that for hepatitis B
- Active immunization not available

Management of patients who are Positive for HBsAg and HBeAg
- All dental staff should be vaccinated against hepatitis B.
- Persons with anti HBsAb should carry out treatment on patients with hepatitis B surface antigen positive.
- Persons who are HBsAg positive can also have HIV and hepatitis C positivity.
- Persons are asymptomatic but HBsAg positive (but negative for HBeAg) may not develop liver disease. If person is HBeAg positive, he should be treated with special facilities.
- Avoid dental treatment in persons who are having acute viral hepatitis. Virus is usually cleared within 3 months.

Precautions during Dental Treatment of Viral Hepatitis or HIV Positive Patients
- Treat the patient at the end of the session or day.
- Provide gloves, goggles, mask and gown to all dental staff.
- If the dental staff is having the skin wound cover it adequately.

Dental Equipments
- Cover the working area with plastic sheets or cling film.
- Use only disposable instruments
- Needle should not be bent, broken or removed from disposable syringes to present needle stick injuries

Dental Radiographs
- Take the intraoral radiograph with each film pack wrapped in a sealable plastic envelope before use.

Suction System
- Use a portable suction system and use metal container.

Dental Laboratory and Dental Impressions
- Take the dental impressions using silicone based material
- Dental lab should have the notice of the high risk patients.
- Dental impressions should be soaked in 2% glutaraldehyde for 1 hour, rinsed and then immersed in 2% glutaraldehyde for further 3 hours.

Sterilisation
- Needles and instruments are placed in a container which is labelled as infective and may be sterilised or incinerated
- Incinerate disposable instruments and dressings, etc.

Non Disposable Instruments
- Instruments which can be sterilised:

- First rinse it in hypochlorite (10%) or glutaraldehyde (2%) and sterilise immediately by autoclaving (134°C for 3 min) or hot air (160°C for 1 hour). Boiling instruments in a dental boiling water for 30 minutes is ineffective.

Non-disposable instruments and dental impressions which cannot be sterilised by heat
- Disinfect them by immersing for at least 1 hour (ideally overnight) in 2% glutaraldehyde.
- Remove the debris by washing in warm water and soak in glutaraldehyde for 3 hrs.

Disinfection of Working Areas
- Working areas are disinfected with 2% glutaraldehyde or hypochlorite 1%.

Spillage of Blood Over the Working Area
- Area should be thoroughly flooded with 2% glutaraldehyde (HBsAg remains stable in the blood for 6 months at room temperature).

Protection for Dental Staff
- Education about hepatitis B and HIV should be given to all dental staff.
- Prevent accidental cuts, injuries from instruments and needles.
- Protective clothing, surgical gown, gloves, masks, eye shield or spectacles should be used all the time throughout treating the patient, cleansing and during disinfection.
- *Injury to the skin by the instrument:* Rinse the area with water and consult the health authorities if the patient is HBsAg, Delta virus and HIV positive.

CHRONIC HEPATITIS

Definition
Chronic hepatitis is defined as a group of liver disorders characterised by inflammation and necrosis of the liver continuing for a minimum period of 6 months.

Aetiology
- Viral hepatitis B and D

- Viral hepatitis C
- Unknown viruses
- Autoimmune hepatitis
- Drug induced, e.g. methotrexate
- Cryptogenic

Features of Chronic Hepatitis

Chronic Persistent Hepatitis
Features
- Minimal evidence of hepatitis
- Fever, bodyache and loss of appetite
- Enlarged tender liver
- Minimal raise of liver enzymes.
- Liver biopsy will show evidence of hepatitis
- Completely recover or may progress to chronic active hepatitis

Chronic Active Hepatitis
Features
- Signs and symptoms of liver disease like fever, jaundice, edema, and signs of liver cell failure.
- Hepatosplenomegaly
- Raise in liver enzymes, decrease of albumin and prolonged prothrombin time.
- Usually progresses to cirrhosis and hepatoma.

Dental Aspects of Chronic Hepatitis
- Avoid hepatotoxic agents, aspirin and paracetamol
- Person may be HBsAg positive

Cirrhosis of Liver

Definition
Chronic parenchymal disease of the liver characterised by distortion of architecture, fibrosis, formation of regenerating nodules with vascular derangement.

Causes

Common causes
- Chronic alcohol consumption
- Hepatitis B and hepatitis C
- Biliary cirrhosis
- Cryptogenic
- Drugs like methotrexate
- Autoimmune diseases

Rare causes

- Cardiac cirrhosis
- Haemochomatosis
- Wilson's disease
- Alpha -1 antitrypsin deficiency

Clinical Features

- Middle aged/elderly
- Anorexia and weight loss.
- Signs of liver cell failure (see under clinical examination of liver in GIT-I) (Fig. 5.20)
- Hepatosplenomegaly
- Ascites
- Signs and symptoms of portal hypertension, hemetemesis, malena and splenomegaly

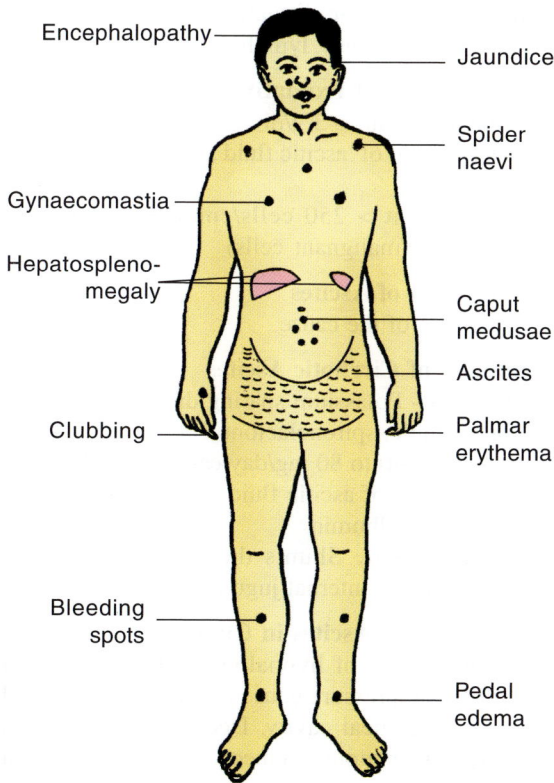

Fig. 5.20 Signs of liver cell failure

- *Alcoholics:* Parotid swellings and Dupuytrens contracture

Lab Investigations

- Minimal raise of liver enzymes and bilirubin
- Decrease of albumin and increase of globulin and reversal of A:G ratio.
- Prolonged prothrombin time

For Portal Hypertension

- *Ultrasound abdomen:* Detects coarse architecture of liver and nodularity, dilated portal vein and splenomegaly.
- *Upper GIT endoscopy:* For detection of oesophageal varices due to portal hypertension.

Tests for Aetiology of Cirrhosis

- Viral markers for hepatitis B and C
- Investigations for rarer causes
  - Serum copper, serum ceruloplasmin-for Wilson's disease
  - Serum iron profile for hemochromatosis
  - Alpha-1 antitrypsin level
- Liver biopsy for confirmation of cirrhosis

Complications of Cirrhosis

- Hepatic encephalopathy
- Upper gastrointestinal tract bleed due to rupture of oesophageal varices
- Spontaneous bacterial peritonitis
- Hepatocellular carcinoma
- Renal failure

Treatment of Cirrhosis

- Salt and fluid restriction
- Potassium sparing diuretics/frusemide
- Albumin infusion
- Treatment of the cause
- Liver transplantation
- Treatment of complications

Treatment of cirrhotic ascites (see above)

Dental Aspects of Cirrhosis

- There is increases tendency for bleeding during dental extraction
- Hepatotoxic drugs, NSAIDS to be avoided
- Person may be HBsAg/HCV positive

- Surgery under general anesthesia is hazardous and requires expert management.

Treatment of Portal Hypertension

Medical Therapy

β blockers and nitrates: Produce splanchnic vasoconstriction and decrease cardiac output with reduction of portal pressure.

For example, propranolol/nadalol, isosorbide mononitrate.

Surgical: Placement of portosystemic shunt, i.e. transjugular intrahepatic portosystemic shunt (TIPS).

Treatment of the Cause

In patients with extrahepatic portal hypertension, it can be cured with splenectomy.

In suitable patients liver transplantation can be done in cirrhotic patients.

Treatment of Acute Variceal Bleed

- IV Blood transfusion
- IV vasopressin/Octeoticle infusion
- Balloon tamponade of the oesophageal varices with Sengstaken - Black More tube.
- Endoscopic sclerotherapy of oesophageal varices.
- Surgical creation of porto-systemic shunt.

Ascites

Accumulation of free fluid in the peritoneal cavity is called ascites.

Causes

Transudative (Non infective/non inflammatory)
- Cirrhosis of liver
- Nephrotic syndrome
- CCF

Exudative (Infective / inflammatory / neoplastic)
- TB peritonitis
- Pyogenic peritonitis
- Malignancy of the peritoneum (carcinoma and lymphoma)
- Pancreatitis
- Collagen disease

Clinical Features
- Abdominal distention
- Fullness in the flanks
- Eversion of umbilicus
- Abdominal striae
- Divarication of rectii
- Shifting dullness
- Fluid thrill
- Right sided pleural effusion (if massive ascites)

Investigations
- Total WBC count and ESR is increased in infective and inflammatory disorders.
- Ultrasound abdomen to detect ascites
- Ascitic fluid tap and ascitic fluid analysis (for exudative and transudative causes)
- Laparoscopic examination of the abdomen and peritoneal biopsy for the aetiology.
- Investigations for exudative causes like tuberculosis, malignancy, lymphoma, pyogenic causes.

Characteristics of Exudative Ascites
- Protein content: > 3 g/dl
- LDH – Ratio of ascitic fluid LDH to serum LDH > 0. 6
- Cell content > 250 cells/cmm (lymphocytes/neutrophils/malignant cells)

Management of Ascites
- Treatment of the cause

Treatment of Cirrhotic Ascites
- Diuretics - Potassium sparing diuretic
  For example, spironolactone 100 to 400 mg/day
  Frusemide 40 to 80 mg/day can be added
- Paracentesis of ascitic fluid
- Infusion of albumin
- *Leveen shunt:* Shunts the ascitic fluid from peritoneum to internal jugular vein

Pathogenesis of Ascites in Cirrhosis
- Combinations of hypoalbuminemia, increased hydrostatic pressure cause accumulation of fluid in the peritoneal cavity. Decreased renal blood flow, renin angiotensin mechanism with retention of sodium and water also play role in the genesis of ascites.

- Infective, inflammatory and neoplastic disorders of the peritoneum cause exudation of fluid into the peritoneal cavity causing ascites.

HEPATIC ENCEPHALOPATHY

Definition
Neuropsychiatric syndrome caused by acute or chronic liver disease.

Aetiopathogenesis
- Liver failure and portosystemic shunting of blood are important factors in causing hepatic encephalopathy
- Ammonia, false neurotransmitters and disruption of blood brain barriers play important role in causing encephalopathy.

Precipitating Factors for Encephalopathy
- Sedative hypnotic intake
- Gastrointestinal bleed
- Hypokalemia
- Excess dietary protein intake
- Infection
- Trauma/surgery
- Renal failure
- Alcohol consumption

Clinical Features
- Altered sensorium/confusion/disorientation
- Inversion of sleep rhythm
- Personality changes
- Flapping tremor
- Fetor hepaticus
- Constructional apraxia
- Extensor plantar response
- Evidence of liver disease

Investigations
- Abnormal liver function tests
- Elevated serum ammonia level
- Characteristic EEGs changes with delta waves.

Management
- Remove precipitating factors.
- No protein intake orally

- Treatment of GI bleed.
- Syrup lactulose - 30 ml tid to induce minimum of 3 loose stools/day.
- Adequate calories and nutrition
- Correction of hypokalemia
- Neomycin 1 g QID orally to sterilise the gut
- Treatment of renal failure and sepsis
- Liver transplantation.

Drug Induced Liver Disease

Tetracycline in massive doses causes liver damage.

Erythromycin
Erythromycin stearate is not hepatotoxic. Erythromycin estolate is hepatotoxic (causes cholestasis) but effect is reversible when the drug is stopped.

Halothane: Can occasionally cause hepatitis

Aspirin
- Aspirin should not be given to children with viral fever as it may cause liver damage and encephalopathy (Reye's syndrome).

Paracetamol
- Large doses (5 g–10 g/day) can cause liver necrosis.

Drugs which can cause dose related liver damage
- Tetracyclines
- Paracetamol
- INH
- Methyldopa, anabolic steroids

Drugs which cause non dose related liver damage
- Halothane
- Sulphonamides
- Antithyroid drugs
- Diphenyl hydantoins
- Nitrofurantoin.

Inflammatory Bowel Disease

Ulcerative Colitis and Crohn's disease
Ulcerative colitis and Crohn's disease are chronic inflammatory diseases of the intestine with recurrent exacerbations and remissions.

Ulcerative Colitis

- Involves only the large intestine. Inflammation usually involves only the rectum (proctitis) or spreads to sigmoid colon (proctosigmoiditis) or may involve the whole of colon.
- Only the mucosa is involved with infiltration of acute and chronic inflammatory cells
- Dysplasia, nuclear atypia may suggest the possibility of malignant transformation.

Clinical Features

- Pain abdomen
- Fever, arthralgia
- Diarrhea, bleeding from GIT
- Clubbing
- Erythema nodosum

Investigations

- *Severe anemia:* Due to iron, folic acid and B_{12} deficiency as a result of gastrointestinal tract bleeding and malabsorption.
- ESR is significantly raised
- Stool culture to exclude infection.

Endoscopy

- Sigmoidoscopy and colonoscopy for evidence of inflammation and biopsy of the colon for the pathological diagnosis and for evidence of malignancy.
- Barium studies, plain radiographs, radionuclide scans and MRI may be required in the diagnosis and for detecting the complications.

Complications

- Severe inflammation of the colon with the development of toxic megacolon.
- Perforation of the colon.
- Severe hemorrhage
- Carcinoma colon

Treatment

- For severe colitis
  - Corticosteroids: Oral/parenteral/retention enema.
  - Tab: Prednisolone; 1 mg/day for 6 to 8 weeks.

- If recurrent relapses azathioprine therapy is recommended.
- For maintenance of remission
  - 5-Aminosalicylic acid is recommended.
- Supportive therapy:
  - Nutritional supplementation
  - Antibiotic for infections
- Surgical resection of colon in severe form of the disease
- Treatment of complications

Dental Aspects

- Inflammatory bowel disease can be associated with chronic oral ulceration, microabscess and glossitis.
- Corticosteroid therapy can cause oral candidiasis.

Crohn's Disease

- Inflammatory disease affecting whole of the gastrointestinal tract.
- Affects all parts of the intestine but predominantly ileocaecal region.
- All layers of the intestine is usually involved.

Pathology

- Ulceration, fissuring, fibrosis of the intestinal wall, chronic inflammation of the submucosa and non-caseating granulomas are predominant features.

Clinical Features

- Presents in identical manner to ulcerative colitis.
- Presence of mass per abdomen, intestinal obstruction, perianal disease and intestinal fistulae are common features of Crohn's disease.

Complications

- Intestinal obstruction
- Fistula of intestine
- Fissuring and abscess formation of intestine

Investigations

- Same as those for ulcerative colitis

Treatment

- Drug treatment is same as that of ulcerative colitis.
- Surgery is required for correction of complications.

Dental Aspects

- Increased incidence of oral ulceration, fissured tongue, cobblestone appearance of oral mucosa.
- Corticosteroid therapy can cause oral candidiasis.

DISEASES OF THE PANCREAS

Acute Pancreatitis

Causes

- Alcoholism
- Gallstone disease
- Hypercalcemia
- Hyperlipidemia
- Mumps
- Corticosteroids
- Trauma
- Idiopathic

Clinical Features

- Pain abdomen: Severe upper abdominal pain radiating to back
- Nausea and vomiting
- Epigastric tenderness
- Paralytic ileus
- Hypotension and shock
- Features of complication
- Acute pancreatitis causes damage to the pancreatic acini and liberation of enzymes causing fat necrosis in the peritoneum.

Complications

- *Intra-abdominal*
  - Pseudocyst formation
  - Pancreatic ascites
  - Pancreatic necrosis
  - Pancreatic abscess
- *Systemic*
  - Hypocalcaemia
  - Hyperbilirubinemia
  - Hyperglycemia
  - Shock
  - ARDS
- *Miscellaneous*
  - Upper gastrointestinal bleed
  - Obstructive jaundice

Investigations

- Raised levels of serum amylase and lipase
- Ultrasound abdomen for evidence of pancreatic pathology
- Serum calcium may be decreased, blood glucose may be increased.
- Serum triglycerides may be increased.
- Blood counts and ESR increase.

Treatment

- Relief of pain with analgesics
- Treatment of shock—IV fluids
- Nasogastric aspiration
- Injectable H_2 receptor/proton pump inhibitors
- Correction of hyperglycemia, hypocalcemia
- Treatment of complications.

Chronic Pancreatitis

Causes

- Same as that for acute pancreatitis
- Chronic pancreatitis causes chronic atrophy of pancreas.

Clinical Features

- Abdominal pain with recurrent exacerbations
- Malabsorption
- Diabetes mellitus

Investigations

- Raised blood glucose
- Ultrasound abdomen and endoscopy to visualize pancreatic pathology

Treatment

- Analgesics
- Treatment of diabetes mellitus.
- Oral administration of pancreatic enzymes
- Surgical treatment if required.

6

Central Nervous System

DISORDERS OF CENTRAL NERVOUS SYSTEM

Headache

Causes of Headache and Facial Pain

Local abnormalities of face and oral cavity:
- Sinusitis and pharyngitis
- Tumors of the paranasal sinuses
- Lesions of the neck
- Disorders of the eye
- Disease of the oral cavity and dental diseases.

Vascular Disorders
- Vascular lesions
- Migrainous headache
- Cluster head ache
- Temporal arteritis

Neurological Disorders
- Intracranial diseases
- Trigeminal neuralgia
- Post herpetic neuralgia
- Glossopharyngeal neuralgia
- Meningitis
- Disease of the skull
- Raised intracranial pressure

Physiological Disturbances
- Atypical facial pain
- Tension head ache

Miscellaneous
- General medical conditions, e.g. febrile states
- Referred pain from ear
- Trauma to the head / face
- Drug induced, e.g. nitrate therapy

Migraine

Migraine is a form of paroxysmal benign headache associated with nausea, vomiting and other symptoms of neurological dysfunction.

Features
- Recurrent headache
- Attacks decrease in intensity and frequency with increasing age.
- Spontaneous remissions are common.
- Attacks appear due to vasodilatation of extra cranial arteries.

Precipitating Factors for Migraine
- Hunger
- Sleep deprivation
- Depression
- Menstrual periods
- Red wine consumption
- Contraceptive pills
- Chocolate consumption

Pathophysiology of Migraine

Mechanisms proposed in the pathogenesis of migraine are following:
1. Genetic factors
   - Mutation in the chromosome 19 (related to calcium induced neurotransmitter release/ smooth muscle contraction).
   - Modification of DRD2 allele (D_2 dopamine receptor) increases the susceptibility to migraine.
2. Alteration in the cerebral blood flow
3. Activation of brainstem structures
4. Serotonin (5- HT tryptophan) plays a significant role.

5. Activation of sympathetic nervous system

6. Dopaminergic stimulation

Classical Migraine

- Headache is preceded by warning symptoms (aura)
- Headache is severe, usually unilateral (hemicrania) and lasts for hours to days.
- Headache is usually associated with photophobia, nausea and vomiting.

Aura - Usually lasts for 15 minutes.

Aura may be - visual - zigzag color lines and vision defect.

- Sensory - paraesthesia of contralateral face and limb
- Motor - weakness of contralateral limb
- Speech disturbance

Headache

- Throbbing type with facial pallor, photophobia and nausea.

Common Migraine

- Unilateral headache without preceding aura.

Migranous Neuralgia

- Pain around the eye with headache

Facial Migraine

- Affects lower half of face

Hemiplegic Migraine

- Rare, hemiparesis is more common than headache.

Ophthalmoplegic Migraine

- Pain behind the eye with impaired eye movement

Vertebrobasilar Migraine

- Presents with ataxia, vertigo, diplopia and occipital headache.
- Loss of consciousness at the onset can occur.

Complicated Migraine

- Migraine is complicated by neurological deficit.

Management

Non drug therapy

- Avoid precipitating factors
- Avoidance of stress

Drug therapy

Acute attack

Mild attack: NSAIDS, for example, aspirin/paracetamol

Severe attack:

- 5-HT agonists: Sumatryptan: available as oral, sublingual, subcutaneous or nasal spray

Dose

Oral

- Tabs: 50 to 100 mg
- Inj- 6 mg subcutaneous repeat dose after 1 hour may be required.

  Ergot derivatives: Oral tabs - 1 mg, ergotamine 1 mg + caffene 100 mg.

Oral/parenteral dopamine agonists, e.g. metoclopramide/prochlorperazine may be used along with the above therapy.

Prophylactic Medication

Indications

- Significant functional disability
- More than 3 attacks/ month

Drugs Used

- Propranalol 80–160 mg/day
- Pizotifen 1.5–3 mg/day
- Amitriptyline 10–50 mg at night
- Sodium valoproate 300–600 mg/day
- Prophylactic medications should be continued for minimum of 6 months and then gradually tapered and stopped.
- Taking contraceptive pills and smoking increases the risk of stroke in patients with migraine.

Cluster Headache (Migranous Neuralgia)

- Treatable vascular headache less common than migraine.
- Disorder results from activation of hypothalamic structures.
- Abnormal serotononergic transmission plays a role in the pathogenesis of cluster headache.

Features

- Localized pain around the eye, forehead, cheeks

and temporal areas. Males are affected more than females.

- Pain occurs usually in the early hours of the morning. Head ache lasts for 30 minutes to 2 hours. Clusters of attacks of head ache occur for weeks and then headache free intervals for months.
- Headache is usually associated with conjunctival ingestion, lacrimation (unilateral), nasal congestion and Horner's syndrome. Heavy smoking and consumption of alcohol precipitate headache.

Management
- Acute attack: Inj. sumatryptan (6 mg subcutaneous)/inhalation of 100% oxygen.

Prophylaxis
- Verapamil 80–120 mg 8th hlry
- Methysergide 4–10 mg × 3 months
- Corticosteroids
- Severe chronic attack: Lithium therapy (600 to 900 mg/day) is beneficial.

Tension Headache

- Common type of headache.
- Females are more affected than males. Headache may be episodic/chronic.
  Generalised, constant type of headache, feeling like a tight band like sensation around the head.
- Headache starts in the occipital region and radiates to the front.
- Headache is not associated with vomiting or photophobia.
- Pain is worse in the evening and may persist for few hours.
- Headache is supposed to be due to muscle spasm and is usually associated with anxiety and depression.

Treatment
- Reassurance and NSAIDs
- Physiotherapy for muscle contraction
- Amitryptaline 10–25 mg /day

Glossopharyngeal Neuralgia
- Less common than trigeminal neuralgia
- Pain is throbbing type affecting that ear

- Pain is triggered by swallowing and eating
- Carbamezapine is not as effective as for trigeminal neuralgia

Note: Occasionally glossopharyngeal neuralgia can be due to tumor in the jugular foramen.

Postherpetic Neuralgia
- Herpes zoster can be preceded by and accompanied by neuralgic pain. Pain may be present after the rash has subsided and may continue for a long time.
- Usually affects elderly persons and pain is of severe burning type.
- Carbamazapine and antitryptaline may help.

Trigeminal Neuralgia
- Age group involved: Middle aged and elderly
- Trigeminal neuralgia is a paroxysmal lancinating type of pain in the distribution of trigeminal nerve.

Pathogenesis
- Pain occurs due to stimulation of sensory (pain carrying) fibers of 5th cranial nerve due to the generation of action potentials.

Features
- Pain is confined to mandibular/maxillary division of Vth cranial nerve.
- Severe stabbing type of pain for few seconds. Recurrent attacks can occur. Pain is associated with spasm of muscles of face. This is called Tic douloureux.
- Stimulus applied to the trigger zones can produce pain.

Trigger Zones of Pain in Trigeminal Neuralgia
- Stimulus near alae nasi
- Gingival touching
- Tooth brushing
- Chewing

Signs
- Evidence for neurological deficit is usually absent.
  – Other causes like multiple sclerosis, posterior fossa tumors should be ruled out (may be associated with sensory loss over the face) in patients with trigeminal neuralgia

Management

1. Rule out secondary causes.
2. Spontaneous remissions are occasionally possible
3. Tab. Carbamezapine 100 mg 1-0-1 and then increase to 200–400 mg /day

Or

Tab. Phenytoin 100 mg 3 HS (at night)/day

Or

Tab. Gabapentin 300 mg to 900 mg/day. Long term medication is required

Pain will not subside when given at the time of attack.

Other Forms of Treatment

- Injection of alcohol or phenol into a peripheral branch of the trigeminal nerve.
- Percutaneous placing of a radio frequency lesion in the nerve near the Gasserian ganglion.
- Vascular decompression of the nerve.

PYOGENIC MENINGITIS

Acute infection of the meninges and subarachnoid space caused by pyogenic organisms.

Common Organisms Causing Pyogenic Meningitis

- Pneumococcal (*Streptococcus pneumoniae*)
- *Neisseria meningitides*
- *Hemophilus influenzae*
- *Listeria monocytogenes*
- Strepto/staphylococci
- Gram negative bacilli

Predisposing Factors for Pyogenic Meningitis

- Bacteremic illness, e.g. Pneumonia
- Spreading infection from the ear
- Skull fracture (maxillofacial injury with fracture of cribriform plate by ethmoid bone).

Pathology of Pyogenic Meningitis

- Pia Arachnoid layers will be covered with thin layer of pus
- May produce intracranial adhesions
- Can result in endarteritis obliterans causing neurological deficit
- Causes cerebral edema

Clinical Features

- Acute onset of fever, chills and rigors
- Headache, vomiting and convulsions
- Neck stiffness and kernig's sign
- Focal neurological deficit, e.g. hemiplegia and cranial nerve palsy
- Altered sensorium and coma
- Meningococcal meningitis can be associated with purpura.
- CT head scan to exclude cerebral abscess.

Investigations

- High WBC count with neutrophilia in the blood
- Blood culture and sensitivity may be positive for the organisms.
- CSF analysis
  - Pressure is raised
  - Protein is increased
  - Glucose is reduced (< 60% of blood glucose
  - Neutrophilia
  - CSF - Gram stain and culture sensitivity may be positive for the organism.
  - CSF - polymerase chain reaction to detect the organism. Antibiotic can be changed according to the culture and sensitivity of the organism in the CSF.
  - CT scan to exclude cerebral abscess.

Complications of Pyogenic Meningitis

- Septicemia : Meningococcemia can cause shock and death.
- Focal neurological deficit due to endarteritis: deafness, blindness cranial nerve palsy, hemiplegia
- Cerebral abscess
- Cerebral edema and effect
- Convulsions
- Mental retardation in children.

Treatment

Symptomatic

- For fever, headache
- Paracetamol
- Adequate hydration
- Treatment for cerebral edema: IV mannitol, hyperventilation

Specific Therapy

Empirical therapy: Not knowing the organism

- Inj. crystalline penicillin 2 to 4 g IV 6th hrly 7–10 days.

Or

- Inj. cefatoxime 2 g IV 6th hrly 7–10 days (4 times)

Or

- Inj. ceftriaxone 2 g 2 times × 7–10 days
- Associated conditions like pneumonia, suppurative otitis media to be treated.

Tuberculous Meningitis

Organism: *Mycobacterium tuberculosis*
Tuberculosis is common in developing countries. Tuberculosis has increased in incidence due to increased incidence of HIV infection.

Pathology

- Can occur after childhood primary infection
- May also be due to disseminated TB
- There is usually submeningeal caseous focus adjacent to CSF pathway
- Meninges will be infected with tubercles.

Clinical Features

Symptoms

- Low degree of fever
- Weight loss
- Headache, vomiting
- Altered sensorium
- Convulsions
- Symptoms of neurological deficit

Signs

- Altered conscious level
- Neck stiffness
- Cranial nerve palsy
- Focal neurological deficit, e.g. hemiplegia

Complications

- Tuberculoma presenting as intracranial space occupying lesion
- Obstructive hydrocephalus
- Basal meningitis causing cranial nerve palsy
- Endarterins can cause hemiplegia

Investigations

- ESR is increased
- CSF analysis
- Protein is increased
- Chloride is decreased
- Pressure is increased
- WBC count is increased with lymphocytosis.
- CSF may show fine clot (cob web) formation after 24 hours of collection due to high protein content.
- CSF should be examined for AFB and culture and sensitivity of tuberculous bacilli.
- CSF can be examined for PCR for mycobacterial DNA.
- CT/MRI can detect meningeal enhancement, tuberculoma (see Chapter 4 Section on tuberculosis) and obstructive hydrocephalus.

Treatment

- Anti TB drugs for 9 months (see Chapter 4 Section on tuberculosis)
- Corticosteroids, e.g. prednisolone-30 mg/day for 6 weeks.
- Anti cerebral edema measures
- Surgical treatment for obstructive hydrocephalus

CEREBRAL ABSCESS

Formation of an abscess in the brain may be due to

- Spread of infection may be directly from middle ear and paranasal sinuses
- From hematogenous spread: Lung abscess and infective endocarditis
- From penetrating head injury

Common Organisms causing Cerebral Abscess

- Streptococci
- Staphylococci
- Anaerobes
- Gram negative organisms e.g. Pseudomonas

Clinical Features

- Fever
- Headache, vomiting and convulsions
- Altered sensorium
- Focal neurological deficit, e.g. hemiplegia
- Evidence of septic focus, e.g. sinusitis middle ear disease /lung abscess or endocarditis

Investigations
- Total WBC count and ESR are increased
- Blood culture and sensitivity for the organism
- CT head scan may show ring enhancing lesion
- CSF analysis—hazardous can result in cerebral coning.
- Chest X-ray and Echocardiogram for pulmonary and cardiac lesions.

Management
- Anti cerebral edema measures, e.g. Inj. Mannitol (20%) - 100 ml
- Anti convulsants, e.g. phenytoin
- Antibiotics: Depending on the organism injectable for 2–3 weeks
- Surgical aspiration of the abscess
- Removal of source of infection like middle ear disease

   Brain abscess can manifest as space occupying lesion in the brain and should be treated with antibiotics and surgical aspiration.

Dental Aspects of Cerebral Abscess
Anaerobic infection in the periodontal pocket can cause brain abscess. Inhaled tooth fragments or materials used in dentistry can be aspirated into the lungs and can produce lung abscess which can metastasize to brain and can cause brain abscess.

CEREBROVASCULAR ACCIDENT (CVA)

Cerebrovascular accident (stroke) is defined as the neurological deficit caused by decreased blood supply to the brain.

Main Types of Cerebrovascular Accidents (CVA)
- Transient ischemic attack (TIA)
- Intracerebral hemorrhage
- Cerebral thrombosis
- Cerebral embolism
- Subarachnoid hemorrhage

Risk factors for CVA
Factors which are irreversible
- Elderly age
- Hereditary factors
- Previous history of stroke and myocardial infarction
- Male sex

Preventable and Modifiable Risk Factors of CVA
- Cigarette smoking
- Alcoholism
- Increased blood viscosity, e.g. polycythaemia
- Contraceptive pills
- Hypertension
- Hyperlipedemia
- Diabetes mellitus
- Cardiac disease (CCF, atrial fibrillation, endocarditis)

Common Features of CVA
- Headache, vomiting and loss of consciousness
- Weakness of one half of the body (hemiplegia)
- Loss of speech, upper motor neuron facial palsy
- Sensory loss and other cranial nerve dysfunction.

Transient Ischemic Attack (TIA)

- Ischemic neurological deficit recovering totally within 24 hours.
- Indicates transient decrease of blood flow to the brain; may be due to embolic occlusion of the cerebral vessel.
- TIA can occur due to the occlusion of carotid and vertebrobasilar system
- TIA is a warning symptom for the occurrence of major stroke.

Cerebral Hemorrhage
Most dangerous form of stroke.

Features
- Common in patients with hypertension and atherosclerosis
- Sudden onset of headache, vomiting and altered sensorium, usually occurs when the patient is active.
- Progressive neurological deficit, e.g. hemiplegia
- Carries bad prognosis
- Brain matter gets destroyed and cerebral edema can occur.

Cerebral Thrombosis

Features
- Hypertension and atherosclerosis are main risk factors
- Previous history of transient ischemic attack of the brain usually present.
- Gradual onset and progressive neurological deficit over 2–3 days.
- Death can occur within 7 days.

Cerebral Embolism
- Sudden onset of headache and neurological deficit
- May affect younger people
- There will be history suggestive of source of embolism like mitral valve disease with atrial fibrillation
- Rapid recovery/recurrent attack can occur

Subarachnoid Hemorrhage

Risk factors
- Hypertension
- Atherosclerosis
- Rupture of congenital berry aneurysm of artery of circle of Willis.
- Physical and emotional stress
  Blood from the ruptured aneurysm leaks into the subarachnoid space and then spreads into ventricles.

Clinical Features
- Can affect any age but berry aneurysms are common in young.
- Sudden onset of severe headache, neck stiffness progressing onto coma and death.
- Classical hemiplegia may be absent
- Carries poor prognosis if not intervened immediately and recurrences can occur
- Neurosurgical intervention may be required

Investigations of CVA
- Routine blood examination - blood counts, ESR, ANCA (antineutrophil cytoplasmic antibody), ANA (antinuclear antibody)
- Blood sugar, lipid profile
- ECG, chest X-ray, ECHO cardiogram

- Blood VDRL, ELISA for HIV
- CT scan, MRI brain and cerebral angiogram.

General Management of CVA
- Care of breathing
- Control of blood pressure
- Control of cerebral edema - by intravenous mannitol and frusemide dexamethasone.
- Urinary catheterisation and nasogastric feeding.
- Treatment of risk factors

Thromboembolic Stroke
- Embolic stroke: anticoagulation and antiplatelet drugs.
- Surgical intervention if required
- Physiotherapy to the affected part, speech therapy and rehabilitation

Dental Aspects of CVA
- Patient can have speech difficulty and communication difficulties.
- Drooling of saliva, bad oral hygiene may be present.
- Local anaesthesia with noradrenaline should be avoided in patients with hypertension.
- Opiates and barbiturates should be avoided in patients with stroke as they can cause hypotension and respiratory depression.

Dental Management may have Following Difficulties in Patients with CVA
- Bleeding due to anticoagulation
- Patient may be immobile
- Patient is usually having hypertension, diabetes mellitus and cardiac disease.

CRANIAL NERVES

Functions of Cranial Nerves
There are 12 pairs of cranial nerves with 12 cranial nerves on each side originating from the brain.

Olfactory Nerve
- Carries sense of smell
- Defect causes anosmia (loss of smell)
  Olfactory nerve damage occurs due to head injury/meningioma of brain.

Optic Nerve
- Responsible for vision
- Defect causes
  - Decrease of vision
  - Decrease field of vision
  - Decrease of color vision
  - Abnormal pupillary reactions.

Causes of 2nd nerve palsy
- Retrobulbar/optic neuritis
- Toxin induced

Oculomotor Nerve
- Supplies all extraocular muscles except superior oblique and lateral rectus muscles.
- Stimulation causes pupillary constriction

Paralysis of oculomotor nerve causes
- Ptosis (drooping of upper eyelid)
- Dilated pupil
- Lateral squint
- Diplopia (double vision on looking medially).

Trochlear Nerve
- Supplies superior oblique muscle
- Paralysis of trochlear nerve causes double vision on looking downwards and medially

Causes of 3rd, 4th and 6th nerve palsy
- Cavernous sinus thrombosis
- Diabetes mellitus

Trigeminal Nerve
- Parts of trigeminal nerve (Fig. 6.1).
  - *Ophthalmic division:* Sensory supply to the upper part of face.
  - *Maxillary division:* Sensory supply to the middle part of face.
  - *Mandibular division:* Sensory supply to the lower part of face.
  - Trigeminal nerve also supplies mucosa of oral cavity, nose, tympanic membrane and conjunctiva.
- *Motor part:* Mandibular division-supplies muscles of mastication.
- *Muscles of mastication:* Masseter, pterygoids, temporalis, anterior belly of digastric.

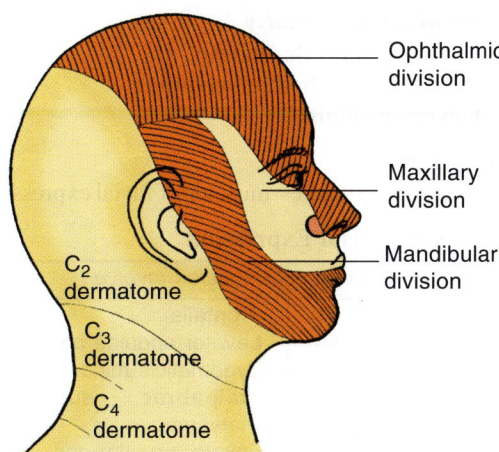

Fig. 6.1 Sensory supply of the face

Taste and Glandular Supply
- Taste from anterior 2/3 of tongue travel via lingual nerve (branch of trigeminal) to end up in chordatympani nerve (branch of facial nerve).
- Trigeminal nerve also carries secretomotor fibers to submandibular and lacrimal glands.

Damage to Sensory Division of Trigeminal Nerve results in
- Corneal anaesthesia of trigeminal nerve
- Loss of sensation over the face except over the angle of the mandible.

Taste sensation: Tested by putting different types of taste – like sweet, salt, sour and bitter substances over the tongue.

Causes of 5th Nerve Palsy
- Cerebellopontine angle tumor
- Infarction or demyelination of pons
- Meningioma of sensory ganglion of trigeminal nerve.

Abducens Nerve
- Supplies lateral rectus muscle
- Abducens nerve paralysis causes paralysis of lateral movement of eye.
- Diplopia occurs on looking laterally to the affected side
- Results in medial squint

Causes of 6th nerve palsy
- Cavernous sinus thrombosis
- Superior orbital fissure syndrome
- Diabetes mellitus

Facial Nerve
Motor supply: Supplies muscles of facial expression.

Muscles of Facial Expression

Facial expression	Muscles involved
Surprise/horror	Frontalis
Sorrow/seriousness	Levator angulae oris/
	Zygomaticis minor, Levator
	palpabrae superioris
	Platysma
Smiling	Levator angular oris
Langtring	Zygomaticus major
Expression of doubt	Mentalis
Grinning	Risorius
Superior	Frontalis
Sorrow/ seriousness	Levator angular oris,
	Zygomatic minor Levator
	palpabral superiors
	Platysma
Smiling	Levator angular oris
Laughing	Zygomatic major
Expression of doubt	Mentalis
Grinning	Risorius

Sensory and secretomotor fibres of facial nerve
- Ant 2/3 of tongue via chorda tympani carries taste sensation.
- Secretor motor fibers to submandibular, sublingual glands and to lacrimal glands
- Nerve to stapidius in the middle ear.

Features of Facial Palsy (Figs 6.2 and 6.3)
1. Absence of furrows over the forehead on the affected side - when the patient is asked to look upwards. Muscle tested - occipito frontalis (LMN facial palsy)
2. Inability to close the eye on the affected side. Eye ball appears to be rolling upwards (Bell's sign) (Fig. 6.2). Muscles tested: Orbicularis oculi (LMN facial palsy)
3. Obliteration of nasolabial fold on the affected side.
4. Rolling of tears over the cheek causes epiphora on the affected side.
5. Deviation of angle of mouth to the normal side on asking the patient to show the teeth (Fig. 6.3).
6. Dribbling of saliva from the affected side.
7. Collection of food on the affected side of the mouth and formation of plaques over the teeth.
8. Hyperacusis and loss of taste over the anterior 2\3 of tongue (LMN facial palsy).

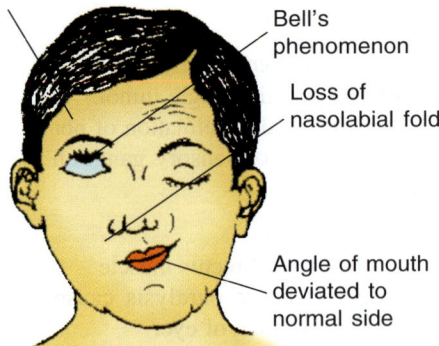

Fig. 6.2 Lower motor neuron lesion of facial nerve on the right side

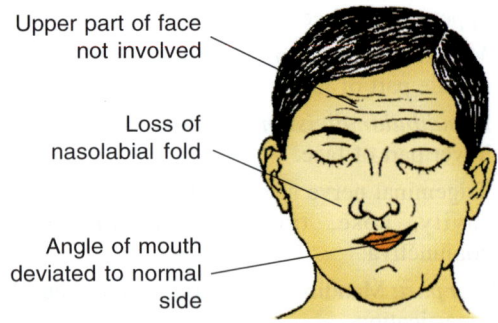

Fig. 6.3 Upper motor neuron lesion of facial nerve on the right side

Types of Facial Palsy

Upper Motor Neuron Facial Palsy (Fig. 6.3)
- Caused by the lesion in the cortex or internal capsule.
- Only lower part of the face on the affected side is affected opposite to the lesion.
- Usually associated with hemiplegia (weakness on the same side of facial palsy).

Voluntary movements on one side are affected. But facial movements can occur on emotional movements (e.g. laughing).

> *Note:* Upper part of face receives supply from both sides of cortex. As a result upper part of face is not involved in UMN facial palsy.

Lower Motor Neurone Facial Palsy (LMN facial palsy)
- All the muscles of facial expression on the affected side are paralysed including the upper part of the face on the same side of the lesion.
- Voluntary and emotional movements are affected.

Facial Palsy

Upper Motor Neuron (UMN) Facial Palsy

Causes
- Cerebrovascular accident affecting the brain stem.
- Trauma to the head
- Supratentorial tumors
- Encephalitis

Part of the face involved
- Lower part of the face on the opposite side of the lesion

Function not involved
- Taste
- Lacrimation
- Emotional movements of face

Associated abnormalities
- Hemiplegia on the same side of facial palsy
- Central speech defect

Abnormalities detectable at different levels of lesions in LMN facial palsy (Fig. 6.4)
At the level of facial nucleus (at PONS)

Abnormalities
- Total facial involvement on the same side of lesion – Involvement of pontine structures.
- Taste and lacrimation may also decrease

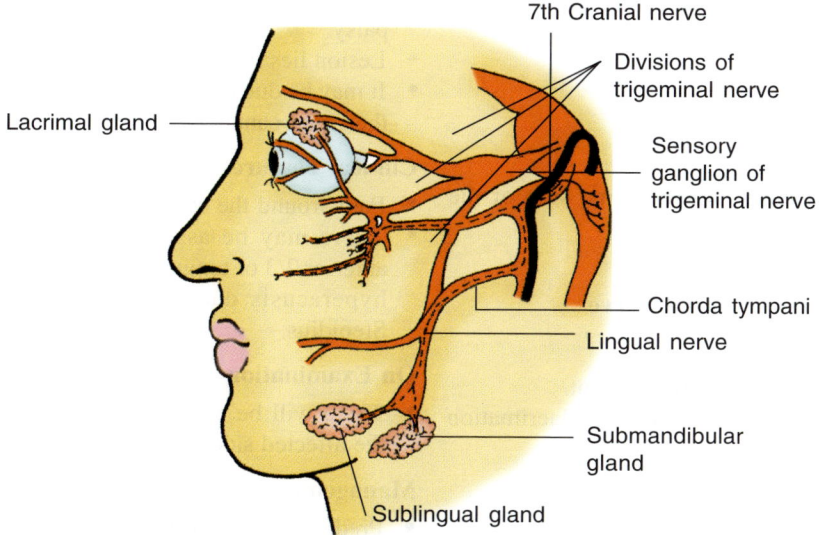

7th Cranial nerve

Divisions of trigeminal nerve

Lacrimal gland

Sensory ganglion of trigeminal nerve

Chorda tympani

Lingual nerve

Submandibular gland

Sublingual gland

Fig. 6.4 Lower motor neurone distribution of facial nerve

Causes
- Cerebrovascular accident
- Pontine tumors
- Multiple sclerosis

Between the Muscles of Facial Nerve and Geniculate Ganglion

Abnormalities
- Total facial involvement on the same side of lesion
- Loss of taste and lacrimation, 8th nerve may also be involved

Causes
- Cerebellopontine angle tumor
- Fracture base of skull.

Between Geniculate Ganglion and Stylomastoid Foramen

Abnormalities
- Total facial involvement on the side of lesion.
- Lacrimation and decrease of taste sensation.
- Hyperacusis (due to involvement of nerve to stepidius).

Causes
- Mastoiditis, middle ear infection
- Ramsay-Hunt syndrome (Herpes zoster of geniculate ganglion)

At Stylomastoid Foramen
Cause: Bell's palsy

Features
- Total facial weakness on the same side of the lesion.
- Lacrimation and tastes are spared.

Lesions of Branches of Facial Nerve

Abnormalities
- Individual facial muscle involvement.
- There is no involvement of taste and lacrimation

Causes
- Injection of local anaesthetics
- Trauma
- Parotid tumor and surgery

Causes of Lower Motor Neuron Facial Palsy
- Diabetes mellitus
- Leprosy
- Bell's palsy
- Parotid tumor, parotid surgery
- Guillain Barrè syndrome
- Lymphoma
- Sarcoidosis

Bell's Sign
- On attempted closure of eyelid on the affected side of facial palsy - patient is unable to close the eye, instead eyeball appears to move upwards and outwards.

Epiphora
- Tears will be rolling on the cheek due to eversion of lacrimal puncta in patients with LMN facial palsy.

Taste Loss
- Ant 2/3 of tongue can have taste loss due to the lesion in the geniculate ganglion of the facial nerve.

Bell's Palsy
- Bell's palsy is an idiopathic type of LMN facial palsy.
- Lesion lies in the facial canal
- It may be due to herpes simplex virus infection in the facial canal

Clinical Features
- Pain around the ear for few hours.
- There may be associated taste loss over the anterior 2/3 of tongue. Occasionally there may be hyperacusis due to involvement of nerve to Stepidius.

On Examination
- There will be evidence of LMN facial palsy on the affected side (see LMN facial palsy).

Management
- Prednisolone 40–60 mg × 1 week.
- Use of acyclovir may be helpful.

- Use of artificial eye drops, prevention of exposure keratitis.
- 70–80% recover within 2–12 weeks

Aberrant reinnervation of 7th nerve can cause abnormal facial movements like in a patient of Bell's palsy

- Eye closure on closing the mouth
- Tearing during salivation (crocodile tears).

Other Modes of Treatment for Bell's Palsy
- Decompression of facial canal
- Physiotherapy to the face
- Anastomoses between facial and hypoglossal nerves

Dental Aspects of Facial Palsy
- There will be accumulation of food materials in the vestibule of the mouth on the affected side.
- Increased tendency for formation of plaques on the teeth.
- There will be dribbling of saliva from the affected side of the mouth and formation of angular stomatitis.
- A splint may be required to support the angle of the mouth

Ramsay-Hunt Syndrome
Herpes zoster of geniculate ganglion can cause vesicles over the external ear and anterior 2/3 of tongue along with LMN facial palsy (see LMN facial palsy).

Facial dyskinesias (abnormal facial movements)

Examples
- Facial tics
- Hemifacial spasm
- Facial myokimia

8. Vestibulococlear Nerve

Vestibular component
- Concerned with position of the head and appreciation of movements
- Cochlear component: Concerned with hearing

Lesion of VIII nerve causes
- Loss of hearing
- Vertigo and ringing in the ear

Cause of 8th nerve lesion
- Aminoglycoside toxicity
- Cerebellopontine angle tumor

9. Glossopharyngeal Nerve
- Sensory supply: Posterior 1\3 of tongue and pharynx and taste sensation from posterior 1\3 of tongue
- Motor supply: Stylopharyngeus muscle
- Secretomotor fibres: For parotid gland

10. Vagus Nerve
- Vagus nerve supplies parasympathetic supply to viscera of thorax, upper abdomen and motor supply to soft palate, pharyngeal and laryngeal muscles.

10th Nerve palsy causes
- Loss of gag reflex
- Soft palate does not move on the affected side and uvula will be deviated to the normal side.
- Hoarseness of voice
- Bovine cough

11. Accessory Nerve
- Accessory nerve is made up of cranial and spinal part.
- Cranial part supplies along with vagus nerve to palate and pharynx and spinal part supplies trapezius and sternomastoids.
- Involvement of spinal part of accessory nerve causes weakness of sternomastoid and trapezius muscles.

Causes of 9th, 10th and 11th nerve palsy
1. Bulbar palsy
2. Lateral medullary syndrome

12. Nerve (hypoglossal nerve)
- Motor supply: To the muscles of tongue

12th Nerve palsy
- Causes difficulty in speaking - dysarthria to lingual sounds (t, d)
- On protrusion the tongue will deviate to the affected side.

- UMN paralysis of 12th nerve - Tongue will be spastic.
- LMN paralysis of 12th nerve - Tongue will be wasted with fasciculations.

Epilepsy

Definition

Disorder of neuronal function which causes episodic disturbances of consciousness and usually motor or sensory function.

Classification of Seizures

a. Generalised seizures (primary)
- Grandmal - tonic clonic
- Absence - petitmal
- Tonic
- Clonic
- Atonic
- Myoclonic

b. Partial seizures
- Simple partial
- Complex partial

c. Other types
- Infantile spasms
- Seizures in neonates

Grandmal Epilepsy (major epilepsy)

Starts at childhood/puberty
- Sequence of events of grandmal epilepsy
  – Aura
  – Loss of consciousness
  – Tonic phase
  – Clonic phase
  – Recovery after sometime

Aura
- Change of mood, irritability, hallucinations, headache

Tonic phase
- Characterised by tonic spasm of whole body.
- Associated with pupillary dilatation, facial pallor, glottis and respiratory muscle spasm causing cry and cyanosis. Urinary incontinence, frothing from the mouth and tongue biting are usually associated.

Clonic Phase
- Starts after tonic phase in less than a minute. There will be repetitive jerking movements of different parts of the body.

After Clonic Phase
- Patient becomes flaccid and comatose for 10–15 minutes.

Post ictal Phase
- Characterised by headache, confusion. Occasionally there may be transient paralysis (Todd's paralysis).

Major convulsions can cause trauma to the body, respiratory difficulty and brain damage.

Petitmal Epilepsy (minor epilepsy)
- Sudden loss of consciousness / transient loss of movements /speech.
- It is usually described as absence seizure
- It may be confused for abnormal behaviour
- It may progress to grandmal epilepsy.

Temporal Lobe Epilepsy (psychomotor epilepsy)
- Patient will have hallucinations, illusion of taste, smell, sight and hearing. There may be smacking of lips and chewing movements.

Focal Epilepsy
- Involuntary movements affects parts of the body. Involvement of part of limb or part of face, arm or leg. It can spread to different parts of the body (Jacksonian march of events).

Causes of Epilepsy
1. Primary or idiopathic epilepsy
2. Secondary causes
   – Intracranial disorders: Head injury, cerebrovascular accident, meningoencephalitis, e.g. HIV / TB / viral, space occupying lesions
   – Metabolic disorders: Hyponatremia, hypoglycemia, hypocarcemia, hyperglycemia, hypoxic brain damage
   – Systemic diseases: SLE, multisclerosis, hepatic and renal disorders

Table 6.1 Antiepileptic drugs and their side effects

	General side effects	Oral side effects
Phenobarbitone	Sedation, rashes	Bullae Erythema multiforme
Phenytorn sodium	Hirsutism Cerebellar dysfunction Generalised lymphadenopathy	Gum hypertrophy Dental anomalies
Sodium valoproate	Drowsiness Hepatic dysfunction	
Ethosuximide	Renal damage Eosinophilia	
Primidone	Drowsiness Ataxia Megaloblastic anemia	Oral changes due to Megaloblastic anemia
Carbamazepine	Leukopenia	Dry mouth Erythema multiforme

– Drugs and alcohol: Alcohol withdrawal, quinalone therapy

In children
- Birth injury
- Cerebral palsy
- Febrile convulsions

Management

Investigations of epilepsy
- For infective and inflammatory disorders
  – Complete blood picture and ESR
  – Chest X-ray
  – CSF analysis
  – Serology for HIV/syphilis/SLE
  – Antinuclear antibodies
- For metabolic disorders
  – Blood sugar, serum calcium, magnesium and electrolytes
  – Liver and renal function tests
- For structural CNS disease: CT/MRI/angiogram
- For the type of epilepsy: EEG

Treatment
Epileptic disorders require long term medications

Drug therapy
- Phenytoin sodium: 100 mg 0-0-3/day

or
- Carbamezapine 200 mg to 400 mg/day

or
- Sodium valoproate 500 mg to 1500 mg/day may be required
- Temporal lobe epilepsy can be controlled with Carbamezapine
- Petitmal epilepsy can be controlled with ethosuximide/sodium valoproate
- Plasma level of antiepileptic drug should be monitored.
- Drug treatment is usually continued for 3–5 years and then depending on the occurrence of convulsions and EEG changes drugs can be tapered and stopped.

Status Epilepticus
- Recurrent attacks of convulsions without regaining consciousness in between. It can result in severe hypoxia and can cause significant mortality. Seizure activity lasting for 15 to 30 minutes satisfies the definition of status epilepticus but requires anticonvulsant therapy if it continues for 5 minutes.

Causes
- Abrupt stoppage of antiepileptics
- Metabolic disturbances

- CNS infections and tumors
- Head injury
- Refractory epilepsy

Clinical Features
- Continuous attacks of abnormal movements/ seizures
- Altered consciousness
- Tachycardia
- Pupillary dilatation and Respiratory depression

Management
- Medical emergency

General Measures
- Move the patient from danger (machines, furnitures, water and fire)
- Establish/ensure clear airway
- Oxygen administration
- IV access to draw the blood for investigations, metabolic parameters (blood glucose, electrolytes, calcium and magnesium), level of antiepileptic drugs and for drug administration.

Drug Therapy
- IV Diazepam 10 mg (or Lorazepam 4 mg IV) - repeat if required after 15 minutes.
- If seizure persists after 30 minutes IV Phenytoin sodium - 20 mg/kg at 50 mg/ minute.

- If seizure persists IV Phenobarbitone 5 to 10 mg/ kg at 100mg/minute
- If seizure persists after 30 to 60 minutes: intubate, ventilate and administer anesthesia with profofol, midazolam or thiopentol and search for the cause and treat.
- Take care of the hydration, hyperthermia and hypoglycemia.

Dental and Oral complication of Epilepsy and its Treatment

1. Injuries caused by convulsions
- Injuries to the tongue and oral mucosa
- Person may fall down and may sustain injury to the face including fracture of facial bones
- Loss of teeth, subluxation and fracture of teeth
- Occasionally there may be dislocation of temporomandibular joint.

2. Complications due to treatment
- Phenytoin: Gum hyperplasia (interdental papillae particularly)
  – Megaloblastic anemia due to folic acid deficiency with recurrent aphthous ulcers.
  – Cervial lymphadenopathy
- Phenobarbitone therapy
- Causes erythema multiforme with bullous eruptions in the oral cavity

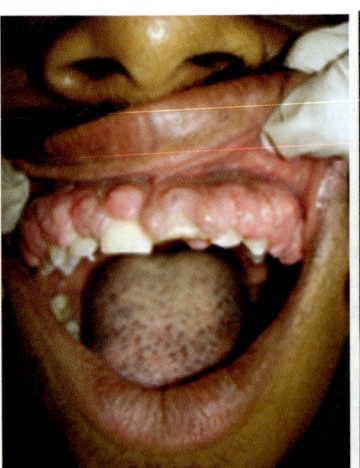 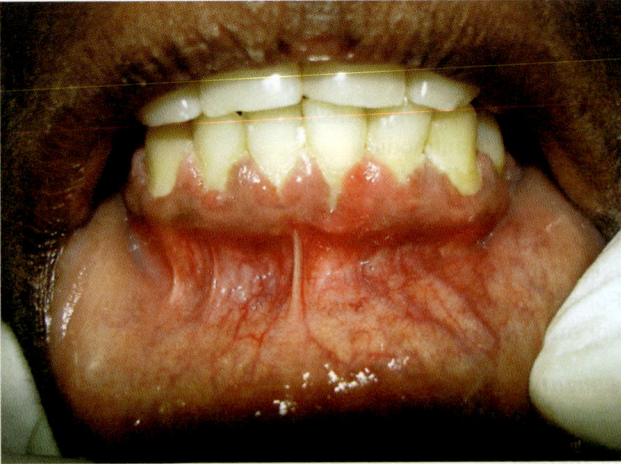

Figs 6.5a and b Phenytoin-induced gum hyperplasia

Dental Surgeons must be Aware of the following Factors which Precipitate Epilepsy

a. Sudden stoppage of antiepileptic drugs
b. Drug which induce epilepsy:
   Quinalones, e.g. ciprofloxacin
   Theophylline
   Tricyclics
   Alcohol
c. Hypoglycemia and starvation
d. Infection
e. Flickering lights
f. Sleep deprivation

Dental Treatment in an Epileptic

- Avoid dental treatment just immediately after convulsions.
- Large doses of lignocaine can cause convulsions.
- During dental treatment oral cavity should be kept free of debris.
- Keep all the apparatus away from the patient to avoid injuries in case he develops convulsions.

Management of an Attack of Convulsion in a Dental Clinic during Dental Treatment

- Keep the patient on sides to maintain the airway and avoid injuries.
- Avoid aspiration by keeping the mouth downwards.
- Keep the instruments and furnitures away from the patient to avoid injuries.
- Person may be drowsy and comatose for 30-60 minutes after an attack of convulsion.
- O_2 inhalation is required to avoid cerebral hypoxia during an attack of convulsion.
- If the attack of convulsion does not stop within few minutes slow IV diazepam 5–10 mg to be given and if required can be repeated and additional medical help should be sought.

SYNCOPE

Definition

Transient loss of consciousness with postural collapse. Loss of consciousness lasts for only 30 seconds.

Presyncope

A state of dizzy feeling with weakness and tendency to develop loss of postural tone. Consciousness is not lost.

Causes

1. Vasovagal syncope (common faint)
2. Cardiovascular
   - Severe aortic stenosis, obstructive cardio-myopathy.
   - Complete heart block
   - Arrhythmias
3. Drug induced antihypertensives.
4. Respiratory cause, severe coughing
5. Brainstem dysfunction
   - Cerebrovascular disease, migraine and seizure.
   - Micturition syncope
   - Postural hypotension - severe blood loss, hypoadrenalism.
   - Hypoglycemia, hypoxia
   - Anxiety disorders

Approach to a Patient of Syncope

Causes of syncope depending on the onset of syncope:
Sudden onset: Stoke-Adam's attack (complete heart block), ventricular tachycardia, seizure disorder.
Gradual onset of syncope: Hyperventilation, hypoglycemia.

Syncope on Movement of the Head and Neck may Indicate

- Hypersensitive carotid sinus (especially in elderly)
- Vertebro basilar insufficiency (due to cervical spondylosis)

Syncope Occurring at any Body Position may be due to

- Complete atrioventricular block (stokes-Adam's attack)
- Hypoglycemia
- Hyper ventilation disorder
- Seizure disorder

Syncope related to Exertion

Exertional syncope is a symptom of severe aortic

stenosis and obstructive cardiomyopathy can cause postexertional syncope.

Following symptoms alongwith an attack of syncope may suggest the attack may be seizure disorder rather than syncope.
- Clouding of conscious for a longer duration.
- Urinary incontinence
- Tongue biting and body injury
- Preceding aura.

Syncope which occurs on different body positions.
- On standing for a longer duration: Vasovagal attack (common faint)
- Immediately after getting up from lying down position.
  Occurs due to postural hypotension: due to antihypertensive medication, autonomic neuro-pathy, volume depletion

Significance of associated symptoms alongwith an attack of syncope
Intake of insulin - suggests hypoglycemia
Intake of antihypertensive medication causes postural hypotension.
Occurance of chestpain - Acute myocardial infarction and pulmonary embolism causing syncope.
Occurance of neurological deficit - cerebrovascular accident causing syncope.
After micturition in elderly - micturition syncope.
Syncope after severe bout of coughing - cough syncope.

For details on cardiac cause of syncope (see Cardiovascular system).

For details on vasovagal attack (common faint - see Medical emergencies in dental practice).

Facial Sensory Loss

Sensation of the Face
- Supplied by trigeminal nerve except over the angle of the mandible. Skin over the angle of the mandible is supplied by C2 dermatome.

Causes of Sensory Loss Over the Face
Damage to maxillary division of trigeminal nerve due to:

- Fracture of middle 1\3 of facial bones
- Carcinoma of maxillary atrium
Damage to mandibular division
- Injection of local anesthesia to inferior dental branch
Infiltration of mandibular division
- By nasopharyngeal carcinoma
Inferior dental nerve involvement due to
- Osteomyelitis
- Tumor deposits

Intracranial causes of facial sensory loss
- Cerebrovascular disease
- Cerebral tumors
- Tuberculosis
- Multiple sclerosis
- Neurosyphilis

DISEASES OF MUSCLES

Muscular Dystrophies
Genetically determined muscle disorders char-acterised by progressive degeneration of muscle since childhood leading on to muscle weakness, respiratory difficulty and death.

General Features of Muscular Dystrophies
- Symmetrical weakness and wasting of muscles.
- Strong family history
- Absence of sensory loss
- Fasciculations are not present
- Preservation of tendon reflexes till late.

Examples of Muscular Dystrophies
- Duchenne muscular dystrophy
- Becker's muscular dystrophy
- Limb girdle dystrophy
- Facioscapular dystrophy
- Oculopharyngeal dystrophy
- Myotonic dystrophy

Duchenne Muscular Dystrophy
- X- linked recessive disease begins in childhood and starts as girdle muscle weakness.
- Child has difficulty in walking, waddling gait and difficulty in standing.
- Calf muscles appear enlarged (pseudo-

hypertrophy) due to fat and fibrous tissue content and weakness spreads to all other muscles.

- Child becomes wheel chair bound before puberty and death occurs around twenties due to cardio respiratory complications.
- General anesthesia is contraindicated in patients with muscle dystrophy.

Myotonic Disorders

Myotonic dystrophies are characterised by slow relaxation of muscles after muscle contraction.

Different types of myotonic dystrophies

- Myotonia congenita (Thomson's type, Becker's type)
- Paramyotonia congenita
- Myotonia dystrophica

Myotonic dystrophy patients can have muscle weakness, cataract, facial weakness, frontal baldness, conduction defects in the heart and impaired respiratory function.

Polymyositis and Dermatomyositis

- Immunologically mediated inflammatory diseases of muscles .
- Usually affects females more than males around 5th decade and occurs.
- May be acute/insidious onset and presents with proximal muscle weakness and painful dysphagia.
- It may be associated with skin rash around the upper eyelid (heliotroph rash) in a condition called dermatomyositis.
- There can be systemic disturbances and patient slowly develops muscle weakness and respiratory impairment.
- Polymyositis can be associated with other collagen vascular diseases and may also be associated with internal malignancy.
- There will be significant increase of muscle enzymes (CK) and it effectively responds to corticosteroids and immune suppression.

Temporal Arteritis (Cranial arteritis)

- Form of vasculitic disorder and affects craniofacial region.

- Presents with severe throbbing headache unilaterally in the temporal region.
- Females are affected more than males and occurs after 5th decade.
- Patient presents with fever, malaise and palpable superficial temporal artery. Artery is usually tender tortuous and prominent.
- ESR is significantly elevated and artery biopsy confirms the diagnosis
- Blindness may occur due to optic nerve ischemia and early administration of corticosteroids is mandatory.

Dental Aspects of Temporal Arteritis

1. Jaw claudication - pain during mastication can occur due to ischemia of muscles of mastication
2. May be confused with temporal mandibular pain dysfunction syndrome (no increase of ESR and no signs of inflammation).

Temporal arteritis should be differentiated from trigeminal neuralgia.

Myasthenia Gravis

- Rare form of muscle weakness due to auto antibodies against acetyl choline receptors and disturbed function of neuromuscular junction.
- Commonly associated with thymic hyperplasia and removal of thymus can cure the disease.
- Women are more commonly affected than males and muscle weakness develops after using the muscle.
- Disability of the muscles is more characteristically develops towards the end of the day.
- Classical features like ptosis, dysphagia, neck muscle weakness and weakness of masticatory muscles (causing hanging of jaw) occur after sustained use of these muscles. Respiratory muscle involvement can occur due to disease itself or due to cholinergic drugs (cholinergic crisis).
- Eaton-Lambert syndrome: Myasthenic type of muscle weakness occurs due to internal malignancy. For example, Small cell carcinoma of lung.

Management
- Treatment with neostigmine/pyridostigmine
- Corticosteroids
- Thymectomy

Dental Aspects of Myasthenia Gravis
- Avoid general anaesthesia and intravenous sedation in patients with myasthenia gravis.
- Patient can develop oral candidiasis (with thymectomy and steroid therapy).
- Cholinergics can increase salivation.
- Perform dental procedures under local anaesthesia (lignocaine) immediately after morning medication for myasthenia gravis.
- Avoid aminoglycosides, suxamethonium and other neuromuscular blocking drugs in patients with myasthenia gravis.
- Paracetamol is the safest analgesia in patients with myasthenia gravis.

7a Hematological Disorders I

Approach to a Patient of Anemia and other Hematological Disorders

Physiological Adaptation to the Development of Anemia

1. Symptoms of anemia depend on the rate of development of anemia and person's cardio-vascular status.
2. Younger age and slower development of anemia are better tolerated.
3. Decrease in the oxygen carrying capacity of blood and tissue hypoxia (Hb% < 5 gm) leads to increase in the level of circulating 2–3 di-phosphoglycerate (2-3DPG) resulting in increased release of oxygen from the RBCs.
4. There will be increase in the circulating plasma volume with redistribution of blood flow to the vital organs.
5. Increased flow of blood and increase in the stroke volume occurs as a result of compensatory mechanisms.

History taking of Anemia and other Haematological Disorders

Symptoms due to the Manifestations of Anemial Fatigue
- Dizziness
- Syncope
- Headache
- Blurring of vision

Cardiovascular Symptoms
- Chest pain
- Palpitation
- Dyspnea
- Pedal edema

Gastrointestinal Symptoms
- Appetite loss
- Abdominal pain
- Jaundice
- Diarrhea
- Dysphagia
- Constipation

Neurological Symptoms
- Tingling and numbness
- Swaying while walking, weakness of limbs
- Altered sensorium

Miscellaneous Symptoms
- Fever
- Bleeding tendencies
- Bony pain

Symptoms Attributable to the Cause of Anemia
- History of blood loss
- Nutritional intake
- History suggestive of malabsorption
- History suggestive of worm infestations.

Past History
- Drug intake
- Exposure to chemicals and radiation
- Anemia since childhood, recurrent jaundice and recurrent blood transfusions.

Personal History
- Appetite loss, weight loss
- Alcohol intake
- Smoking
- Urine output
- Bowel habits

Family history: Anemia in the family members.

Menstrual history: Details of menstrual blood loss.

SYMPTOM ANALYSIS OF AN ANAEMIC DISORDER

Non Specific Symptoms

Fatigue, dizziness, headache and syncope may be due to severe anemia causing tissue hypoxia.

Cardiovascular Symptoms

- Symptoms like chest pain, dyspnea and palpitation are due to hypoxia of the myocardium.
- Anemia can cause aggravation of preexisting heart disease (due to high cardiac output state).
- Dyspnea occurs usually on exertion (when Hb% < 3 gm/dl). Dyspnea can also occur at rest especially in individuals with anemia causing cardiac failure.
- Chest pain: Elderly persons with pre-existing coronary heart disease will have aggravation of chest pain with development of significant anemia.

Gastrointestinal Symptoms

Loss of Appetite

Severe anemia can cause appetite loss. Appetite loss may also be a manifestation of systemic disease causing anemia.

Iron deficiency anemia can be associated with pica (see below).

Jaundice

Jaundice may be the manifestation of the hepato-biliary disease causing anemia or may be due to hemolytic anemia.

Dysphagia

Chronic severe iron deficiency can cause dysphagia due to post cricoid web. For example, Plummer Winson syndrome—combination of iron deficiency, glossitis and dysphagia due to post cricoid web.

Abdominal Pain

Abdominal pain with anemia may due to peptic ulcer disease, gastrointestinal malignancy or due to *Ancylostoma* infestation.

Diarrhea

Diarrhea may be a manifestation of malabsorption syndrome. Megaloblastic anemia itself can be associated with diarrhea.

Pica

Person eats persistently non-nutritive substances like soil, leaves, pastes, etc. Pica is usually associated with iron deficiency anemia.

Neurological Symptoms

Paresthesia

Folic acid and vitamin B_{12} deficiency leads on to peripheral neuropathy causing tingling and numbness of hands and feet.

Weakness of Limbs

Vitamin B_{12} deficiency can also result in subacute combined degeneration of the spinal cord. This causes pyramidal disturbance with weakness of lower limbs and also swaying while walking in the dark due to posterior column disturbance.

Severe anemia can cause altered sensorium due to hypoxic encephalopathy.

Miscellaneous Symptoms

Fever

- Severe anemia itself may be associated with mild fever.
- Pyrexia in a patient of anemia may be due to associated systemic disease like:
  - Infections, e.g. malaria
  - Lymphoma
  - Leukemia
  - Endocarditis
  - Collagen vascular disease
  - Pancytopenia conditions are associated with fever due to sepsis.

Bleeding Tendencies and Bony Pain

Hematological malignancies like leukemia, myeloma or lymphoma can cause bony pain and bleeding tendencies.

Bleeding tendencies may also be due to platelet/clotting disorder.

Symptoms due to Systemic Illness

Chronic renal, hepatic, musculoskeletal and other systemic disorders can cause severe anemia.

All persons with severe anemia should be evaluated for associated systemic illness.

> **SYMPTOMS ATTRIBUTABLE TO THE CAUSES LEADING ON TO ANEMIA**

History of Blood Loss

- Enquire the history of haematemesis, malaena, haemoptysis and menstrual blood loss in all patients with anemia.
- Recurrent small amount blood loss can cause severe anemia (occult bleeding from gastrointestinal tract).
- Enquire also symptoms like heartburn, altered bowel habit and abdominal pain for ruling out chronic occult gastrointestinal tract blood loss.

Nutritional Intake

1. Details of nutritional intake should be enquired. Inadequate dietary intake causes iron, folic acid and vit. B_{12} deficiency. Strict vegetarians have more chance of developing vit. B_{12} deficiency.
2. Symptoms of malabsorption like diarrhea, steatorrhoea should be enquired in all patients with unexplained anemia.

Worm Infestation

- Hookworm infestation is an important cause of iron deficiency.
- *Ancylostoma duodenale* can cause 0.2 ml blood loss/worm/day.
- *Nicator americanus* can cause 0.03 ml blood loss/worm/day.

- Person with roundworm infestation gives history of passing worms in the stool.
- Poor hygiene and poor toilet facilities give an indirect indication of worm infestation.
- Person with hookworm infestation may have epigastric pain and inflammatory diarrhea.

Past History

- Anemia since childhood with recurrent history of blood transfusion is a feature of congenital hemolytic anemia or a bleeding/clotting disorder since childhood.
- Intrauterine and childhood death can be due to Thalassemia disorders.
- Exposure to chemicals like benzene and exposure to radiation may be responsible for the development of aplastic anemia.

Importance of Drug History in a Patient of Anemia

- Long term intake of NSAIDS and corticosteroids cause erosive gastritis and chronic blood loss.
- Chloramphenicol, cytotoxics, oxyphenbutazones, gold salts can cause bone marrow suppression and aplastic anemia.
- Primaquine intake causes hemolysis in patients with GOPD deficiency.

> *Note:* Previous history of jaundice due to viral hepatitis may be responsible for the development of aplastic anemia.

Personal History

Appetite loss due to anemia itself or systemic disease causing anemia.

Weight loss suggests systemic disease and decreased nutritional intake.

Alcohol can cause erosive gastritis, bleeding due esophageal varices. Alcoholics can have associated nutritional deficiency.

Smoking causes peptic ulcer and reflux esophagitis causing blood loss.

Family History

- Congenital hemolytic anemia can involve several members of a family.

- History of consanguinity between parents should be enquired in all patients with hereditary disorders of haemoglobin and also disorders like haemophilia.
- Worm infestation can affect several family members causing anemia.
- People of low socioeconomic groups will have decreased nutritional intake causing anemia affecting several family members.

Menstrual History

Excessive menstrual loss of blood is an important cause of anemia in females.
Repeated childbirth is also a contributory factory for the development of anemia.

EXAMINATION

Scheme of Examination

General Physical Examination
Pallor   Clubbing
Jaundice   Lymphadenopathy
Cyanosis   Edema
Vital Signs: Pulse, blood pressure, respiratory rate and temperature.

Other Specific Examination Related to Anemia
Examination of face/oral cavity/skin/nails/leg ulcers/ bone tenderness/bleeding spots.

Systemic Examination
- *Cardiovascular system:* Cardiomegaly/murmurs/ cardiac failure/venous hum
- Respiratory system: Evidence of pulmonary disease.
- *Gastrointestinal tract:* Mass lesion/hepato-megaly/ splenomegaly/ascites.
- *Central nervous system:* Motor, sensory and cranial nerve deficits.
- Urogenital, musculoskeletal, hepatobiliary system and other systemic examination wherever necessary.

General Physical Examination

Build and Nourishment
1. Chronic anemic disorders are associated with stunted skeletal growth, e.g. hemolytic anemias.

2. Persons with deficiency anemias like iron, folic acid are usually poorly nourished with decreased muscle bulk and subcutaneous fat due to associated calorie deficiency.

Pallor
Conjunctival pallor may be mild or severe. Iron deficiency may be associated with pearly white sclera (see also general examination).

Icterus
Hemolytic anemias are associated with mild icterus (lemon yellow tint).
Hemolytic anemias with pigmented gallstones can have severe icterus.

Cyanosis
Severe anemia (Hb% < 5 gms/dl) is usually not associated with cyanosis.
Cyanotic patients will be polycythemic with suffused conjunctiva.

Clubbing
Presence of clubbing may suggest associated systemic disease in an anemic patient.

Lymphadenopathy

Causes of lymphadenopathy with severe anemia
a. **Supraclavicular lymphadenopathy:** GIT malignancy (left supraclavicular)/bronchogenic carcinoma.
b. **Generalised lymphadenopathy:** Acute and chronic leukemia/ lymphomas/systemic causes of generalised lymphadenopathy.
See also general examination for details on lymphadenopathy.

Edema

Pedal Edema in an Anemic Patient may be due to
- Severe anemia itself (due to renal retention of salt and water and also may be due altered capillary permeability).
- Congestive cardiac failure.
- Systemic causes like renal and hepatic diseases.
- Associated hypoalbuminemia.

Non - pitting edema - myxedema can be associated with severe anemia.

Examination of Face and Oral Cavity

Facial abnormality-look for pallor/puffiness of face. **Chip-monk facies:** frontal bossing, malar prominence with protuberant teeth. Seen in patients with thalassemia major.
Oral cavity examination (Table 7.1): check for the following abnormalities.
Agranulocytosis will result in ulcers in the oral cavity and pharynx.

Bony Tenderness

Bony tenderness is detected by applying pressure on the body of the sternum (often-lower end)/part of the sternum corresponding to the 5th intercostal space.
Common sites for bony tenderness—body of sternum, ribs, clavicles, pelvic bones and skull.

Causes of Bony Tenderness

Common causes: Acute leukemias, multiple myeloma, chronic leukemia
Rare causes: Severe anemia, osteomalacia and osteoporosis.

Note: Bony pain and tenderness is usually due to the expansion of the marrow and sub periosteal leukemic infiltration. Focal bone tenderness is due to secondary deposits in the bone.

Bleeding Spots

* Common sites: oral cavity, conjunctiva, gum (gum hypertrophy and bleeding is common in case of AML), limbs
* Associated conditions: Bleeding and clotting disorders
* Systemic causes like vasculitis
* Leukemic disorders
* Aplastic anemia

Skin Examination

For pallor, bleeding spots, pigmentation (megaloblastic anemia, Addison's disease).

Nails

Platynychia (flat nails) and Koilonychia (spoon-shaped): Iron deficiency anemia
Brittle nails and Longitudinal ridges: Severe chronic anemia

Retinal Examination : Check for
* Pallor (severe anemia)
* Hemorrhages (severe anemia, bleeding disorder).
* Roth spots (infective endocarditis)
* Hypertensive and chronic renal failure changes.
* Papilledema (severe anemia can cause papilledema).

Leg Ulcers

Site : medial aspect of tibia above the ankle.

Characteristics
* Chronic ulcers
* Single or multiple
* Unilateral or bilateral
* Only scarring of healed ulcers may be present.

Table 7.1 Oral cavity examination

Site	Abnormality
1. Oral mucosa	• Pallor
2. Tongue	
– Pale and bald (Atrophy of papillae)	– Iron deficiency
– Beefy red appearance	– Niacin deficiency
– Magenta colored	– Riboflavin deficiency
3. Palate and gum	• Bleeding spots (bleeding and clotting disorder. Gum hypertrophy and bleed-Acute Myeloid leukemia.
4. Angular stomatitis	• Iron and B complex deficiency

Significance: Commonly associated with sickle cell anemias and hereditary spherocytosis

Mechanism of leg ulcers: Leg ulcers are due to ischemia and super-added infection in the distal circulation.

VITAL SIGNS

Vital sign changes in anemic disorders
Pulse: Severe anemia causes tachycardia and high volume pulse.

Blood pressure: Wide pulse pressure occurs due to anemia.

Temperature: Minimal raise of temperature due to severe anemia itself.

Severe rise of temperature: Suggestive of systemic illness.

SYSTEMIC EXAMINATION

Clinical findings on systemic examination

Cardiovascular System

- Cardiomegaly with hyperdynamic apex.
- Murmurs - Ejection systolic murmur at the left sternal border (pulmonary area); murmur occurs due to the increased velocity of blood flow with decrease in the viscosity of blood.
  Murmurs may also be due to underlying heart disease.
- Congestive cardiac failure
- Venous hum

Note: In patients with chronic anemia, who are adjusted to very low Hb concentration , sudden transfusion of blood can expand the intra vascular volume and increase in the LV filling pressure can precipitate cardiac failure.

Gastrointestinal Tract

- Oral cavity (see above)
- Abdomen: Check for
  – Epigastric tenderness - peptic ulcer
  – Epigastric mass - carcinoma stomach

- Right iliac fossa - carcinoma caecum
- Retroperitoneal mass: Secondary carcinoma, chronic lymphatic leukemia, lymphoma.
- Hepatomegaly: Due to anemia itself. Anemia with CCF. Systemic disease involving the liver; leukemia, lymphoma, cirrhosis etc.
- Splenomegaly: Due to anemia itself, e.g. hemolytic anemia. Systemic conditions like leukemia, lymphoma, etc.
- Ascites: Due to anemia with congestive cardiac failure. Anemia with hypo- albuminemic states. Exudative causes of ascites associated with anemia.

Respiratory System

Check for evidence of tuberculosis, malignancy, chronic suppurative lung disease which can cause significant anemia.

Central Nervous System

Severe Anemia may be Associated with
- Altered sensorium (severe anemia with encephalopathy).
- Peripheral neuropathy: Loss of sensation (glove and stocking type), loss of deep reflexes (ankle jerks) folic acid and B_{12} deficiency.
- Subacute combined degeneration of spinal cord (patients with chronic vit B_{12} deficiency): Pyramidal tract abnormality and posterior column disturbance.

Examination of Other Systems

- Systemic examination should also include examination of hepatobiliary, musculo-skeletal and other systems in relevant cases.
- Patients of anemia should undergo per rectal examination.
- Perrectal examination may reveal - haemorrhoids, rectal bleeding, occult blood loss.
- Per-vaginal examination is helpful to find the etiology of anemia in female patients.

Differential Diagnosis and Investigations of Hematological Disorders

Iron Deficiency Anemia

Features
- History of blood loss
- Dietary lack of iron
- Occasionally dysphagia and pica

Signs
- Severe anemia
- Pale and bald tongue
- Koilonychia and platynychia

Investigations

For evidence of iron deficiency
- Peripheral smear: Microcytic hypochromic anemia
- Serum iron decrease with increase in the iron binding capacity.
- Bone marrow iron stores depleted (stained by Prussian blue).

For the cause of iron deficiency
- Stool for ova, cyst and occult blood.
- Upper and lower GIT endoscopy and barium studies for evidence of blood loss.
- Gynecological evaluation for evidence of blood loss.

Folic Acid Deficiency

Clinical Features
- Poor dietary intake, symptoms of malabsorption
- Anemia, red bald tongue
- Peripheral neuropathy - rare

Investigations
- Macrocytic anemia, hypersegmented neutrophils
- Megaloblastic marrow and low serum folate level

Vitamin B_{12} Deficiency

Clinical Features
- Strict vegetarians, diarrhea may be present.
- Disease of terminal ileum, previous gastrectomy
- Pallor, mild icterus (lemon yellow)

- Peripheral neuropathy, subacute combined degeneration of spinal cord.

Investigations
- Macrocytic anemia, megaloblastic marrow
- Serum B_{12} level very low
- Abnormal B_{12} absorption test (Schilling's test)

Aplastic Anemia (Primary)

Clinical Features
- Infection, pharyngeal ulcers,
- Bleeding tendencies, anemia, no organomegaly

Investigations
Pancytopenia, hypoplastic/aplastic bone marrow (dry tap)

Hemolytic Anemia

Features
- Anemia, jaundice since childhood
- Positive family history
- Severe anemia, mild jaundice and splenomegaly

Evidence of Hemolysis
- Reticulocyte count ↑↑
- RBC enzyme LDH ↑↑
- Urine urobilinogen increased
- Marrow-erythroid hyperplasia

Hereditary Spherocytosis

Features
- Anemia, jaundice, splenomegaly, leg ulcers.
- Evidence of hemolysis, osmotic fragility ↑↑ 51-chromium (^{51}Cr) labeled RBCs destroyed in the spleen.

Sickle Cell Anemia

Features
- Anemia, aplastic and infarction crises
- Splenomegaly and later autosplenectomy
- Leg ulcers

Investigations
- Sickle cells in the smear
- Sickling phenomenon demonstrated by adding sodium metabisulphite

- Hb electrophoresis-HbS (beta chain of Hb-at 6th position-valine is replaced by glutamic acid).

Thalassemia Major (β)

Features
- Anemia since childhood
- Incompatible without recurrent transfusion or marrow transplant
- Splenomegaly

Investigations
- Microcytic hypochromic anemia.
- Hb electophoresis:Hb-A_1(alpha$_2$ and beta$_2$) is decreased and Hb F(alpha$_2$ and gamma$_2$) is increased.

Thalassemia Minor (β)

Features
- Anemia and splenomegaly
- Not responding to iron therapy

Investigations
- Microcytic and hypochromic anemia
- HbA$_2$ (alpha$_2$ and delta$_2$) is ↑↑
- Osmotic fragility of RBCs ↓

Autoimmune Hemolysis

Features
- Anemia at any age
- Hepatosplenomegaly
- Microspherocytes and polychromasia in the peripheral smear
- Positive Coombs' test

Polycythemia Vera

Features
- Suffused conjunctiva with plethoric appearance
- Splenomegaly
- Hb%↑↑ and RBC mass ↑↑

Marrow: hypercellularity of all marrow elements
- ↑↑ Neutrophil ALP (alkaline phosphatase)
- ↑↑ Serum B$_{12}$ level
Decrease in the erythropoietin level.

Agranulocytosis

Features
- Severe opportunistic infection
- Mouth and pharyngeal ulcers
- Sepsis syndrome
- Granulocytes decreased, marrow-granulocyte precursors decreased.

Acute Lymphoblastic Leukemia (ALL)

Features
- Younger age
- Acute onset - anemia, bleeding and infection
- Bone tenderness
- Generalised lymphadenopathy and hepato-splenomegaly

Investigations
- Severe anemia
- Peripheral smear - Very high WBC count (> 50000 cells/cu) with blast cells
- Marrow - 20% lymphoblasts.

Acute Myeloblastic Leukemia (AML)

Features
- Acute onset- anemia, bleeding and infection.
- Lymphadenopathy - less common compared to ALL
- Hepatosplenomegaly

Investigations
- Bleeding due to DIC-common with M3 (pro-myelocytic)
- Gum hypertrophy-common with M4 (myelo-monocytic)

Investigations
- Very high WBC count (> 50000 cells/cu)
- Marrow - myeloblasts 20%, myeloblasts-auerrods+, myeloperoxidase stain +ve.

Chronic Myeloid Leukemia (CML)

Features
- Third to fifth decade
- Anemia with massive splenomegaly

Investigations

- WBC count > 50000 cells/cu, platelet count is increased.
- Peripheral smear - myelocytes, metamyelocytes with matured neutrophils.
- Marrow ↑↑cellularity of myeloid series, blasts-normal or mild (5%), 90%.
- Marrow cells Philadelphia chromosome +ve.
- Serum B_{12} is increased and leukocyte alkaline phosphatase is decreased.

Chronic Lymphocytic Leukemia (CLL)

Features

- Age: 45 to 65 years, slowly progressive anemia
- Generalised lymphadenopathy, hepatospleno-megaly.

Investigations

- WBC counts 50000/cu, small lymphocytes.
- Marrow - cellularity of lymphoid series

Multiple Myeloma

Features

- Elderly age group
- Bone pain and pathological fracture
- Anemia and renal failure

Investigations

- Urine - presence of Bence-Jones protein
- Serum protein electrophoresis - presence of 'M' band
- Marrow - malignant plasma cells

Hodgkin's Lymphoma

Features

- Early adolescence and later age group
- Lymphadenopathy with hepatosplenomegaly
- B symptoms - fever (> 38°C), weight loss, itching.

Investigations

- ESR, lymph node biopsy - Reed Sternberg cells

Non-Hodgkin's Lymphoma

Features

- At any age usually at later ages
- More common with HIV positives
- Waldeyer's ring and epitrochlear nodes commonly involved
- Abdomen and tissue involvement - more common
- Lymph node biopsy - Abnormal lymphocytes depending on the histological type.

Anemia Associated with Bleeding Disorder
(Table 7.2)

	Table 7.2 Differences between bleeding disorders and clotting disorders	
	Bleeding disorder *(defect of primary hemostasis)*	*Defects of secondary hemostasis* *(clotting defect)*
Site of bleed	Superficial skin and mucosa	Deep muscle, joint etc.
Family history	May not be present	Usually present
Sex involved	Females/males occasionally	Males
Bleeding after trauma	Immediate	Delayed (hours to days)
Findings	Petechiae and ecchymoses	Muscle hematomas, hemarthroses
Treatment	Local measures effective	Requires systemic treatment

7b Hematological Disorders II

Causes of Iron Deficiency

Due to increased loss of iron from the body
- Acute blood loss and chronic blood loss
- Gastrointestinal blood loss
- Hook worm infestation
- NSAID induced GIT bleeding
- Menstrual blood loss
- Repeated blood donation

Due to excess demand for iron
- Children and adolescents
- Pregnancy and breast feeding

Due to defective absorption of iron or decreased intake of iron
- Dietary deficiency
- Intestinal disease and malabsorption
- Acute or chronic disease and inflammation

Hook worm infestation and nutritional iron deficiency are the common causes of iron deficiency in tropics.

Clinical Features of Iron Deficiency Anemia
- Fatigability
- Dyspnea
- Chest pain, palpitation

Specific Features of Iron deficiency
- Pale bald tongue (Fig. 7.1)
- Platynychia and koilonychia
- Pica - altered craving for food.

Associated Features
- Tachycardia, cardiomegaly, systolic murmurs and
- Congestive cardiac failure.

Plummer Winson syndrome
(Postcricoid Dysphagia)

Combination of iron deficiency, glossitis and post cricoid dysphagia due to post cricoid web is called Plummer-Vinson syndrome. Post cricoid web is premalignant.

Investigations for Iron Deficiency

Confirmation of Iron Deficiency
- Serum Iron is decreased
- Total Iron binding capacity is increased
- Serum Ferritin level is decreased.

Blood smear: Shows microcytic hypochromic anemia.

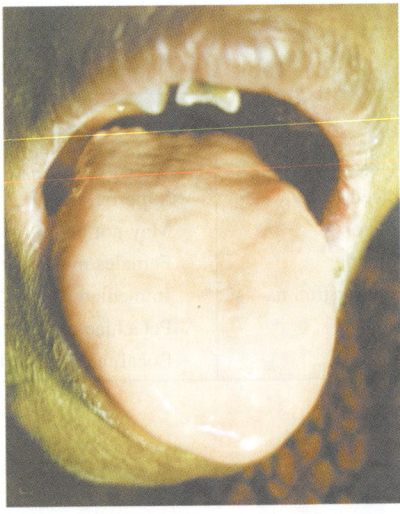

Fig. 7.1 Pale and bald tongue in iron deficiency anemia

238

Investigations for the Cause of Iron Deficiency

- Stool - for ova, cyst and occult blood
- Upper and lower gastrointestinal tract studies and barium studies for the gastrointestinal tract cause of blood loss
- Tests for evidence of malabsorption
- Gynaecological evaluation in females for blood loss

Management

- Oral iron therapy:
  – Ferrous sulphate 200 mg 1-1-1 for 3 to 6 months.
- If the patient is intolerant to oral iron or malabsorption, parenteral iron IM\IV can be administered.
- If iron deficiency is associated with congestive cardiac failure blood transfusion may have to be given.
- Treatment of the cause
- Dietary supplementation of iron

Megaloblastic Anemia

Megaloblastic anemia occurs due to the deficiency of Vit B_{12}\folic acid.

Causes of Vit B_{12} Deficiency

Due to intrinsic factor deficiency

- Total gastronomy
- Pernicious anemia

Due to Defective Cobalamin Release from Food

- Partial gastrectomy
- Gastric achlorhydria

Due to Disorders of Terminal Ileum

- Intestinal resection
- Non tropical sprue
- Tropical sprue
- Neoplasms and granulomas
- Fish tapeworm
- Bacterial overgrowth in the intestine

Due to Drugs

- Neomycin, PAS and colchicine

Clinical Features

Vitamin B_{12} deficiency results in anemia and neurological involvement.

Pernicious Anemia

- Deficiency disease caused by a specific defect of absorption of Vitamin B_{12}.
- There are antibodies to intrinsic factor and parietal cells.
- Coexisting endocrine disorders are usually present like hypothyroidism, Addison's disease, diabetes mellitus type I and vitiligo.
- Atrophic gastritis, achlorhydria (failure of gastric acid secretion with intrinsic factor deficiency)
- Associated with increased risk of development of gastric malignancy.
- Development of megaloblastic anemia - slow to occur.
- Patient will have usual symptoms and signs of anemia with neurological manifestations (peripheral neuropathy and subacute combined degeneration of spinal cord) causing paraplegia.

Diagnosis

- Peripheral smear
  – Macrocytic anemia
  – Hypersegmented neutrophils in the peripheral smear
- Serum Vit. B_{12} is decreased
- Pancytopenia can occur
- Schilling test to detect the site of malabsorption of B_{12}
- Antibodies to intrinsic factor

Treatment

- Injection Vit. B_{12} (cyanocobalamin): Inj. B_{12} (1000μg) every week × 2 months and then Inj. B_{12} every month/once in 3 months life long.
- Oral B_{12} supplementation in the tablet form.

Folate Deficiency

Site of absorption of folic acid: Throughout small intestine

Source: Fruits and vegetables

Causes of Folic Acid Deficiency

- Increased demand
  - Infancy
  - Pregnancy
  - Malignancy
  - Chronic hemodialysis
- Inadequate intake (alcoholics, teenagers)
- Malabsorption
  - Tropical sprue
  - Non tropical sprue
- Drug induced
  - Alcohol
  - Barbiturates
  - Phenytoin
  - Methotrexate
  - Pentamidine
  - Cotrimoxazole

Clinical Features

- Patients are usually malnourished.
- Diarrhea, cheilosis and glossitis are common.
- Neurological abnormalities do not occur.

Investigation

- Hb% is decreased
- Macrocytic anemia with hypersegmented neutrophils
- Serum folate is decreased
- Serum B_{12} level is normal

Treatment of Foliate Deficiency

- T. Folic acid 5mg/day
- Dietary supplementation containing folic acid

Hemolytic Anemias

Features of Hemolysis

- Increased reticulocyte count
- Increased level of indirect bilirubin
- Decreased level of haptoglobins
- Increased LDH level
- Positive urinary hemosiderin

Classification of Hemolytic Anemia

Hemolysis Due to Defects in the RBC Membrane

- Hereditary spherocytosis and elliptocytosis

- Paroxysmal nocturnal hemoglobinuria
- Anemia due to spur cells

Hemolysis due to Abnormal hemoglobin and RBC Enzyme Defect

- Hemoglobinopathies, e.g. Thalassemias and sickle cell anemia
- Enzyme defects, e.g. G-6-PD and pyruvate kinase deficiency

Hemolysis due to Defect Outside the RBCs

- Toxins and infections
- Hypersplenism
- Microangiopathic hemolysis
- Antibody mediated hemolysis

Investigations of Hemolytic Anemia

Features of hemolysis

- Reticulocyte count is increased
- RBC enzyme - LDH is increased
- Increased level of indirect bilirubin
- Decreased haptoglobin level
- Urine contains excess urobilinogen
- Hb % is decreased

Peripheral Smear

Features in hemolytic anemia

- Spherocytes - Hereditary spherocytosis
- Micro spherocytes - Autoimmune hemolysis
- Microcytic hypochromic anemia- Thalassemias
- Sickled cells - Sickle cell anemias

Other Tests

- Osmotic fragility is increased in spherocytosis
- Coombs test is positive in autoimmune hemolysis
- Bone marrow shows erythroid hyperplasia
- G - 6 PD and pyruvate kinase levels are decreased in enzyme deficiency

Hb Electrophoresis

- ↑ Hb F (Foetal haemoglobin) - Thalassemia major
- ↑ Hb A2 - Thalassemia minor
- Presence of Hb S - Sickle cell anemia

Hereditary Spherocytosis

Hereditary disorder associated with RBC membrane defect.

Commonest abnormality is the deficiency of β-spectrin or ankrynin causing defective RBC membrane.

- Commonly presents with chronic hemolytic state with spherocytes in the blood and reticulocytosis may be since childhood.
- Anemia, jaundice and splenomegaly are the dominant clinical features.
- Complications like megaloblastic crises, hemolytic crises, aplastic crises and pigment gall stones can occur.

Investigations
- Features of hemolysis
- Peripheral smear shows presence of spherocytes.
- Direct - Coombs' test negative
- Osmotic fragility of RBCs is increased.

Management
- T. Folic and 5 mg/day life long
- If severe - Splenectomy

Haemoglobinopathies

General Aspects
- Each of the hemoglobin peptide chain has amino acid sequences. Amino acid sequence can be altered as a result of DNA mutations and lead to variant hemoglobins.
- These disorders are hereditary and are grouped under hemoglobinopathies.

Sickling Disorders
Sickling disorders result from substitution of glutamic acid to valine at position 6 of β chain of hemoglobin resulting in abnormal HbS.

Sickling Disorders Include
- Heterozygous sickle cell trait (HbAS)
- Sickle cell anemia (HbSS)
- Heterozygous sickling trait associated with another hemoglobinopathy.

Pathogenesis
During hypoxia HbS precipitates to structures called tactoids. These distort the RBC membrane producing sickled RBCS. Tactoids result in microvascular occlusions and undergo premature RBC destruction.

Clinical Features of Sickle Cell Anemia
Person suffers from chronic anemia and intermittent crises

Features
- Anemia
- Impaired growth
- Skeletal deformities
- Jaundice
- Dactylitis
- Painful and aplastic crises
- Susceptibility to infection
- Skin ulcers - lower limb
- Gallstones
- Infarction of CNS, lungs, kidney and spleen

Crises of Sickle Cell Disease
Painful crises
- Crises is precipitated by
  - Infection
  - Dehydration
  - Hypoxia
  - Acidosis/cold exposure

Crises occurs due to infarction as a result of sickling causing severe bony pain and fever. Infarction can cause abdominal, pulmonary, renal or neuro- logical damage.

- Hematological crises: 3 types
  - Hemolytic
  - Aplastic
  - Sequestration crises

Anemia and infarction can be severe but cause of death is usually infection due to salmonella/pneumococci.

Recurrent infarction of spleen results in auto-splenectomy.

Lab Investigations
- Anemia with reticulocytosis
- Peripheral smear: Sickled erythrocytes

Demonstration of Sickling of RBCs
By adding a reducing agent like sodium meta-bisulphate.

Hb electrophoresis demonstrates predominantly HbS and a small amount HbF.

General Management of Sickling Disorders
- Daily folic acid supplementation
- Prophylaxis against pneumococci with oral penicillin and vaccination against pneumococci and *Haemophilus influenzae.*
- Painful crises: Treatment with oxygen, rehydration, analgesics and if required transfusion of blood.
- Regular blood transfusion may also be required.
- Hydroxyurea to increase the HBF level and there by reduce HbS and sickling of RBCs.
- Bone marrow transplantation

Dental Aspects of Sickle Cell Anemia
- Patients with sickle cell disease have got increased susceptibility to dental infection.
- Bone infarction of mandible can occur and may predispose to osteomyelitis

Dental Management
- Preventive dental care is very important.
- Routine dental conservation can be carried out under local anesthesia and analgesia.
- Acute dental infection should be treated properly or otherwise they may precipitate crises.

All surgical procedures should receive antibiotic coverage.

Surgical Management
- Before general anesthesia anemia should be corrected and Hb% should be 10 g/dl.
- Nitrous oxide administration may be hazardous as it increases oxygen affinity of hemoglobin and causes hypoxia
- Hypoxia, acidosis, volume depletion should be avoided during surgery. Bloodless surgery using vasoconstrictors may prove hazardous.

Oxygen should be administered during the time of sickle cell crises.

Heparinisation is beneficial if there is abdominal or limb pain during a crisis to prevent pulmonary embolism.

Thalassemias

General Aspects
- Thalassemias are inherited disorders of Alpha or Beta goblin chain of hemoglobin biosynthesis
- There will be decreased hemoglobin production and hypochromic microcytic anemia.

Unaffected goblin chains are produced in excess and precipitate within the RBCs and predispose to hemolysis.

Alpha Thalassemias
Alpha thalassemias are characterised by decrease or absence of alpha chain synthesis (alpha chain includes 4 alpha genes).
- If all 4 genes are deleted - baby will be stillborn (hydrops foetalis).
- If 3 genes are depleted person will have HbH disease.
- If 2 genes are deleted person will have mild hypochromic microcytic anemia.

Treatment
- Hydrops foetalis - no specific therapy
- HbH - avoid iron therapy.
- Folic acid supplementation may be required.

Beta Thalassemia
- Beta thalassemia is characterised by failure to synthesize beta chains.
- *Beta Thalassemia minor*
  – Heterozygous state of thalassemia.
  – Usually asymptomatic except for mild hypochromic anemia.
  – There in increase in the level of HbA2.
- *Beta Thalassemia major*
  – Homozygous state of thalassemia

Features
- Severe anemia since childhood
- Failure to thrive
- Hepatosplenomegaly
- May be associated with skeletal deformities

Affected children are susceptible to infection and folate deficiency.

Because of recurrent blood transfusions patient can develop iron deposition in the heart, liver and pancreas resulting in hemosiderosis and organ dysfunction.

Investigations
* Hb% is decreased
* Peripheral smear
  – Hypochromic microcytic anemia, aniso-poikilocytosis, target cell formation.
* Serum iron and ferritin levels are normal.
* Significant increase in the level of HbF.

General Management
* Recurrent blood transfusion
* Folic acid supplementation
* Iron chelation with desferrioxamine
* Splenectomy if hypersplenism
* Allogenic bone marrow transplantation

Dental Aspects of Beta Thalassemia
* Radiological aspects
  – Enlargement of maxilla caused by bone marrow expansion (chipmonk facies).
  – Alveolar bone rarefaction in the X-ray .
  – Delaying of pneumatization of sinuses.
  – Hair on end appearance of skull on lateral view of skull X-ray due to expansion of diploe of the skull.
* Dental management
  – Painful swelling of parotid can rarely occur due to hemosiderosis.
  – Glossitis due to folate deficiency requires therapy.
  – General anesthesia is difficult due to severe anemia and intubation may be difficult due to maxillary enlargement.
  – Recurrent transfusions carry the risk of Hepatitis B, C and HIV transmission.
  – Prophylactic antibiotics are recommended before surgery in splenectomised patients.

PANCYTOPENIA

Pancytopenia is the term used to describe the combination of anemia, leucopenia and thrombocytopenia.

Causes of Pancytopenia
* Idiopathic
* Constitutional: Fanconi's anemia
* Systemic disorders
  – Hypersplenism
  – SLE
  – Sarcoidosis
* Infections
  – Tuberculosis
  – Brucellosis
  – Viral hepatitis
* Hematological disorders
  – B_{12} and folic acid deficiency
  – Acute leukemias
  – Myelodysplasia
  – Lymphomas
  – Paroxysmal nocturnal hemoglobinuria
* Drug induced
  – Chloramphenicol
  – Phenylbutazone
  – Cytotoxics
  – Sulpha drugs
  – Anticonvulsants
  – Gold
* Exposure to chemicals
  – Heavy metals
  – Benzene
  – Toluene

Approach to a Patient of Pancytopenia

Bleeding is the most common manifestation of thrombocytopenia due to associated thrombocytopenia. Bleeding usually manifests as petechiae, easy bruisibility, gum bleed, excessive menstrual flow or systemic bleed.

Symptoms of anemia like easy fatigability, breathlessness and symptoms of leucopenia leading onto sepsis can also be the manifestations of pancytopenia.

Previous history of chemicals and drug exposure, previous viral illness should be enquired for the secondary causes.

Family history of blood disorder may indicate genetic or constitutional disorder of pancytopenia.

History of weight loss, joint pain point to the systemic causes of pancytopenia.

Clinical Examination in a Patient of Pancytopenia

- Look for pallor, bleeding spots, gum bleeding and presence of sepsis (gum, pharynx, etc.).
- Organomegaly, lymphadenopathy are absent in patients with primary aplastic anemia.
- Hepatosplenomegaly and lymphadenopathy are usually associated with lymphomas and leukemias along with pancytopenia .
- Leukoplakia and nasal abnormalities are characteristic features of dyakeratosis congenita along with pancytopenia.

Investigations of Pancytopenia

- Hb %, total WBC count, platelet count to know the severity of pancytopenia.
- Reticulocyte count is decreased in conditions associated with marrow hypoplasia and reticulate count is increased in patients with peripheral destruction of RBCs.

Peripheral Smear

- *Macrocytic anemia:* Due to B_{12} and folic acid deficiency causing pancytopenia.
- *Abnormal cells:* In leukemias associated with pancytopenia.

Bone Marrow : may be Acellular/hypocellular

Other tests like serological markers for hepatitis, anti nuclear antibodies, cytogenetic study, serology for HIV, and tests for tuberculosis should also be done while investigating for pancytopenia.

Aplastic Anemia

Aplastic anemia is due to bone marrow aplasia causing refractory normochromic normocytic anemia, leucopenia and thrombocytopenia.

Causes

- Primary - Idiopathic
- Secondary:
  - *Radiation*
  - *Drugs* - NSAIDS, cytotoxics, chloramphenicol, chemicals - Benzene

- *Viruses* - Hepatitis, HIV infection
- Paroxysmal nocturnal hemoglobinuria.
- Inherited - Fanconi's anemia

Features

- Symptoms and signs of severe anemia.
- Infection due to leucopenia.
- Thrombocytopenia causes bleeding tendency and purpura.
- No organomegaly in patients with primary aplastic anemia.
- History suggestive of predisposing causes may be present.

Investigations

- All blood counts are decreased
- Peripheral smear - shows pancytopenia
- Bone marrow - shows hypoplasia/aplasia

Management

- Blood transfusion and treatment of infection.
- Removal of precipitating cause.
- Younger patients (20 yrs of age) - Bone marrow transplantation - ideal.
- Older patients - immune suppressive therapy with cyclosporine and antithymocyte globulin.
- Anabolic steroids - not much beneficial.
- Prognosis is poor in patients, managed with supportive care alone.

Dental Aspects of Aplastic Anemia

Oral manifestations of aplastic anemia can be due to:

- Severe anemia
- Hemorrhagic tendencies
- Liability to infection
- Effect of corticosteroid therapy
- Risk of hepatitis B, C and HIV infection due to blood transfusion

AGRANULOCYTOSIS

Clinical syndrome due to reduction in the granulocytes (mostly neutrophils) causing increased susceptibility to infection.

Causes: Same as that for pancytopenia

Clinical Features

- Sudden onset of fever, fatigability and sore throat
- Ulceration and pseudomembrane formation over the oral and pharyngeal mucosa including the gum.
- Cervical lymphadenopathy.
- Hemorrhagic necrosis of the mucosa, respiratory infection.
- Septicemia

Investigations

- Decreased total WBC count with decreased neutrophils.
- Bone marrow will confirm the diagnosis with decrease of myeloid serius.

Management

- Stop the offending drug if it is due to drug induced agranulocytosis.
- Control the infection with non bone marrow toxic antibiotics.

Dental Aspects

- Agranulocytosis can cause oral infection and ulcers
- Minor oral infection can result in gangrenous stomatitis.
- Septicemia can be caused by various oral micro organisms.

Oral Manifestations of Common Hematological Disorders

1. **Glossitis**
   - Pale bald tongue (atrophy of papillae) can occur in iron deficiency anemia.
   - Red smooth tongue can occur in B complex deficiency.
   - Magenta colored tongue can occur in riboflavin deficiency
   - Red beefy tongue can occur in niacin deficiency Soreness of tongue without color change/ depapillation can occur in B_{12} deficiency.
2. **Oral candidiasis:** Can occur due to severe anemia.
3. **Angular stomatitis and cheilitis**
   - Can occur in iron deficiency
   - Staphylococci and candidiasis can also cause angular stomatitis.

- Apthous stomatitis may also be a mani-festation of folate deficiency.
4. **Leukemias**
   - Acute myeloid leukemia can cause gum hyperplasia and bleed.
   - Leukemias, thrombocytopenias and coagulation defects can present with bleeding into the oral cavity.
   - Neutropenia causes oral infections and recurrent oral ulcerations.
5. **Hemolytic anemias:** Beta thalassemias results in enlargement of maxilla and rarefaction of alveolar bone.
6. **Plasma cell disorders:** Plasma cell disorders like multiple myeloma results in osteolytic lesions of the jaw, gingival bleeding and amyloid deposition in the oral soft tissues.
7. **Lymphomas**
   - Lymphomas can cause cervical lymph-adenopathy, oral ulcerations.
   - Herpes, simplex, zoster infections, oral candidiasis and bleeding tendencies in the oral cavity.

LEUKEMIAS

Leukemias are a group of malignant disorders of hematopoietic system characterised by increased number of abnormal white cells in the peripheral blood and or bone marrow.

Etiology of Leukemias

Following are the factors associated with the development of leukemias.

Heredity

Increased incidence of leukemia occurs in identical twins. Leukemia incidence also increases in patients with Down's syndrome and other genetic abnormalities.

Immunological abnormalities

Leukemia disorders are increased in persons with immunodeficiency and hypogammaglobulinemic states.

Viral

Retroviruses appear to be associated with rare form of T cell leukemia - lymphoma.

Exposure to chemicals

Exposure to benzene, petroleum products, smoking, paint, pesticides have been associated with increased incidence of leukemias.

Radiation

Ionizing radiation exposure increases incidence of leukemias.

Drugs

Alkalizing agents therapy can induce leukemias, may be after long duration of exposure..

Classification of Leukemias

- Acute
  - Lymphoblastic
  - Myeloblastic
- Chronic
  - Lymphocytic
  - Myeloid

Acute lymphoblastic

- Common (preB)
- T cell
- B cell
- Undifferentiated

Acute myeloid (French, American, British classification)

- M0-Undifferentiated
- M1-Minimal differentiation
- M2-differentiated
- M3-Promyelocytic
- M4-Myelomonocytic
- M5-Monocytic
- M6-Erythrocytic
- M7-Megakaryocytic

Chronic lymphocytic

- B cell - common
- T cell-rare

Chronic myeloid

- Ph - positive

- Ph - Negative
  - BCR - Abl positive
- Ph - Negative
  - BCR - Abl negative
- Eosinophilic leukemia

> *Note*
> - Ph -Philadelphia chromosome
>   - BCR - Break point cluster region
> - Abl - Abelson oncogene

Acute Leukemias

General Features

Age: Acute lymphoblastic leukemia is common in pediatric age group. Acute myeloblastic leukemia - common in adults.

Symptoms and Signs

- Pallor
- Generalised lymphadenopathy
- Bleeding tendencies
  - Purpura
  - Mucosal bleeding
- Weight loss
- Fever
- Bony pain
- Hepatosplenomegaly
- Infection
- Organ dysfunction
- Acute lymphoblastic leukemia (ALL)
  - Common in children
  - Generalized lymphadenopathy and hepato-splenomegaly
- Acute myeloblastic leukemia (AML)
  - More common in adults
  - Can have hepatosplemomegaly
  - Lymphadenopathy less common compared to ALL
  - Bleeding tendencies are commonly associated with Type - M3
  - Gingival infiltration is more commonly associated with type M4 and M5

Investigations

- Hb% - decreased

- WBC count > 50,000 cells to 1,00,000 cells/ cmm.
- Peripheral smear: Appearance of blast cells
  – Platelet count is decreased
- Bone narrow - Blast cells>20% of cells
  – Normal elements are reduced.
- Presence of Auer rods in the cytoplasm of blast cells suggest leukemia is of AML type.
- Renal function tests, liver function tests and coagulation profile may be abnormal.

Management

General Measures
- Psychological support
- Blood transfusion\platelet transfusion.
- Treatment of infection with appropriate antibiotics, antiviral and antifungal drugs.
- Monitoring of hepatic, renal function and treatment of hyperuricemia with allopurinol.

Specific Therapy Acute Leukemia
Chemotherapeutic agents used in the treatment of acute leukemia:
- IV Vincristine
- IV Daunorubicin
- IV L. Asparginase
- IV Cytarbine/IV Etoposide
- For intrathecal administration - Methotraxate
- For IV or oral route - Prednisolone

Different phases of chemotherapy in the treatment of acute leukemia
- *Induction of remission:* Combination of chemotherapeutic agents is used to destroy the tumour cells.
- *Consolidation of remission:* Combination of chemotherapeutic agents is administered to maintain the remission.
- *Period of remission maintain:* Requires repeated drug administration upto 2 years to maintain the remission.
- *Definitive therapy:* Bone marrow transplantation is a definitive form of therapy in acute leukemias.

Note
- Chemotherapeutic agents are administered in cycles.
- Dangerous cytopenia and infection can occur during chemotherapy which requires supportive care.

- Nervous system involvement requires therapy with intrathecal methotrexate and irradiation of the cranium.

CHRONIC LEUKEMIAS

Chronic Myeloid Leukemia (CML)
- CML is characterised by excessive proliferation of myeloid cells.
- Age: Involves 30–80 years of age.

Cytogenetics
- CML is associated with philadelphia chromosome (shortened chromosome 22 and is due to reciprocal translocation of material with chromosome 9).
- Break on chromosome 22 occurs at break point cluster region (BCR).
- Fragment of chromosome 9 that joins BCR carries an oncogene called - Abelson oncogene (ABL). Fusion of BCR with Abelson oncogene can transform hematopoetic progenitor cells.

Clinical Features
- May be asymptomatic
- Massive splenomegaly
- Anemia and hepatomegaly
- Weight loss
- Loss of appetite

Investigations
- Normocytic normochromic anemia
- WBC count > 50,000 to 1,00,000 cells/cmm.
- Platelet count may be increased
- Peripheral smear - Increased number of myelocytes and metamyelocytes

Bone Marrow
- Shows increased cells of myeloid series and few blast cells with presence of Philadelphia chromosome.
- Leucocytes Alkaline phosphatase score is decreased.
- Serum B_{12} level is increased

Different Phases of CML
- Chronic phase
- Accelerated phase
- Blast crisis

Treatment
- Chemotherapy with hydroxy urea/busulphan till total count is < 20,000 cells/cmm
- Alpha interferon therapy
- Imatinib mesylate inhibits Abelson oncogene action. Imatinib can cause remission of CML.
- Bone marrow transplantation

Chronic Lymphocytic Leukemia

- Most common type of leukemia
- Male to female ratio is 2:1
- Age group involved: 45–65 years of age

Clinical Features

May be asymptomatic and disease may remain asymptomatic for a long duration of time.

Other Features
- Anemia
- Weight loss
- Fever
- Generalised lymphadenopathy
- Hepatosplenomegaly

Investigations
- Anemia
- Coombs positive hemolytic anemia may be present
- WBC count > 50,000–1,00,000 cells/mm
- Bone marrow - High number of lymphocytes with abnormal markers.
- Immunoglobulin level is increased.

Staging

Clinical stage A: No anemia\thrombocytopenia, less than 3 areas of lymph node involvement

Clinical stage B: No anemia/thrombocytopenia three or more areas of lymph node involvement

Clinical stage C: Anemia + thrombocytopenia

regardless of lymphadenopathy

Treatment

Stage A
- No treatment is required
- Reassure and follow up

Stage B
- Chemotherapy with chlorambucil
- Local radiation to lymph nodes

Stage C
- Blood transfusion, corticosteroids

Other treatment like treatment of infection, splenectomy for hemolytic anemia may be required.

Dental Aspects of Leukemias

Predominant Oral Manifestations of Leukeimias
- Cervical lymphadeopathy
- Gingival swelling and bleeding
- Purpuric spots in the oral cavity
- Oral ulcerations
- Membrane formations over the tonsills

Oral Infections
- Candidiasis
- Aspergillosis
- Herpes virus infections

Due to Drug Therapy
- Cytotoxics - oral ulceration

KEY POINTS 7.1

Oral infections in acute leukemia

- Severe infections with gram negative organisms or candida can complicate many oral lesions
- Patient may require isolation.
- Oral lesions can lead onto systemic infection.
- Usage of soft nylon tooth brush and 0.2% chlorhexidine mouth wash is used to keep the oral hygiene.
- Herpes virus infection requires treatment with acyclovir.
- Prophylactic acyclovir may have to be given especially in patients who have undergone bone marrow transplantation.

- Busulphan - oral pigmentation
- Antibiotics - candidiasis
- Adriamycin - dry mouth, cardiac side effects

Most of the patients of acute myelomonocytic leukemia have oral manifestations.

Mandibular and parotid swelling can occur in certain leukemias.

Loss of alveolar crest bone, destruction of crypts of developing teeth can occur in leukemias and may be reversible after chemotherapy.

Dental Problems in Acute Leukemias

Predominant problems which come across in dental practice in an acute leukemia patient.
- Bleeding
- Infection in oral cavity
- Associated with severe anemia
- Complication of steroid and cytotoxic therapy
- DIC (disseminated intravascular coagulation)
- Hepatitis B and C and HIV infection
- Complications of bone marrow transplantation

Dental Treatment in Acute Leukemia
- Conservative management is always beneficial.
- Surgery is to be carried out only in emergency situations. (e.g. fracture, hemorrhage, potential airway obstruction and severe sepsis).
- Local anesthetic injection is not recommended as it can cause bleeding.

Bleeding from Oral Cavity
- Requires blood transfusion

Oral Ulceration
- Common with methotrexate treatment
- Concomitant usage of folinic acid is beneficial.

Dental Aspects of Chronic Leukemias
- Palatal, mucosal swelling, gingival bleeding, oral petechiae, and oral ulceration can occur but less common compared to acute leukemias.
- *Herpes simplex, Herpes zoster* and candidiaces can occur in chronic leukemia patients.
- Platelet deficiency can cause oral hemorrhage. Leukemia infiltration of lacrimal and salivary glands can occur.

- It is advisable not to carry out dental extraction - may precipitate bleeding /Infection.
- Platelet\blood transfusion is indicated before surgery and also in severe anemia. Adequate antibiotic coverage is given after surgery. Packing of sockets should be avoided as it predisposes to infection
- Screening for HBsAg and HIV is indicated before surgery.
- NSAIDS are not indicated as they may precipitate bleeding.

Dental Treatment of Chromic Leukemia is Complicated by
- Predisposition to infection
- Anemia
- Bleeding tendencies
- Susceptibility to Hepatitis B and HIV infection
- Side effects of drug therapy

Dental Aspects of Leucopenia
- In patients with severe neutropenia mild periodontal disease may result in gangrenous stomatitis.
- Cyclical neutropenia may result in recurrent ulcers. Various oral microorganisms can cause septicemia.

Oral Complications of Cytotoxic Chemotherapy
Oral ulcers and mucositis
- Ulcers
  - Shallow, painful affecting lateral and faucial mucosa.
  - Ulcers usually heal within 2 weeks of stoppage of cytotoxic therapy.
- Bleeding
- Platelet deficiency due to drug toxicity can cause oral cavity bleeding.

Infections
Anti malignant therapy can predispose to:
- Oral - candidiasis and mucormycosis
- *Herpes zoster* and simplex infection
- Staphylococci and gram negative oral infections

Dry Mouth (Xerostomia)
Chemotherapy drug especially like adriamycin can cause dry mouth.

HEMORRHAGIC DISORDERS

- Significant and prolonged bleeding can occur after dental extraction and may be a first manifestation of hemorrhagic disorder.
- Bleeding after dental extraction most commonly occurs due to local cause.
- Hemorrhagic disease can be caused by disorders of platelet, vascular or clotting mechanism.
- Platelet and vascular disorders produce minor superficial bleed like petechiae, ecchymosis over the skin mucosa and gingival bleed.
- Coagulation defects cause significant bleeding into the tissues and hematuria, severe prolonged bleed after injury/surgery and can be fatal.

Approach to a Patient of Bleeding Disorder

- Enquire previous episodes of bleeding after dental extraction\tonsillectomy may be suggestive of congenital bleeding disorder.
- If previous episodes of bleeding after dental extraction are controlled by local measures it is usually suggestive of local cause.
- If multiple transfusions are required person may be having major bleeding disorder.
- Positive family history is suggestive of usually a coagulation disorder.
- Enquire the history of taking drugs like anticoagulants, liver disease, AIDS which can cause bleeding tendencies.

Screening Tests Done for Bleeding and Coagulation Disorders.

1. **Platelet count:** Thrombocytopenia (decreased platelet count) < 1.5 lakhs/cmm.
2. **Bleeding time (BT)**
   - Normal bleeding time: Less than 8 minutes
   - Prolonged bleeding time:

   Causes of prolonged bleeding time
   - Vascular abnormalities
   - Platelet function abnormalities
   - Thrombocytopenia
   - von Willebrand factor deficiency

3. Prothrombin time (PT)
   - Normal prothrombin time: 12–15 seconds
   - Prolonged prothrombin time

   Causes of prolonged PT
   - Liver disease
   - Factor deficiency: VII, II, V or X
   - DIC
   - Warfarin therapy

4. Activated partial prothrombin time (APTT)
   - Normal (APTT): 30–40 seconds
   - Prolonged APTT

   Causes of prolonged APTT
   - DIC
   - Standard heparin therapy
   - Deficiency of factors V, VIII, IX and X
   - Antibodies against clotting factors
   - Presence of lupus anticoagulant

5. Estimation of fibrinogen level
   - Decreased fibrinogen level : DIC

Thrombocytopenia

- Normal platelet count - 1.5 lakhs to 4.5 lakhs\cmm
- Bleeding can occur when the platelet count is less than 1,00,000/cmm

Causes of thrombocytopenia

- Due to increased destruction of platelets
- Immunologically mediated
  - Idiopathic thrombocytopenic purpura
  - Drug induced
  - Sepsis
- Non immunological
  - Disseminated intravascular coagulation
  - Aplastic anemia
  - Marrow infiltration with tumor and fibrosis
- Due to splenic sequestration
  - Hypersplenism.

Idiopathic Thrombocytopenic Purpura (ITP)

ITP is a disorder of platelets caused by the auto-antibodies directed against the platelet membranes resulting in macrophage induced platelet destruction.

Clinical Features

- In children

– Occurs after 2–3 weeks of viral illness
– Sudden onset of purpura and oral and nasal bleeding
- In adults
  – Insidious onset
  – Female > males
  – Purpura and petechiae
  – Becomes chronic with exacerbations and remissions
  – May be a manifestation of SLE

Investigations

- Platelet count is reduced
- Bleeding time is prolonged
- Bone marrow-shows megakaryocytic hyperplasia
- Anti platelet antibodies are present.

Rule out HIV infection/SLE and drug induced thrombocytopenia in all patients with ITP.

Management

- Children
  – Platelet transfusion
  – Corticosteroids: Tab prednisolone 1 mg/kg for 4–6 wks and taper and stop.

  If recurrent thrombocytopenia small dose of maintenance steroid for a longer duration.
  – IV immunoglobulins
- Adults
  – Platelet transfusion
  – Corticosteroids
  – IV immunoglobulins
  – Splenectomy

Dental Aspects of Thrombocytopenias

- Minor dental surgery may be tolerated if the platelet count is around 50,000 cells/cmm and platelet transfusion is required for major dental surgery (platelet count should be > 80,000 cells/cmm).
- Platelet transfusions should be given immediately before surgery and to be replaced immediately after surgery.
- Use platelet transfusion within 6–24 hours of collection. Platelet rich concentrate or platelet rich plasma can be used as platelet replacements.

- In patients with ITP, corticosteroids/splenectomy is more beneficial than platelet transfusions.
- Recurrent transfusions of platelet carry the risk of hepatitis B\C and HIV transmission. Local measures and use of tranexamic acid (antifibrinolytic agent) may be helpful in stopping minimal bleeding.

von Willebrand's Disease

- Mild form of a bleeding disorder inherited usually as an autosomal dominant pattern due to the deficiency of Von Willebrand factor.
- von Willebrand factor is a protein synthesized by endothelial cells and platelets.

Functions of von Willebrand Factor (vWF)

- Acts as a bridge between platelets and collagen
- Acts as a carrier protein for factor VIII

Deficiency of von Willebrand Factor Results in

- Defective adherence of platelets to collagen
- Secondary reduction in the factor VIII level
- vWF deficiency leads to prolonged primary bleed following trauma.

Clinical Features

- Both sexes are equally affected
- Presents as bleeding after trauma or surgery
- May present with epistaxis, purpura, menorrhagia and GIT bleed.
- Presentation may vary from milder to severe form.
- Less common to present with hemarthrosis.

Investigations

- Bleeding time and activated partial thromboplastin time is prolonged.
- Low von Willebrand factor level
- Normal platelet count
- Low Ristocetin cofactor level

Management

- *Milder form:* Desmopressin administration will control the bleed.
- *Severe bleed:* Facter VIII administration (contains von Willebrand factor).

Dental Aspects
- Patient can have profuse bleed after tooth extraction.
- Avoid aspirin/NSAIDS.
- Minor bleeding can be controlled with desmopressin
- Severe bleeding is to be controlled with factor VIII concentrate.

CONGENITAL COAGULATION DISORDERS

Most important hereditary coagulation disorders are hemophilia A and hemophilia B.

Hemophilia A
- Hemophilia A is due to the deficiency of coagulation of factor VIII. Affects males and inherited as x linked recessive disorder. Females act as carriers. Positive family history is always present.

Clinical Features
- Presents in childhood as muscle/joint hematomas following trauma.
- Bleeding after dental extraction may be the only sign or first sign of hemophilia.
- Bleeding into the joints (hemarthroses) can cause joint damage.
- Bleeding into the vital organs including brain can cause fatal complications.
- Pharyngeal and laryngeal complication can occur following bleeding into the neck and can be fatal.

Lab Findings
- Prolonged activated partial thromboplastin time (APTT)
- Normal prothrombin time (PT)
- Normal bleeding time (BT)
- Reduced factor VIII level

Treatment of Hemophilia
- Avoiding trauma
- Fresh frozen plasma infusion
- Cryoprecipitate of factor VIII infusion
- Human fresh dried factor VIII concentrate infusion

KEY POINTS 7.2

- Persistant oozing after dental extraction can occur over for days or weeks in hemophiliacs.
- Pressure has no effect on the bleeding. Even if the clots are formed it has no lasting effect.
- Bleeding may stop temporarily after trauma, but recurs after an hour or more and may be severe.
- Severity of bleeding in hemophilia depends on level of factor VIII activity and extent of trauma.
- At factor level of 5–25% even minor trauma can lead to prolonged bleeding.

Dental Management
Hemophiliacs can have following problems during dental management:
- Frequent dental infections due to improper dental care.
- Bleeding during and after surgery
- Hematoma formation occurs due to IM injections and hazards of anesthesia.
- Risk of hepatitis B, hepatitis C and HIV infection due to transfusion of blood and blood products.
- Psychological upset

Hazards of Anesthesia and IM Injections in Hemophilias
- Conservative dental treatment can be carried out occasionally without anesthesia.
- Local anesthetic infiltration in the papillary or periodontal region can cause sufficient analgesia without severe bleeding.
- Regional blocks or injections into the floor of the mouth can cause severe hemorrhage allowing tracking down of blood causing airway obstruction. Massive hematomas may result from submucosal injections.
- If regional anesthesia is to be used, factor VIII replacement is required.
- During endotracheal incubations severe bleeding can occur and adequate factor VIII replacement is required. Oral latex cuffed endotracheal tube is preferred as it causes minimal trauma.
- Severe anemia due to blood loss requires blood transfusion.

- IM injections should be avoided as it can cause massive hematomas.

Difficult Dental Extractions
- Factor VIII replacement, removal of minimal bone and remaining teeth should be sectioned for removal whenever possible.
- Occasionally packing of sockets with Tranexamic acid soakings may be required.
- All patients require antibiotics preferably oral b-lactams for a full duration of 7 days. All patients after oral surgery require follow up for post operative bleed/hematoma formation.

Head and Neck Injuries in a Hemophilia
- Replace factor VIII in any case of head and neck injuries.
- Root canal treatment, scaling of teeth, minor orthodontic procedure may not cause bleeding and if necessary, factor VIII should be replaced.

Miscellaneous Problems in Hemophiliacs
Consider always possibility of presence of inhibitors for factor VIII in all patients with hemophilia requiring factor VIII replacement.

Postoperative Period
Amount of factor VIII to be given depends on the level of factor VIII and type of surgery. Factor VIII infusion must be continued for longer duration to prevent post operative bleeding.

Antifibrinolytic Agents
- Trenexamic acid 1g 6th hly can be used to reduce factor VIII requirement. But if bleeding recurs\persists factor VIII should be transfused.
- DDAVP - Desmopressin intranasally or infusion can temporally correct the deficit in hemophiliacs.

Surgery and Postoperative Hemorrhages
- Assess the patient before surgery for APTT, platelet count, factory VIII assay and factor VIII inhibitors.
- Blood grouping, cross matching and Hb% should be estimated and blood transfusion may be required. Recurrent transfusions carries the risk of transmission of hepatitis B and C and HIV infections.
- Administer anti hemophiliac factor one hour before surgery. Bleeding can occur 4–10 days after surgery.

Importance of Preventive Dental Care in Hemophiliacs
- Patient education and preventive dentistry should be started as early as possible.
- Uses of fluorides, decreased sugar in the diet, regular dental inspections are mandatory in all patients with hemophilia.

Local Measures During Surgery in the Oral Cavity in Hemophilia
- Induce minimal trauma to the bone and soft tissues.
- Suturing with non-restorable sutures is preferred to stabilize gum flaps.
- Sutures can be removed after one week.
- If significant bleeding occurs factor VIII replacement is required.
- NSAIDs are preferably to be avoided in hemophiliacs. Paracetamol, propoxyphene are preferred analgesics.

Hemophilia B (Christmas Disease)

Features
- Characterised by deficiency of factor IX
- Clinical features are indistinguishable from factor VIII deficiency.
- Factor IX deficiency can be treated with transfusion of fresh frozen plasma or plasma fraction enriched with prothrombin complex protein.

Disseminated Intravascular Coagulation (DIC)
- DIC is also called consumption coagulopathy.
- DIC is a complex process in which there is activation of haemostatic related mechanisms with consumption of platelets and coagulation factors.

Effects of DIC
- Bleeding tendencies
- Occurs due to consumption of platelets and

clotting factors and activation of fibrinolytic system
- Thrombosis phenomenon
  - Clotting in capillaries cause major vital organ damage
- Hemolysis
  - Damage to RBCs due to changes in the capillaries (microangiopathy hemolytic anemia).
- Shock
  - Due to adrenal damage or obstruction of the pulmonary circulation by fibrin deposits.

Causes of DIC
- Infections
  - Bacterial, viral and parasitic like malaria/rickettsial.
- Damage to the endothelium
  - Aneurysum of aorta, hemolytic uremic syndrome, acute glomerulo nephritis
- Malignant diseases
  - Bronchogenic, pancreatic and prostatic malignancies
- Obstestric causes
  - Abruptio placentae
  - Retained dead fetus
  - Pre-eclampsia
  - Amniotic fluid embolism

Management
- Treatment of the cause
- Treatment of hypoxia, acidosis
- Heparinisation, platelet and clotting factor replacement and antifibrinolytic therapy.
- Dental treatment cannot be carried out when the person has DIC.

LYMPHOMAS

Hodgkin's and Non-Hodgkin's Diseases

Lymphomas are clinically and histopathologically divided into:
- Hodgkin's and non Hodgkin's lymphomas
- Lymphomas are malignant tumors of the lymphatic tissue.

Hodgkin's Lymphoma
- Age group involved
  - Bimodal presentation
  - 1st peak around 20–35 years and second peak around 50–70 years of age.

Pathological classification
- Lymphocyte predominant
- Nodular sclerosis
- Mixed cellularity
- Lymphocyte depleted

Pathological hallmark

Presence of Reed-Stern berg cells-large malignant lymphoid cells of B cell origin.

Clinical features
- Lymphadenopathy
  - Painless, rubbery lymphadenopathy usually in the neck. Lymph nodes are firm discrete and not attached to the skin.
  - There will be generalized lymphadenopathy involving cervical, mediastinal, epitrochlear, inguinal, para-aortic and Waldeyer's ring.
- B-Symptoms
  - Fever> 38°C
  - Weight loss, night sweats and itching.
  - Fever - Pel Ebstein type - Fever for few days to weeks, afebrile intervals with recurrent development of fever.
- Younger patients usually develop nodular sclerosing type of lymphoma and elderly patients develop mixed cellularity type.
- Hodgkin's lymphoma can spread to other structures by contiguous spread.
- Pain in the region of lymph mode after alcohol intake can occur.
- Fungal, and viral infection can occur due to impaired immunity and compressive effect of lymph node mass can cause pressure effect over the trachea, oesophagus, major blood vessels and spinal cord.

Investigations
- Full blood count-May have lymphocytosis
- ESR is significantly elevated (> 100 mm/hr)

- LFT may be normal, alkaline phosphatase can raise in cases of hepatic infiltration
- Chest X-ray, ultrasound, CT scan can be utilized for evidence of involvement of mediastinal, para aortic lymph nodes and visceral involvement.
- Lymph mode biopsy for histopathological evidence of lymphoma and the presence of Reid-Sternberg cells.

Staging and Treatment of Hodgkin's Disease

Stage I: Involvement of a single lymph mode region -I or extralymphatic site (A1).

Stage II: Involvement of two or more nodes or extra lymphatic site on the same side of the diaphragm.

Stage III: Involvement of lymph nodes on both sides of diaphragm with or without splenic involvement or other site involvement.

Stage IV: Diffuse involvement of one or more extra lymphatic site or lymph nodes.

Stage A: Absence of symptoms

Stage B: Presence of fever, weight loss and night sweats.

Management

- Radiotherapy
  - For stage I disease
  - For stage IIA disease with three or fewer areas are involved
  - After chemotherapy to sites where there was originally bulk disease.
  - For compressive symptoms by lymph nodes.
- Chemotherapy
  - For patients with B symptoms.
  - For stage II disease with more than 3 or more areas of lymph nodes involved
  - For stage III and IV disease

Non-Hodgkin's Lymphoma (NHL)

- Occurs as a result of mononuclear proliferation of B cell (70%) and T cell (30%).
- Clinically NHL is graded into high grade lymphoma and low grade lymphoma.

Clinical Features

- Age of involvement: 65 to 70yrs.
- Lymphadenopathy: Waldeyer's ring and epitrochlear nodes are more likely to be involved.
- Symptoms like fever, night sweat, weight loss and itching may be present.
- More likely is to be associated with extranodal involvement (bone marrow, gut, skin), etc.
- Compression syndromes, gut obstruction, ascites can occur and HIV infected patients are more likely to develop NHL.

Investigations

- Complete blood tests, T and B cell markers, immunoglobulin levels, HIV testing and lymph mode biopsy
- High ESR, lymphocytosis, raised immunoglobulin levels and abnormal lymph node biopsy.

Treatment of Non Hodgkin's Lymphoma

- Combination chemotherapy and radiotherapy
- Low grade lymphoma:
  - If the patient is asymptomatic: No treatment is required.
  - For stage-I disease: Radiotherapy.
  - Chemotherapy: Oral therapy with chlorambucil
  - Monoclonal antibodies and autologus stem cell transplantation
- High grade lymphoma
  - Chemotherapy:
  - IV chemotherapy with CHOP regime. (Cyclophosphamide, doxorubicin, vincristine and prednisolone).
  - Radiation-for debulking of tumor
  - Autologus stem cell transplantation and Monoclonal antibodies are other forms of therapy.

Dental Aspects of Lymphomas

- Oral lymphadenopathy can occur as a part of cervical lymphadenopathy.
- NHL often causes Waldeyer's ring enlargement.
- Oral candidiasis, herpes zoster and herpetic gingivostomatitis occur in patients with lymphomas especially after chemotherapy.

Factors that influence Dental Treatment in Patients of Lymphoma

- Anemia
- Viral and fungal infection of the oral cavity

- Chemotherapy induced oral ulceration
- Bleeding tendencies
- Side effect of corticosteroid therapy

Oral Complications of Cytotoxic Chemotherapy in a Patient of Lymphoma

- Cracking of lips
- Oral ulceration
- Drug induced thrombocytopenia with bleeding into the oral cavity
- Cytotoxic drugs can predispose to infection with candida, herpes and pseudomonas, etc.
- Dry mouth (xerostomia) especially due to adriamycin toxicity.

BLOOD TRANSFUSION

ABO Antigens and Antibodies

Major blood groups
- A, B, AB and O Blood group depends on the RBCS containing different antigens.
- A, B, and O system contains antigens which are of carbohydrate in nature.

Blood group type A
- Type A individuals produce anti B antibodies (antibodies against antigen B).

Blood group type B
- Type B individuals produce anti A antibodies.
- There are no antibodies in Type AB persons. So they are universal recipients of blood.
- Persons with blood group O are universal donors because their cells are not recognized by any antibodies in the recipient (they have both anti A and anti B).

Rh system

- Second most important blood group system.
- Rh antigens are proteins in nature.
- Person with D antigen makes the person Rh positive.
- Persons with lack of D antigen become Rh negative.

Bombay Blood Group

- Rare form of blood group
- Individuals produce antibodies to H substance on RBCs except Rh phenotype individuals. They also produce antibodies to Group A and Group B antigens. They can be transfused only with hh phenotype donors.

Pre Transfusion Testing

- Pretesting of a recipient consists of type and screening of blood.
- Pre transfusion testing determines blood group ABO and Rh phenotype of the recipient and determines cross matching with the donors blood group antigens.
- Blood of the donor is also screened for hepatits B, hepatitis C, VDRL and HIV infection.

Transfusion Therapy

- Blood products for transfusion are collected as 450 ml of whole blood with anticoagulation (acid citrate dextrose).
- Following blood/blood products can be transfused:
  - Whole blood
  - Packed red blood cells
  - Platelets and white blood cells
  - Fresh frozen plasma - for correction of coagulopathies
  - Cryoprecipitate - source of factor VIII and von willebrand's factor

Plasma derivatives contain albumin, immunoglobulin and coagulation factors.

Adverse Reactions to Blood Transfusion

- Immune mediated reactions
  - *Acute hemolytic transfusion reactions:* Due to ABO incompatibility
  - Delayed hemolytic transfusion reaction
  - Occurs in patients who have been previously sensitive to RBC allo-antigen
  - Febrile reactions
- *Allergic reactions:* Due to urticarial rashes to plasma proteins.
- *Anaphylaxis:* Occurs immediately after starting the transfusion.
- *Graft vHost disease:* Can occur after receiving the

blood from family members.
- Transfusion related acute lung injury.

Non immunological Complications
- Hyperkalemia
- Fluid overload
- Iron overload
- Hypotension
- Hypothermia

Transmission of Infections
- Viruses: Hepatitis B, hepatitis C, HIV virus, cytomegalovirus
- Bacterial contamination
- Infections like malaria, babesiosis and Chaga's disease

Lymphadenopathy and Disorders of Spleen

Approach to a Patient of Lymphadenopathy
- Children and young adults have invariably benign causes of lymphadenopathy, where as in persons above the age of 50 years there is increased incidence of malignant disorders causing lymphadenopathy.
- Localised lymphadenopathy suggests involvement of a single anatomical area.
  Involvement of 3 or more non contiguous areas of lymphadenopathies is defined as generalized lymphadenopathy.
- Lymphadenopathy of less than 1 cm size in the submandibular area in children and young adults and < 2 cm size of inguinal lymph nodes are clinically not significant.
- Coexistance of splenomegaly along with lymphadenopathy is invariably associated with systemic disease.
- Lymphadenopathy of < 1 cm size requires follow up and > 1 cm size requires detail evaluation.

Significance of Different Localized Lymphadenopathies
- *Occipital lymphadenopathy:* Suggestive of infection of the scalp.
- *Preauricular lymphadenopathy:* May be due to conjunctival infection.

Cervical Lymphadenopathy
Causes of cervical lymphadenopathy
- Local infection in the oral cavity, pharynx, Tonsil
- Tuberculosis
- Lymphomas/leukemias
- Secondaries in the neck from primary malignancies from:
  – Head and meek
  – From GIT
  – Lungs
  – Thyroid, etc.
- *Scalene lymphadenopathy:* May be due to secondary from lungs
- *Supraclavicular lymphadenopathy:* (Virchow's) - secondaries from gastrointestinal tract, genitalia and lungs

Clinical Aspects of Lymphadenopathy
- Matted groups of lymph nodes are suggestive of Tuberculosis and neck is the common site of TB lymphadenopathy.
- Lymphoma lymph nodes are discrete, large, rubbery, firm, mobile and non tender.
- Metastatic deposits in the lymph nodes cause hard, non tender and fixed lymphadenopathy.

Important Causes of Generalised Lymphadenopathy (see general physical examination)

SPLEEN

Spleen is a reticuloendothelial organ which is present in the left hypochrondrium

Physiological Functions of Spleen
- Removes older and defective erythrocytes
- Splenic white pulp is a site for antibody synthesis
- Spleen removes antibody coated bacteria and antibody coated blood cells.

Functions of Spleen
- *Culling:* Removal of dead and damaged blood cells.
- *Pitting:* Removal of Heinz and Howell-Jolly bodies

Splenomegaly

- Splenomegaly can cause pain and heaviness in the left hypochondrium.
- Early safety may be a manifestation of massive splenomegaly.
- Palpable spleen suggests splenomegaly and usually indicates diseases affecting the spleen

Causes

Due to Congestive splenomegaly
- Cirrhosis of liver
- CCF
- Portal vein and splenic vein obstruction

Due to Infiltrative disorders of spleen
- Leukemias
- Lymphomas
- Myeloproliferative disorders
- Storage diseases

Due to reticuloendothelial hyperplasia
- Hemolytic anemias
- Nutritional anemias
- Paroxysmal nocturnal hemoglolinuria

Due to immune hyperplasia
- Tuberculosis
- Malaria
- AIDS
- SLE
- Rheumatoid arthritis

Causes of massive splenomegaly

(Enlargement>8cms from costal margin)
- Chronic malaria
- CML
- Lymphomas
- Polycythemia Vera
- Myelofibrosis

Effects of splenectomy

- Increased susceptibility to infection, e.g.
  1. Infection with capsulated organisms like pneumococcus, Hemophilus, Influenzae and enteric gram negative organisms.
  2. Infection with the Parasite Babesia
- Splenectomised patients blood smear shows presence of denatured hemoglobin (Heinz bodies) and nuclear remnants of RBCs (Howell-Jolly bodies).

Note

All patients who undergo splenectomy should receive vaccine against pneumococci and *Neisseria meningitidis* 2 weeks before the surgery.

Hypersplenism

Combination of cytopenia, enlargement of spleen with bone marrow being normal or hyperplastic while splenectomy will reverse the abnormality.

8 Endocrine Disorders

DIFFERENT HORMONES PRODUCED BY THE ENDOCRINE SYSTEM

Hormones from Hypothalamus
- GHRH - Growth hormone releasing hormone
- CRF - Corticotrophin releasing hormone
- Prolactin inhibitory factor
- TRH - Thyrotrophin releasing hormone
- GnRH - Gonadotrophin releasing hormone
- Vasopressin (Antidiuretic hormone-ADH) and oxytocin (stored in the posterior pituitary)
- Somatostatin

Trophic Hormones from Pituitary
- ACTH - Adrenocorticotrophic hormone
- MSH - Melanocyte stimulating hormone
- TSH - Thyroid stimulating hormone
- FSH - Follicle stimulating hormone
- LH - Luteinising hormone
- GH - Growth hormone
- Prolactin (Fig. 8.1).

Physiological Control of Endocrine System
(Fig. 8.2)

Hypothalamus secretes releasing hormones which facilitate the secretion of trophic hormones from the pituitary. Trophic hormones in turn facilitate the secretion of corresponding hormone from the peripheral endocrine gland. Prolactin inhibitory factor which is released from the hypothalamus has got negative effect on the pituitary secretion of prolactin. Increase in the level of hormones from peripheral endocrine gland has got negative effect on the pituitary secretion of trophic hormones and increase in the level of trophic hormones have got negative effect on the hypothalamus.

DISORDERS OF PITUITARY

Anterior Pituitary Dysfunction

Hypopituitarism

Causes
- Due to hypothalamic dysfunction
  - Head injury
  - Tuberculosis
  - Sarcoidosis
  - Craniopharyrgioma
  - Surgery
  - Radiation
  - Encephalitis
- Due to pituitary dysfunction
  - Head injury

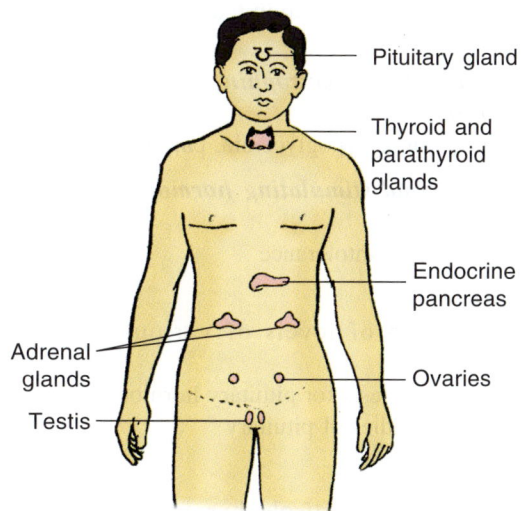

Fig. 8.1 Major endocrine glands

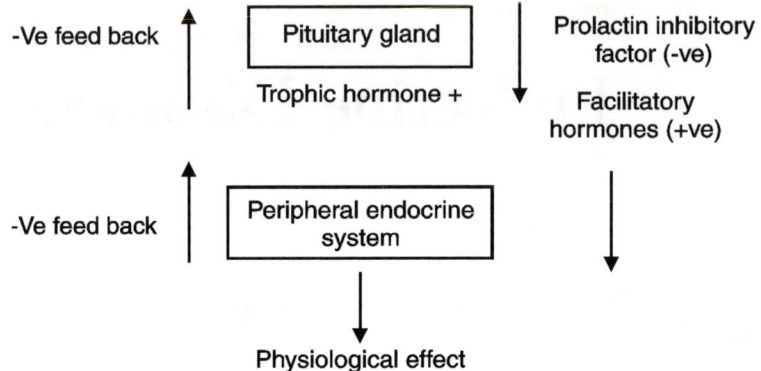

Fig. 8.2 Hypothalamus and pituitary control of endocrine glands

– Hemorrhage into the pituitary
– Postpartum pituitary necrosis
– Surgery, radiation

Clinical Features of Hypopituitarism

Due to growth hormone deficiency
• Short stature
• Muscle weakness

Due to gonadotrophin deficiency (LH and FSH)
• Males: Loss of libido and impotence
• Females: Amenorrhea
• Decreased hair growth in the axilla and pubis
• Skin is wrinkled

Due to adrenocorticotrophin deficiency (ACTH decrease)
• Hypotension, hypoglycemia, pallor

Due to thyroid stimulating hormone deficiency (TSH)
• Apathy, cold intolerance

Investigations

1. Estimation of levels of various pituitary hormones
2. Stimulating tests for pituitary hormones
3. Imaging studies of pituitary

Management

Replacement of cortisol, thyroid hormone, sex steroids and growth hormone.

Dental Aspects

General anesthesia is contraindicated in patients with hypopituitarism and can precipitate coma. Hypopituitary coma can be precipitated by trauma, surgery, general anesthesia and infection. Hypopituitary coma is to be treated in the same way as adrenal crisis.

POSTERIOR PITUITARY DYSFUNCTION

Posterior pituitary stores vasopressin antidiuretic hormone (ADH) and oxytocin which are secreted from hypothalamic nuclei.

Diabetes Insipidus

Diabetes insipidus is a disease characterised by passing of large amount of diluted urine.

Diabetes insipidus occurs due to
• Lack of ADH secretion
  – Central (cranial) diabetes insipidus
• Renal insensitivity of ADH
  – Nephrogenic diabetes insipidus

Cranial Diabetes Insipidus

Causes
• Genetic defect: Didmoad syndrome
• Trauma to the head
• Vascular destruction of hypothalamus/pituitary
• Idiopathic
• Tumor of the pituitary

- Nephrogenic (renal tubules are not responding to ADH)
  - Genetic abnormality
  - Lithium therapy
  - Heavy metal poisoning
  - Hypokalemia

Clinical features

- Poly uria: passage of large amount of dilute urine (15–20 lts./day)
- Polydypsia: Excessive thirst
- Fatiguability
- Severe volume depletion and altered sensorium
- Tumors in the region of pituitary and hypothalamus can cause headache and visual field defects.

Investigations

- Plasma osmolality is increased (> 300 mOsm/kg)
- Urine osmolality < 660 mOsm/kg
- Serum ADH not measurable
- Inability to concentrate the urine during water deprivation test.
- Skull X-ray and MRI of hypothalamus and pituitary.

Treatment of Diabetes Insipidus

- Cranial: Administration of ADH like peptide (desmopressin) administered via nasal mucosa (5 microgram in the morning and 10 microgram at night)
- Nephrogenic: Responds to thiazides
  For example Bendrofluazide 2.5 to 3 mg/day.

ANTERIOR PITUITARY HYPERFUNCTION

Growth hormone (GH) excess causes gigantism and acromegaly.

If growth excess occurs in childhood before epiphyses have fused causes gigantism.

If GH excess occurs in adults causes acromegaly.

Acromegaly

It is caused by macroadenoma of the pituitary causing excess GH secretion.

Clinical features

- Acral (terminal part of the body) enlargement:
  - Large hands, feet and jaw
- Soft tissues abnormalities
  - Excessive sweating and sebum production
  - Thickened skin
  - Nose, lips and tongue enlargement
  - Arthropathy and myopathy
  - Enlargement of heart and liver
  - Increased heel pad thickness
- Other bone abnormalities
  - Prognathism, i.e. enlargement of lower jaw
  - Large frontal sinuses with supra orbital ridges becoming prominent
  - Osteoarthritis
- Metabolic abnormalities
  - Hyperglycemia and hypertension
- Long term complication: Atherosclerosis, colonic cancer
- Local effects of pituitary tumor
  - Headache
  - Visual field defect
  - Raised intracranial pressure

Investigations

- Growth hormone level estimation during oral glucose tolerance test. Growth hormone level fails to get suppressed during the test in patients with acromegaly.
- Visual field testing for evidence of field defects caused by the tumor
- Skull X-ray, MRI pituitary for evidence of adenoma of the pituitary

Treatment

- *Surgical:* Resection of the tumor, curative form of therapy
- *Radiation:* External radiation to the skull after surgery for further reduction in the tumor growth.
- *Medical:* Somatostatin analogues, Dopamine antagonists and growth hormone receptor antagonists are also tried in the treatment of acromegaly.

Dental aspect of growth hormone excess

Mandibular enlargement leads to spacing of teeth and thickening of soft tissues of gum.

Dental management can be complicated by

- Hypertension
- Diabetes mellitus
- Cardiomyopathy
- Thromboembolism
- Narrowing of vocal cords and mobilization of cords reduced.

THYROID DISORDERS

Anatomy and Physiology

- Thyroid gland is present in front of the neck
- Normal thyroid gland produces two main hormones thyroxin (T4) and trio-idothyronine (T3).
- Thyroid hormones are released under the regulatory influence of thyroid stimulating hormone (TSH).
- Thyroid hormones are responsible for carrying out various metabolic activities in the body.

Goitre

Enlargement of thyroid gland is called goitre (Fig. 8.3).

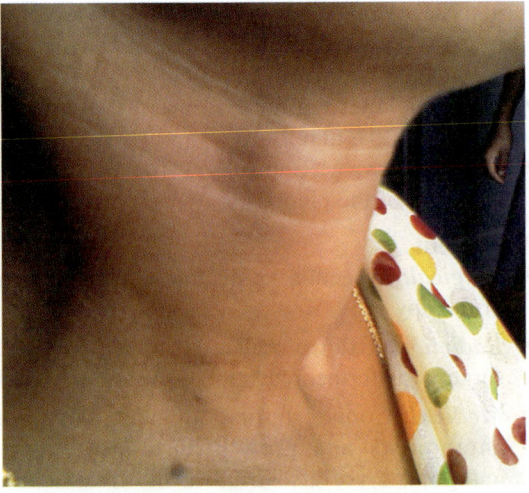

Fig. 8.3 Thyroid enlargement (goitre)

Causes of goitre

- Physiological - puberty, pregnancy
- Grave's disease
- Iodine deficiency (endemic goitre)
- Dyshormonogenesis
- Thyroiditis
- Carcinoma of thyroid

Different types of goitre

- Simple goitre
  - May occur due to iodine deficiency or dyshormonogenesis
  - Thyroid function is within normal limits.
- Simple diffuse goiter
  - Occurs between 15 to 25 years of age.
  - May occur during pregnancy.
  - Soft and symmetrical enlargement of thyroid.
  - Thyroid functions are within normal limits
- Simple multinodular goitre
  - Slowly increasing size of thyroid
  - There will be multiple nodularity
  - Can have thyroid function abnormality.
- Toxic nodular goitre
  - Nodular goitre with thyrotoxicosis
- Thyroiditis and thyroid carcinoma usually present with goitre.

HYPOTHYROIDISM

Decreased functioning of the thyroid gland results in hypothyroidism.

Common Causes of Hypothyroidism

- Primary (disease of the thyroid)
  - Autoimmune thyroiditis
  - Iodine deficiency
  - Radioactive iodine therapy
  - Surgical resection of thyroid
- Secondary (disease outside the thyroid)
  - Hypopituitarism
  - Hypothalamic disease

Clinical Features

- Dry cold skin
- Cold intolerance
- Loss of hair

- Decreased appetite
- Weight gain
- Hoarseness of voice
- Bradycardia
- Angina
- Constipation
- Slow mentation
- Psychosis
- Pleural and pericardial effusion
- Delayed relaxation of ankle jerk.

Myxedema

Severe hypothyroidism causes thickening of subcutaneous tissues due to myxomatous substance deposition resulting in non-pitting edema. This is called myxedema.

Cretinism

Hypothyroidism in infancy results in a condition called cretinism with defective intellectual development and enlarged tongue.

Diagnosis and Management

Thyroid function tests
- Estimation of T3, T4 and TSH and free thyroxin Index
- Elevated TSH with depressed T3 and T4 levels suggest primary hypothyroidism (defect in the thyroid).
- Depressed T3, T4 and TSH suggest secondary hypothyroidism (pituitary hypothalamic cause).
- TPO antibody (thyroid peroxidase antibody) present in autoimmune hypothyroidism.

Treatment

- Daily levothyroxin sodium tablet is required orally, starting with low dose (25 microgram to 50 microgram/day) till the TSH is within normal limits. Treatment should be continued life long.

- Measurement of TSH every year is required.

- In patients with IHD, levothyroxine dose should be adjusted depending on the patient's tolerance.

- Pregnant patients should be given adequate dose of thyroxine to maintain the normal TSH level.

Dental aspects

- Tranquilizers and general anesthetics can precipitate coma in hypothyroid patients.
- Local anesthesia is preferable to general anesthesia.
- Associated hypoadrenalism and hypotension may be associated with hypothyroidism
- Hypothyroidism may be associated with anemia and IHD.

Myxedema Coma

Rare complication of hypothyroidism presenting with depressed level of consciousness. Common in elderly hypothyroid with poor compliance to therapy.

Precipitated by

- Cold exposure
- Myocardial infarction
- Sedatives and antidepressants
- Pneumonia
- CCF
- GI bleed
- Sepsis
- Cerebrovascular accident

Features

- Altered sensorium
- Convulsions
- Hypothermia
- Hypoglycemia
- Hyponatremia

Treatment

- IV/oral levothyroxine 400 to 500 micrograms stat and then 50 to 100 micrograms/day
- Correction of hyponatremia with IV sodium.
- Correction of hypoglycemia with IV glucose
- Inj. Hydrocortisone 50 to 100 micrograms 6th hourly
- Antibiotics for infection
- Ventilatory support

HYPERTHYROIDISM

Hyperthyroidism results from excessive functioning of thyroid gland.

Causes

- Primary (disease of the thyroid)
  - Grave's disease
  - Toxic multinodular goitre
  - Functioning thyroid carcinoma
  - Subacute thyroiditis
  - Drug induced (iodine excess)
  - Amiodarone therapy
- Secondary (disease outside the thyroid)
  - Pituitary adenoma induced TSH excess
  - Hydatidiform mole/choriocarcinoma.

Clinical Features

Symptoms and Signs

- *Goitre:* Thyroid is enlarged (diffuse/nodular)
- *Cardiovascular:* Palpitation, atrial fibrillation, angina pectoris, cardiac failure
- *Dermatological:* Excessive sweating, nail destruction (onycholysis), pretibial myxedema
- *Gastrointestinal:* Increased appetite and weight loss, diarrhoea and vomiting
- *Neuromuscular:* Fine tremors, hyperreflexia, myopathy
- *Ocular:* Exophthalmos, ophthalmoplegia, corneal ulceration
- *Others:* Fatigability, heat intolerance.

Graves' Disease

This is a form of primary hyperthyroidism characterised by diffuse goiter, eye involvement (exophthalmos) and skin involvement (pretibial myxedema).

Diagnosis and Management

Measurement of T3, T4 and TSH levels

- In primary hyperthyroidism T3 and T4 levels are raised and TSH is suppressed.
- In secondary hyperthyroidism T3, T4 and TSH levels are raised (pituitary induced).

Other investigations like radioactive iodine uptake, thyroid scan, fine needle aspiration cytology of thyroid, free thyroxin index are also helpful in the diagnosis of hyperthyroidism.

Treatment

Medical

- Initial therapy of thyrotoxicosis
- Period of therapy : 12 to 18 months

Drugs used

- Antithyroid drugs: Carbimazole (30–60 mg/day). Propyl thiouracil (safer in pregnancy). Dose: 100–200 mg/day,

Duration of therapy

- 6 months to 18 months.
- 50% of patients can have relapse of thyrotoxicosis after stopping antithyroid drugs.
- Carbimazole can cause agranulocytosis.
- Patients of thyrotoxicosis with symptoms of palpitation and sleep disturbance should be given:
  - β-blockers - propranolol - 20 to 40 mg/day (for palpitation).
  - Sedation - Diazepam - 5 mg/day

Surgical

Preferred procedure: Subtotal thyroidectomy.

Indications

- Large-sized goiters with thyrotoxicosis
- Patients under the age of 40 yrs with thyrotoxicosis (patient requires treatment with Lugol's iodine for 2 weeks before surgery to decrease the vascularity of the gland).

Note: Hypoparathyroidism can result from thyroid surgery and recurrent laryngeal nerve paralysis can also occur due to thyroid surgery.

Radioactive Iodine Therapy

Action: Destroys the functioning thyroid cells.

Indications

- For patients with relapse of hyperthyroidism after stopping antithyroid drugs and if patient is not fit for surgery.
- Radioactive iodine therapy can result in hypothyroidism. Radioactive iodine is contraindicated in pregnancy.

Thyrotoxic Crises

Medical emergency occurring due to the excess release of thyroid hormones.

Sudden increase in the manifestations of hyperthyroidism with atrial fibrillation with cardiac failure and hyperthermia.

Precipitates by
- Infection
- Inadequate preparation before thyroid surgery for thyrotoxicosis

Treatment
- Adequate hydration
- Treatment of hyperthermia
- Propranalol IV 80 mg qid
- Sodium Iopodate 50 mg/day
- Carbimazole 40 to 60 mg/day

Dental Aspects of Thyroid Dysfunction

Carbimazole which is used in the treatment of hyperthyroidism can cause agranulocytosis and can result in pharyngeal and oral ulcers.

Uncontrolled hyperthyroidism can result in arrhythmias when general anesthesia is used and there is a risk of development of thyrotoxic crisis during anesthesia.

Adrenaline containing drugs should be used carefully in patients with uncontrolled hyper-thyroidism.

Adrenal Gland

Adrenal glands are present on upper poles of each kidney. Gland consists of 2 parts called outer cortex and inner medulla.

Outer cortex secretes corticosteroids, mineral corticoids and sex steroids. Inner medulla secretes catecholamines.

CUSHING'S SYNDROME

Cushing's disease Occurs due to excess ACTH production by Pituitary adenomas.
- Cushing's syndrome is caused by adrenal adenoma, adrenal carcinoma or other causes of cortisol excess.

Aetiology and classification of Cushing's Syndrome
- Due to excess ACTH
  - Bilateral adrenal hyperplasia due to excess ACTH from pituitary.
  - Paraneoplastic syndrome due to ectopic ACTH production, e.g. small cell carcinoma.
  - ACTH therapy - Iatrogenic
- Non ACTH dependant
  - Adrenal carcinoma
  - Adrenal adenoma
  - Glucocorticoid therapy - Iatrogenic

Clinical Features of Cushing's Syndrome
- Abdominal striae
- Acne
- Hypertension
- Infections
- Moon face
- Menstrual abnormalities
- Osteoporosis
- Peptic ulcer
- Truncal obesity
- Osteoporosis
- Hypertension
- Diabetes mellitus
- Psychosis
- Myopathy/vertebral collapse causes mobility limitation
- Steroid crisis

Investigations
1. Increased serum cortical level with loss of circadian rhythm.
2. ACTH level estimation
   - ACTH level is increased in pituitary induced cushing's syndrome.
   - ACTH is decreased in adrenal disease
3. Dexamethasone suppression test
   - Low dose (0.5 mg) dexamethasone QID -

estimate the cortisol level. In Cushing's syndrome cortisol level is not suppressed.
- A high dose dexamethasone test is required to distinguish pituitary, adrenal and ectopic ACTH induced Cushing's syndrome.
4. MRI pituitary, CT and ultrasound of the abdomen are required for localizing the tumor.

Treatment

- Removal of pituitary adenoma through the transphenoidal route. Removal of the adrenal gland bilaterally is required.
- Medical treatment with antiadrenal drugs may be required before surgery.
- *Adrenal tumor:* Removal of the tumor.
- *Ectopic ACTH syndrome:* Treatment of the cause and medical therapy for Cushing's syndrome.

Dental Aspects of Cushing's Syndrome

Dental treatment in Cushing's syndrome can be complicated by the following.

ADDISON'S DISEASE

Addison's disease occurs due to adrenocortical insufficiency.

Causes of Adrenocortical Insufficiency

Addison's disease (Primary adrenal insufficiency - ACTH excess)

Common causes
- Autoimmune adrenalitis
- Tuberculosis of the adrenal gland
- HIV/AIDS of the adrenal gland
- Bilateral adrenalectomy

Rare causes
- Meningococcal septicemia
- Adrenal hemorrhage
- Lymphoma of adrenal gland
- Congenital adrenal hyperplasia

Secondary Adrenal Insufficiency (ACTH-decrease)
- Hypothalamic pituitary disease
- Withdrawal of steroid long term therapy

Clinical Features

- Anorexia, nausea and vomiting
- Fatigability
- Hypotension
- Hypoglycemia
- Mucosal pigmentation
- Skin pigmentation
- Weight loss

Cortisol deficiency leads to hypoglycemia and hypotension. Skin pigmentation occurs due to increased levels of melanocyte stimulating hormone.

Patients with autoimmune adrenalitis will be associated with other endocrine deficiencies.

Secondary adrenal insufficiency is due to ACTH deficiency due to pituitary disease or due to steroid therapy with sudden stoppage of steroids.

Diagnosis and Management

Investigation
- Serum sodium level and blood sugar is decreased.
- Cortisol level is decreased
- ACTH level is increased in primary adrenal insufficiency

ACTH stimulation test
- 250 mg of synthetic ACTH (synacthen) is injected
- Plasma is collected before and 30 minutes after injection synacthen for cortisol level. Normally cortisol level increases after ACTH level. In primary adrenal insufficiency cortisol level does not increase after ACTH injection.
- Chest X-ray to rule out tuberculosis, CT head scan for pituitary disease may also be required.

Treatment
- Glucorticoid replacement
- T. Prednisolone 7.5 mg in the morning and 5 mg in the evening and adjust the dose with monitoring of cortisol level.
- Replacement with fludrocortisone (mineralo-corticoid) may be required.

Addisonian Crisis (adrenal crisis)
- Addisonian crisis occurs due to acute reduction of cortisol level.
- Addisonian crisis occurs in patients with

Addison's disease either due to infection, surgery, stress or sudden stoppage of intake of steroids.

Features
Severe hypotension, hypotension and shock, hyponatremia and hyperkalemia, hypoglycemia and hypercalcemia.

Treatment
Medical emergency, IV hydrocortisone succinate 100 mg QID, IV dextrose saline, treatment of the cause.

Dental Aspects Addison's Disease
- Oral mucosal and tongue pigmentation can occur due to Addison's disease (Fig. 8.4).
- Dental treatment can cause sudden hypotensive collapse in patients with Addison's disease if preoperative corticosteroids are given.

CORTICOSTEROID THERAPY

Indications
- Replacement therapy in Addison's disease and in adrenocortical deficiency.
- Connective tissue disorders like SLE and rheumatoid arthritis
- Gastrointestinal disorders
- Inflammatory bowel disease
- *Renal disorders:* Nephrotic syndrome
- *Blood disorders:* Leukemias, lymphomas and ITP.
- *Dermatological disorders:* Pemphigus

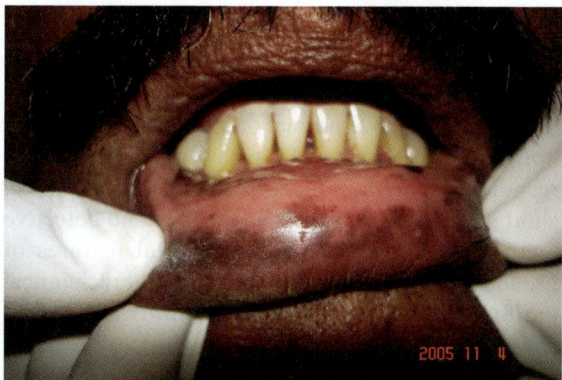

Fig. 8.4 Pigmentation of oral cavity in Addison's disease

- *Allergic disorders:* Bronchial asthma, allergic disorders .

Complications of Corticosteroid Therapy

Metabolic
- Hyperglycemia
- Osteoporosis
- Hypothalamopituitary adrenal suppression
- Growth retardation in children

Immunological suppression
- Susceptibility to infection
- Reactivation of tuberculosis

Cardiovascular
- Hypertension
- Myocardial infarction

Gastrointestinal
- Peptic ulceration
- Neurological
- Psychoses

Dermatological
- Acne, striae
- Hirsutism

Miscellaneous
- Cataract formation
- Proximal myopathy
- Osteoporosis

Dental Aspects of Systemic Corticosteroid Therapy
- Impaired wound healing
- Oral candidiasis
- Patient can go into adrenal crisis after trauma, surgery if corticosteroid supplementation is not given adequately (injection hydrocortisone 100 mg QID).
- General aesthesia should be given by specialized anesthetists with adequate cortisol replacement.

PARATHYROID GLANDS

Parathyroid Glands Secrete: Parathyroid Hormone (PTH)
Parathyroid hormone (PTH) regulates the serum calcium level through its action on the gastrointestinal

tract, kidneys and bone. Decrease in the level of ionized calcium stimulates PTH secretion.

Physiological Aspects of Calcium, Phosphorous and Magnesium

Metabolism of Calcium
Normal calcium level in the blood is 8.5 to 10.5 mg/dL and 50% of it is in the ionised form. Ionised calcium is important as it is responsible for metabolic activity especially neumomuscular function.

Normal serum calcium level is maintained by parathormone (PTH) and active form of Vit. D (1-25 (OH$_2$) cholecalciferol).

When serum ionised calcium level decreases PTH secretion increases. Parathyroid hormone acts synergistically with active Vit. D.

Action of Parathyroid Hormone along with 1-25(OH)$_2$ Cholecalciferol
- Increases gastrointestinal absorption of calcium.
- Increases renal absorption of calcium
- Decreases renal reabsorption of phosphate
- Increases bone resorption

Calcitonin which is secreted by parafollicular cells of PTH and decreases serum calcium level.

Corticosteroids, thyroxine and oestrogen also affect the bone formation and metabolism.

Metabolism of Phosphorous
Normal concentration of phosphorous in blood 2.5 to 4.5 mg/dl.

Phosphorous is mainly present in the blood and also as a component of nucleic acids ATPs and intracellular enzymes.

Active form of vitamin D [1-25 (OH)$_2$D] increases intestinal absorption of phosphorous and reduced by parathyroid hormone. In patients with renal insufficiency increase in the level of phosphorous occurs in the serum. If the serum calcium and phosphorous product becomes more than 50 it will result in metastatic calcification.

Metabolism of Magnesium
- Normal serum concentration of magnesium is 1.5 to 2.4 mg/dl. Extracellular magnesium along with calcium is required for neuromuscular function.

- Intracellular magnesium is required for the action of enzymes, nucleic acid and ATP. 1-25 (OH)$_2$D increases, intestinal absorption of magnesium.
- Decrease in the magnesium level results in decrease secretion of parathyroid hormone (PTH), resistance to the action of PTH and defective synthesis of 1.25 (OH)$_2$D.

Hypoparathyroidism

Causes
- Idiopathic
- Pseudo hypoparathyroidism
- Thyroid surgery
- Hypoparathyroidism results in hypocalcemia.

Clinical Features of Hypocalcemia
- Convulsions
- Cataract formation
- Tetany

Features of Tetany (see below)
- Tingling and numbness of arms and legs
- Facial twitching (Chvostek's sign)
- Corpopedal spasm (Trousseau's sign)
- Laryngeal stridor

Idiopathic Hypoparathyroidism
Characterised by symptoms and signs of tetany, stridor, cataract calcification of basal ganglia, defects of teeth, mucocutaneous candidiasis and other endocrine deficiencies.

Pseudohypoparathyroidism
These patients have normal or increased parathyroid hormone secretion as the tissue receptors do not respond to parathormone. Patient will be having short stature, small fingers and toes but no defective teeth. Patients who have got skeletal features of pseudo hypoparathyroidism but normal biochemical parameters (normal serum calcium) are called pseudohypoparathyroidism.

Dental Aspects of Hypoparathyroidism
Following dental abnormalities can occur
- Enamel hypoplasia

- Short root of teeth
- Delayed eruption of teeth
- Chronic mucocutaneous candidiasis
- Facial paraesthesia and twitching

Treatment of hypoparathyroidism
- Chronic hypocalcemia - replacement of calcium and active vitamin D_3
- Alpha hydroxycholecalciferol (alpha-calcidol) administration
- Treatment of tetany

HYPOCALCEMIA AND TETANY

Causes of Hypocalcemia
Due to hypoparathyroidism
- Idiopathic
- Pseudohypoparathyroidism
- Parathyroid surgery

Due to vitamin D deficiency
- Decrease intake and decrease exposure to sunlight
- Malabsorption
- Anticonvulsant therapy
- Vitamin D dependant rickets
- Chronic renal failure

Miscellaneous causes
- Acute renal failure
- Acute pancreatitis
- Metabolic alkalosis
- Hypomagnesemia

Tetany
Tetany occurs due to increased excitability of peripheral nerves secondary to decreased in the ionized calcium.

Causes
- Hypocalcemia
- Alkalosis
- Hypomagnesemia due to malabsorption, diuretic therapy, alkalosis.

Features
- Carpopedal spasm
- Stridor
- Convulsions

Carpopedal Spasm

Carpal spasm
- Metacarpophalangeal joints are flexed, interphalangeal joints of fingers and thumb are extended with opposition of thumb.

Pedal spasm
- Spasm of feet can occur

Stridor
- Occurs due to spasm of glottis: common in children.
Adults: Tingling of hands and feet and tingling sensation around the mouth.

Latent Tetany
- Signs of manifest tetany are absent.

Signs to Elicit Latent Tetany

Trousseau's sign
- Apply the BP cuff to the upper arm and raise the BP more than systolic BP and keep it for more than 3 minutes. This will elicit carpal spasm.

Chvostek's sign
- Twitching of facial muscles occurs when the facial nerve is tapped as it emerges out of the parotid gland.

Management of Tetany
- Hypocalcemia: Injection of 10% calcium gluconate - 20 ml IV slowly.
- Inj. Magnesium can also be tried if it is not controlled by calcium.
- Alkalosis: Rebreath the expired air in a paper bag or administration of 5% CO_2 in oxygen.

HYPERCALCAEMIA AND HYPERPARATHYROIDISM

Causes of Hypercalcemia
Normal or excess parathormone level
- Primary/tertiary hyperparathyroidism
- Lithium induced hyperparathyroidism
Low paratharmone level
- Multiple myeloma
- Thyrotoxicosis

- Thiazide diuretics
- Addison's disease
- Paget's disease with immobilization

Malignancies: For example, lungs, breast, renal, ovary colon and thyroid

Symptoms and Signs of Hypercalcemia

- Polyuria
- Polydypsia
- Constipation
- Drowsiness
- Altered sensorium
- Ureteric colic
- Anorexia, nausea and vomiting
- Peptic ulceration

Primary Hyperparathyroidism

Features

- Chronic disease
- Symptoms of bony pain, ureteric colic due to ureteric calculus and abdominal pain
- Hypertension
  May be associated with other endocrine diseases in other family member. For example, multiple endocrine neoplasia

Investigations

Increased serum calcium and increased serum alkaline phosphatase level with decreased phosphorous level suggests: primary hyperparathyroidism

Serum parathyroid hormone level is increased in primary and tertiary hyperparathyroidism. If parathyroid hormone is low and if no other cause is found for hypercalcemia internal malignancy may be the cause for hypercalcemia.

Management of Hypercalcemia

Different forms of therapy for hypercalcemia: Mild hypercalcemia (up to 12 mg/dl): Hydration with IV saline.

For more rapid bringing down the serum calcium level. IV saline + frusemide.

- IV calcitonin can act within hours and can bring down the serum calcium level rapidly.

- In several hypercalcemia Ser. Ca >15 mg/dl). Hemodialysis can be performed.
- Biphosphonates like zolendronate can bring down the serum calcium level within 1–2 days and can acts for 3 weeks.
- Corticosteroids act within days to bring down the serum calcium sugar and action will be prolonged for weeks.

Management of the Cause

Surgical removal of the parathyroid gland in primary hyperparathyroidism.

Secondary Hyperparathyroidism

In patients with low serum calcium level like in chronic renal failure with increased parathyroid hormone secretions treatment of the cause.

Tertiary Hyperparathyroidism

Prolonged secondary hyperparathyroidism becomes autonomous hypertrophy of parathyroid gland causes tertiary hyperparathyroidism.

Dental Aspects of Hyperparathyroidism

Hyperparathyroidism can cause generalized rarefaction of bone with giant cell lesions.

Dental Treatment can be Complicated by

- Bone rarefaction
- Hypertension
- Renal disease
- Peptic ulcer
- Cardiac arrhythmias
- Increased sensitivity to muscle relaxants

DIABETES MELLITUS

Diabetes mellitus is one of the most common endocrine disorders. Diabetes mellitus literally means passing sweet urine.

Diabetes mellitus is characterized by persistently raised blood glucose levels (hyperglycemia) either due to absolute or relative deficiency of insulin.

Classification

Primary

Type1: Beta-cell destruction of pancreas causing absolute deficiency of insulin.

Type 2: Associated with predominantly insulin resistance/defect in beta cell function and insulin action.

Secondary
Endocrine disorders
- Cushing's syndrome
- Corticosteroid therapy
- Acromegaly
- Phaeochromocytoma
- Glucagonoma

Pancreatic
- Pancreatitis
- Pancreatectomy
- Cystic fibrosis of the pancreas

Drug induced: Glucocorticoids, diazoxide, phenytoin

Infective
- Coxsackie virus
- Congenital rubella
- Cytomegalovirus

Genetic Syndromes
- Down's syndrome
- Turner's syndrome
- Pregnancy related-gestational diabetes mellitus

Clinical Features of Diabetes Mellitus

Symptoms of Diabetes Mellitus
- Tiredness, fatigue, irritability, loss of weight
- Thirst and dry mouth
- Polyuria and nocturia
- Blurring of vision
- Pruritis vulvae, balanitis and genital candidiasis
- Nausea, headache
- Hyperphagia (excessive hunger and eating)

Classical triad of symptoms of polyuria, polyphagia (excessive hunger) polydypsia (excessive thirst) are prominent in type I diabetes mellitus but not a feature of type 2 diabetes mellitus. Uncontrolled diabetes mellitus can cause genital candidiasis and pruritis vulvae.

Persons with type I diabetes mellitus may not have any clinical signs and may present with significant weight loss or they may present with acute complications of diabetes mellitus like diabetic ketoacidosis.

Type II diabetes mellitus are usually obese, hypertensives and 25% of them may present with chronic complications of diabetes mellitus (Table 8.1).

Maturity Onset Diabetes Mellitus in Young (MODY)

Characterised by
- Autosomal dominant inheritance
- Hyperglycemia
- Impairment in insulin secretion

Diagnoses and Investigations of Diabetes Mellitus

Testing Urine for Glucose
Using glucose strips by dipstick method

Presence of glucose in the urine suggests glycosuria which may not be specific for diabetes mellitus. Requires testing of blood glucose for the diagnosis of diabetes mellitus.

Blood Glucose Measurement
Criteria for diagnosis of diabetes mellitus
- Fasting glucose > 126 mg/dl
- Two hour plasma glucose > 200 mg/dl during oral glucose tolerance test (post prandial blood glucose > 200 mg/dl 2 hours after the main meal).
- Blood sugar testing should be repeated on two occasions.

Urine Ketones
Testing for ketones in urine detected with ketostix is useful in the diagnosis of diabetic ketoacidosis.

Urine Protein
Measurement of albumin in the urine and presence of microalbuminuria is suggestive of diabetic nephropathy.

Glycosylated Haemoglobin
Measurement of glycosylated haemoglobin provides an accurate measurement of glycaemic control over a period of 3 months.

Table 8.1 Clinical features of different types of diabetes milletus

	Type I	Type 2
Age of onset	<40 yrs	>40 yrs
Family history	Uncommon	Common
Body weight	Normal or low	Obese
Duration of symptom	Short in weeks	Long-months, years
Ketosis prone	Yes	No
Death without Insulin	Yes	Less common
Auto antibodies	present	Not associated
Complications of diabetes mellitus at diagnosis	Rare	25% of patients
Other autoimmune diseases	Yes	Uncommon

Blood Lipids

Concentration of serum lipids, total cholesterol, LDL, HDL and triglycerides indicate the metabolic control of diabetes mellitus.

MANAGEMENT OF DIABETES MELLITUS

Nutritional Therapy in Diabetes

Medical nutritional therapy (MNT) includes diet therapy, exercise and insulin therapy.

Exercise

Regular exercise will decrease the obesity and improve the blood sugar control.

Exercise induces weight loss, decreases blood pressure, maintain muscle mass and decreases cardiovascular risk and helps in control of blood sugar.

Diet Therapy in Diabetes Mellitus

- Dietary control is useful in treating obese diabetic patients.
- Should have a regular balanced diet
- To avoid rapidly absorbed carbohydrates
- 30–35 kcalories/kg body weight is the ideal calory requirement depending on the type of life style.

Different dietary recommendations

- Intake of proteins: 15–20% of total calories.
- Carbohydrates: 60–70% of total calories (avoid direct sugar)
- Polyunsaturated fat: Less than 10% of total calories.
- Intake of dietary fibre: 20–30 g/day

- Avoidance of alcohol
- Use of sweetners if required.

Oral Hypoglycemic Drugs

Sulphonyl ureas

- Glybenclamide 5–20 mg/day
- Glypizide (5–20 mg/day)
- Glymepride (1–8 mg/day)
- Glyclazide (40–80 mg/day)
- Sulphonyl ureas stimulate insulin release from beta cells of the pancreas.

  For example, 1st generation sulphonyl ureas: Tolbutamide, chlorpropamide

  2nd generation sulphonyl ureas: Glyclazide, glypizide, glymepride, glybenclamide.
- Sulphonyl ureas are useful in type II diabetes mellitus. They can produce significant hypoglycemia. After initial response to sulphonyl urea patients of type II diabetes mellitus may fail to respond, called-sulphonyl urea failure.

Biguanides

For example, metformin, dosage 1 to 3 g/day

Mechanism of Action

Increases insulin sensitivity and peripheral uptake of glucose.

Indications

In type II diabetics along with sulphonyl ureas especially in obese diabetics.

Contraindications
- Liver and renal dysfunction
- Can cause lactic acidosis

Alpha Glucosidase Inhibitors
- Inhibit carbohydrate absorption in the gut.
- Useful in treating post prandial hyperglycemia, e.g. acarbose.

Thiazolidinediones
- Enhances the action of insulin and useful in patients with insulin resistance, e.g. pioglitazones 15 to 30 mg/day.

Meglutinides
- Stimulate endogenous insulin secretion
- Useful in controlling post prandial glucose, e.g. Repaglanides 0.5 to 1 mg.

Insulin Preparations

Present preparations of insulin are divided from recombinant DNA technology almost resemble endogenous insulin from human pancreas and are called human insulins. They are least antigenic and very effective in controlling blood sugar.

Different Types of Insulin Preparations
Short and rapid acting insulins.
- Regular (crystalline insulin): duration of action 3–4 hrs.
- Insulin analogues (insulin lispro and insulin aspat): start acting within 15 mins. and can act upto 3–4 hrs.

Intermediate Acting
(Addition of zinc): Lente insulin
(Addition of protamine): NPH insulin
Onset of action within 2–4 hrs and duration of action for 10–18 hrs.

Long Acting Insulins
Glargine: Onset of action : 4–10 hrs.
Ultralente: Duration of action : 18–24 hrs.

For initial control of blood sugar premixed insulin (short acting + intermediate acting)/long acting insulin is used.

In all medical emergencies short acting insulin is used.

Indications for Insulin Therapy
- Type I diabetes mellitus
- All acute complications of diabetes mellitus e.g. diabetic ketoacidosis
- Chronic complications of diabetes mellitus
- In type II diabetics with failure of oral antidiabetics.
- Pregnancy with diabetes mellitus
- In the treatment of hyperkalemia

Side Effects of Insulin Treatment
- Hypoglycemia
- Weight gain
- Pedal edema (due to salt and water retention)
- Insulin antibodies
- Insulin allergy
- Insulin lipodystrophy

Complications of Diabetes Mellitus
Acute Complications
- Diabetic ketoacidosis
- Non ketotic hyperosmolar coma
- Lactic acidosis
- Hypoglycemia
- Infections

Diabetic Ketoacidosis (Hyperglycemic Coma)

Diabetic ketoacidosis occurs due to relative or absolute deficiency of insulin.

Factors Precipitating Diabetic Ketoacodsis
- Infection
- Not taking insulin; in type I diabetes mellitus
- Myocardial infarction, stroke
- Pregnancy

Clinical Features
- Usually occurs in persons with type I diabetes mellitus.
- Slow onset of altered sensorium
- Signs of dehydration (weak pulse, dry skin, hypotension, tachycardia)
- Acidotic (Kussmal) breathing-deep rapid breathing
- Vomiting and pain abdomen

- Ketosis - smell of ketone (acetone), and fruity odour to breath

On Investigation
- Blood sugar - very high (200–600 mg/day)
- pH of blood - acidotic
- Urine ketones positive
- Electrolyte abnormalities (hyponatremia, potassium serum) normal or increased.
- Evidence of infection: Urine showing WBCs and chest X-ray - evidence of pneumonia

Treatment of Diabetic Ketoacidosis
- Admission to the intensive care unit.
- Monitor pulse rate blood pressure, respiratory rate and urine output.
- Following biochemical investigations are assessed.
  – Measurement of blood sugar every 1 to 2 hrs.
  – Measurement of urine ketones, urea, creatinine, blood pH, serum electrolytes and b hydroxybutyric acid every 1 to 4 hrs.
- Correction of serum electrolytes - Serum sodium and potassium

Intravenous Fluids
- Replace with 0.9% saline rapidly (about 3 litres of extracellular fluid) in 3 hours.
- Replace with 5% dextrose (about 3 litres of intra cellular fluid)

Insulin Therapy
- Start IV insulin infusion—about 5 units/hr or 0.1U/Kg/hour and then increase/decrease the insulin infusion depending on the blood sugar level till the blood sugar level reaches 250 mg/dl. Make the insulin - short acting 6th hrly. when blood glucose is 250 mg/dl and then change over to longer acting insulin at the time of discharge.
- Correct metabolic acidosis by IV bicarbonate if blood pH is < 7.0.

Following therapeutic measures may be required
- Urinary catheterisation, Ryle's tube aspiration of stomach, central venous pressure monitoring.
- Treat precipitating factors like myocardial infarction, stroke, infection.

- Proper antibiotics if evidence of infection.
- Monitoring of blood sugar, blood urea, creatinine, electrolytes and urine ketones and urine output.

Hyperosmolar Non Ketotic State

Features
- Elderly type 2 diabetic
- Usually precipitated by severe infection, stroke/ acute myocardial infarction.
- Relatively less deficiency of insulin compared to diabetic ketoacidosis which results in hyperglycemia without ketoacidosis.
- Severe hyperglycemia results in severe hyperosmality with dehydration, hypotension, tachycardia and coma.

Lab Investigations
- Severe hyperglycemia (blood sugar 500 to 1000 mg/dl)
- Serum osmolality > 350 mOsmo
- Ketosis and acidosis are usually absent.

Treatment
- IV fluids 0.45% saline if serum sodium is high (1–3 lits in 3 hours). Use normal saline (0.9%) if serum sodium is at a lower level.
- IV short acting insulin depending on the blood sugar level.
- Replace fluid till the serum osmolality and serum sodium is normal.
- Correction of serum potassium and precipitating cause.

Hypoglycemic Coma
(decrease of blood sugar)

Causes
- In a diabetic: Excess of insulin/oral hypoglycemic drugs
- Exercise
- Missing a meal after insulin

In Non Diabetics (rare)
- Hepatic Disease
- Insulinoma
- Hypoadrenalism
- Hypopituitarism

Clinical Features

- Occurs usually in a diabetic either due to failure to take food, over dosage of anti diabetic drugs or alcohol intake (Table 8.2).
- Rapid onset of fainting like symptoms, lack of memory, sweating, palpitation and tremulousness.

Management

- In conscious persons administration of glucose orally.

In Patients with Altered Sensorium

- IV 50% dextrose 100 ml and if necessary, continuous administration of dextrose
  - Stop all the antidiabetic drugs.
  - IM injection of glucagons can be administered

Chronic Complications of Diabetes Mellitus

Cardiovascular
- Ischemic heart disease
- Cerebrovascular accident
- Peripheral vascular disease

Ocular
- Retinopathy
- Cataract

Renal
- Renal failure
- Hypertension

Neuropathies
- Peripheral neuropathy
- Mononeuropathy
- Autonomic neuropathy

Infection
- Candidiasis
- Tuberculosis
- Bacterial infection

Dental Aspects of Diabetes Mellitus

Following oral manifestations may be common in patients with diabetes mellitus
- Periondontitis
- Dry mouth
- Caries tooth
- Mucormycosis of nose and paranasal sinuses
  Hypoglycemia can occur in a diabetic if he is unable to eat properly because of dental disease.

General Anaesthesia in a Diabetic may be Complicated by
- Chronic renal failure
- Ischemic heart disease
- Autonomic neuropathy

Autonomic neuropathy can cause hypotension, mask hypoglycemia and cardiorespiratory arrest during general anesthesia.

Routine Non Surgical Dental Procedures in a Diabetic
- Local anesthetic procedures can be safely carried out.
- Treatment can be carried out after breakfast to avoid hypoglycemia.

Surgical Procedures

Precautions required during oral surgery in a diabetic
- Severity of diabetes mellitus
- Type of anesthetic

Table 8.2 Differences between hyperglycemic and hypoglycemic coma	
Hypoglycemic coma	*Hyperglycemic coma*
Patient is usually a known diabetic	May not be a known diabetic
Excess intake of insulin/anti diabetic drugs or too little food intake or too much of exercise or alcohol	Too little insulin/sepsis or myocardial infarction
Tachycardia, high volume pulse	Low volume pulse
Dilated pupil	Low blood pressure
Administration of IV glucose immediate recovery	No change after administration of glucose

- Extent of surgery
- Extent of interference with oral feeding post operatively.
- Diabetes should be under good control before all surgical procedures.
- If the patient is on insulin, patient can be given morning dose of insulin and breakfast and minor dental procedures can be carried out.

Precautions During Major Dental Procedures in A Diabetic

- Admit the patient a 2–3 days before surgery and do the full medical assessment.

- Put the patient on soluble (short) acting insulin 3 or 4 times a day until the blood sugar is under control.
- Surgery preferably to be carried out as a first case in the morning.
- Skip the dose of insulin on the morning of surgery and start dextrose with neutralising dose of insulin (1 unit of short acting insulin for 2 g of dextrose). Continue the infusion till the patient is taking orally.
- Monitor the blood glucose every 2–4 hours till the patient is taking orally.

Renal, Water, Electrolyte and Acid Base Disorders

Tests for Kidney Function and Urogenital System

Urine Analysis

- Normal volume of urine output/day = 1.5 to 2.5 lits/day
- Polyuria passage of more than 3 litres of urine per day
- Oliguria passage of less than 400 ml/day
- Anuria - total absence of formation of urine

Proteinuria

- Normal excretion of protein in the urine - less than 150 mg/day
- Microalbuminuria - urinary albuminuria excretion > 30 micrograms/day

Different Types of Proteinuria

- *Glomerular proteinuria:* Due to glomerular disease
- Tubular proteinuria: presence of tubular protein called - Tamm Horsfall protein
- *Excretion of abnormal proteins in the urine,* e.g. Light chains in patients of multiple myeloma.
- *Nephrotic range of proteinuria:* Excretion of more than 3.5 g of protein/24 hours.

Causes of Proteinuria

Benign causes: Orthostatic proteinuria / post exercise.

Pathological causes
- Glomerulonephritis
- Bence Jones proteinuria
- Diabetic nephopathy
- Amyloid kidney
  Cellular analysis of urine (see Chapter 16 on normal laboratory data)

Biochemical tests of renal function (see also Chapter 16 on normal laboratory data)

Blood urea: Does not reflect actual kidney function. Blood urea value depends on renal blood flow, liver function and dietary intake of protein.

Serum creatinine
- Significantly reflects renal function
- Serum creatinine level raises only if more than 50% of glomerular function is lost.
- Creatinine clearance value indirectly represents glomerular filtration rate.
- Changes in muscle mass can affect the serum creatinine level.

Radiological Investigations

Ultrasound of the kidney: Ultrasound of the kidney helps in detecting renal tumors, cysts, calculi and chronic renal parenchymal disease.

Renal artery doppler: Detects renal artery blood flow and can detect renal artery stenosis.

CT scan: Useful in detecting cysts, mass lesions and vascular disorders of the kidney.

MRI scan: Because non nephrotoxic contrast (gadolinium based) is used, it is useful in patients with renal dysfunction. Renal blood vessels can be better delineated.

Intravenous Pyelography (IVP)

Serial X-rays are taken after intravenous administration of contrast which is excreted by the kidney. It is helpful in detecting anatomical and physiological function of the kidney. Renal stones, tumors and papillae can be delineated by IVP.

Isotope Study of the Kidney

DTPA (diethylene triamine penta acetic acid) scan of the kidney can detect renal function, vascular disorders of the kidney. It can detect function of each kidney, vesicoureteric reflux and cortical scarring.

Renal Biopsy

Kidney biopsy is performed for accurate diagnosis of acute/chronic parenchymal renal disease and assessing the response to treatment.

SYMPTOM ANALYSIS OF RENAL DISEASE

SYMPTOM ANALYSIS

I. Pain During the Act of Voiding Urine

Pain during the act of micturition may be indicative of pathology in the kidney, ureter, prostate, urethra.

Pain of different Renal and Urogenital Disorders

Characteristic features

1. *Acute glomerulonephritis:* Dull aching pain in the lumbar region.
2. *Acute pyelonephritis:* Renal angle pain on the affected side.
3. *Prostatitis:* Perineal or rectal pain.
4. *Cystitis/urethritis:* Person feels burning or scalding discomfort during or at the end of micturition.
5. *Perinephric abscess:* Causes severe back pain.
   - Tracking of perinephric abscess towards diaphragm: shoulder pain due to diaphragm irritation.
   - Tracking of perinephric abscess towards the Psoas: Extension of hip causes pain.
6. *Loin pain hematuria syndrome:* Intermittent dull aching loin pain associated with hematuria.
7. *Obstruction to the urine flow:* Obstruction to the urine flow may be due to calculus, pus, blood clots, infection.

Note: Acute urinary obstruction causes colicky pain. Chronic obstruction may be painless.

8. *Ureteric colic:*
   - Severe spasmodic pain
   - Starts from the renal angle and radiates up to the groin (testes or medial thigh).
   - *Patient:* Restless associated with vomiting and sweating.
   - Pain increases by jolting or movement and may last upto few hours (common with calculus disease).
9. *Bladder and urethral obstruction pain:* Referred to lower abdomen, perineum and glans penis in the male.
10. *Strangury:* Painful passing of urine drop by drop.
11. *Dysuria:* Difficulty in passing urine may be associated with pain or discomfort.

Note: Grossly enlarged or scarred kidneys may occasionally cause dull aching flank pain. "Progressive and advanced renal disease may be without discomfort".

II. Symptoms Due to Disturbance during the Act of Voiding the Urine

Increased Frequency of Micturition

Causes

1. Due to increased urinary volume (all causes of polyuria).
2. Frequency with normal urinary volume:
   Due to irritation of bladder:
   For example, Calculus, growth, infection or blood clot.
   Due to decreased bladder capacity:
   For example, extrinsic compression of the bladder from a pelvic mass.
3. Neurological disorder affecting the bladder

Nocturia (frequency of Urine more at Night)

Frequency of urine is more easily recognised at night than the day.

Note
- Disturbed sleep leads to decreased ADH level.
- During recumbency renal blood flow increases.
- Above mechanism result in increased urine formation at night.
- All causes of increased frequency can have nocturia.
- *Specific causes of nocturia:* Renal failure, early CCF.

Precipitancy

Person passes urine suddenly without prior warning symptoms. For example, neurological disorders of bladder, occasionally gynecological causes.

Incontinence

Person has difficulty in holding the urine.

Causes

Overflow incontinence
- *Spinal cord damage:* Due to multiple sclerosis/trauma
- *Stress incontinence:* Due to increased abdominal pressure causes incontinence.
  For example, uterine prolapse with cystocoele
- Weakness of pelvic floor
- Vesico vaginal fistula
  Frontal lobe disease: Due to cerebrovascular disease-can also cause incontinence.

Urinary Retention

Person has difficulty in passing urine.

Causes

1. *Obstruction to urine outlfow*
   - Vesical calculus
   - Stricture urethra
   - Prostatic enlargement
2. *Neurological:* Spinal cord or sacral nerve root disease.
   - Preceding to total obstruction of urine flow there may be:
   - Poor stream of urine.
   - Person has difficulty in initiating the act of micturition (hesitancy).
   - Terminal dribbing of urine.

Acute Retention of Urine in Females

Causes
- Retroverted uterus
- Ovarian cyst
- Ectopic pregnancy/rupture of ectopic pregnancy.

III. Alteration in the Color (Appearance) of Urine

Hematuria
- Passing of blood in the urine

- Hematuria may be macroscopic or microscopic (centrifuged urine).

Causes
- Cystitis and urethritis
- Glomerulonephritis
- Carcinoma kidney
- Renal tuberculosis
- Papillary necrosis
- Bleeding into the urinary tract

Causes of Brownish/Reddish Colored Urine

a. *Drugs:* Rifampicin, metronidazole, phenacetin, phenytoin
b. *Vegetables:* Beet root and food coloring materials
c. Haematuria
d. Haemoglobinuria
e. Alkaptonuria
f. Porphyria

Clinical Significance of Different Types of Urine Discoloration

Frothy urine	- Proteinuria
Blue colored urine	- Methylene blue intake
Orange colored	- Rifampicin intake
Dark yellow	- Conjugated bilirubin excess
Pus in the urine	- Urinary infection
Cloudy urine with offensive smell	- Infected urine
White urine	- Phosphaturia, chyluria
Appearance of small tissue pieces in urine	- Papillary necrosis

IV. Change in the Urinary Volume

Normal individual requires to pass minimal 400 ml/day for clearing the metabolic waste products.
Oliguria: Urine output less than 400 ml/day.

Causes
Pre-renal
- Due to decreased renal blood flow
- Hypovolemic shock
- Dehydration
- Congestive cardiac failure

Renal
- Acute glomerulonephritis

Anuria: No urine output within 24 hours. most common cause: obstruction to the urine flow.

Other Causes of Anuria

- **Renal infarction:**
  - Massive embolisation, renal artery occlusion
  - Dissecting aneurysm of aorta.
- **Bilateral cortical necrosis:** Post partum hemorrhage
- Bilateral calculus disease
- **Rarer causes:** Retroperitoneal fibrosis

Polyuria: Passing urine volume greater than 3 litres/day

Causes (common)
- Diabetes mellitus
- Diuretic therapy
- Diabetes insipidus
- Hypercalcemia

Other causes
- Consumption of alcohol, coffee and tea
- Anxiety
- CRF
- Diuretic phase of ARF

V. General Symptoms of Renal Disease

Pedal Edema

Causes
- Acute glomerulonephritis
- Nephrotic syndrome
- Chronic renal failure

Puffiness of Face

Fluid collection in the loose areolar tissue around the eyes causes periorbital edema more common in the early morning hours.

Causes
- Acute glomerulonephritis
- Nephrotic syndrome

Generalised Edema
- Nephrotic syndrome causes generalised edema
- Late stages of CRF with GFR < 5 ml/min and 95% nephron loss will have edema of face and feet.

Symptoms Due to High Blood Pressure

Acute glomerulonephritis causes sudden raise in the blood pressure causing headache, vomiting convulsions (due to hypertensive encephalopathy) and dyspnea due to congestive cardiac failure.

Uremia

Clinical syndrome which develops in a patient with severe renal failure. Uremia develops with 95% loss of renal function.

Non-Specific Symptoms of Uremia

Tiredness	Irritability
Nausea	Confusion
Vomiting	Convulsions
Pruritus	Stupor

Systemic Symptoms

Hematological:	Severe anemia
	Platelet and coagulation defect
Cardiovascular:	Pericarditis pain
	Angina and dyspnea
Respiratory:	Haemoptysis
	Pleuritic pain
	Dyspnea
	Hyperventilation due to metabolic acidosis
Musculoskeletal:	Muscular weakness and bony pain
Nervous system:	Convulsions
	Coma
	CVA
	Peripheral neuropathy symptoms
Eye disturbance:	Blurring of vision due to retinal damage and retinal vascular disease
Urogenital:	Polyuria, nocturia
	Impotence and loss of libido
	Secondary amenorrhea
Gastrointestinal:	Anorexia, nausea and vomiting
	Loss of weight
	Ammoniacal odour of breath

Proteinuria
- Normal protein excretion in the urine/day is less than 30 mg/day.
- More than 30 mg/day called proteinuria

- Microalbuminuria: 30–300 mg/day
- Nephrotic range of proteinuria: 3.5 g/24 hours.

Causes of Proteinuria

Glomerular proteinuria
- Diabetes mellitus
- Minimal change glomerulonephritis
- Focal and segmental glomerulosclerosis
- SLE

Tubular proteinuria
- Hypertension
- Chronic renal failure
- Tubular damage secondary to drugs/toxins

Proteinuria due to abnormal protein excretion
- For example, multiple myeloma

Causes of microalbuminuria
- Early diabetic nephropathy
- Essential hypertension
- Early stages of glomerulonephritis

Physiological causes
- Febrile conditions
- Exercise

HAEMATURIA

Passing of blood in the urine is called haematuria. Table 9.1 lists type of hematuria and associated disorders.

Causes of Haematuria
Renal disorders
- Cysts, tumors
- Clotting disorders
- Vascular malformation

- Glomerular disease
- Inflammatory disease
- Infarction
- Interstitial diseases

Ureteric causes
- Tumors
- Stones

Urinary bladder causes
- Tumors
- Infection

Urethral causes
- Trauma
- Infection

Acute Glomerulonephritis (Nephritic syndrome)

Features of Acute Nephritic Syndrome
- Haematuria
- Oedema
- Hypertension
- Oliguria (urine output<400 ml/day)

Causes
- Viral, bacterial and fungal infections
- Post streptococcal glomerulonephritis
- IgA nephropathy
- Collagen vascular disease
- Vasculitic syndrome.

Clinical Features
- History of streptococcal sore throat and infected wound, 2–3 weeks prior to the onset of pedal edema and puffiness of face in patients with post streptococcal glomerulonephritis.
- History of joint pain, rash, fever in patients with collagen disease/vasculitis

Table 9.1 Approach to a patient of Haematuria

	Types of hematuria	*Associated disorders*
1.	Transient hematuria	Severe exercise
2.	Intermittent hematuria	IgA nephropathy
3.	Passing blood during initial part of micturition	Urethral bleed
4.	Hematuria at mid and later part of micturition	Bladder and prostate bleed
5.	Smoky or tea colored (red brown) urine	Glomerular bleed

- History of pedal edema, puffiness of face, hypertension and decreased urine output for evidence of renal disease.

Signs
- Puffiness of face (early morning hours)
- Pedal edema
- Hypertension
- Person can have left ventricular failure due to hypertension and convulsions due to hypertensive encephalopathy.

Investigations
- For streptococcal infection: ASO titer or C Reactive protein
- Serum complement levels
- Urine-volume, RBCs and RBC casts
- Blood urea, creatinine may be normal or increased
- Ultrasound abdomen - kidney size usually increased.

Complications
- Hypertensive encephalopathy
- Acute renal failure
- Pulmonary edema (left ventricular failure)
- Chronic glomerulonephritis

Treatment
- Absolute bed rest
- Decrease of salt and water intake
- Control of hypertension with diuretics and anti hypertensives
- If streptococcal infection
  Injection penicillin - procaine penicillin-8 lakhs/ day for 7 days.
- Vasculitis, idiopathic glomerulonephritis - Corticosteroids can be administered.
- Treatment of hyperkalemia and dialysis in patients with renal failure.

NEPHROTIC SYNDROME

Criteria for Diagnosis
- Generalised edema (anasarca)
- Massive proteinuria (24 hours urine protein> 3.5 g/day)

- Hyperlipedemia
- Hypoalbuminemia

Causes
- Idiopathic:
  - Minimal lesion glomerulonephritis
  - Membranous and proliferative glomerulo- nephritis
  - Focal and segmental glomerulonephritis
- Collagen disease - SLE
- Metabolic - Diabetes mellitus, amyloidosis
- Drug induced - Captopril, penicillamine, gold
- Infection: Hepatitis B, Leprosy, syphilis and HIV infection

Clinical Features
- Puffiness of face or pedal edema
- Pleural effusion or ascites
- History of intake of drugs, joint pain, rash and diabetes mellitus.
- Hypertension except in minimal lesion glomerulo- nephritis.

Investigations
- 24 hours urine protein estimation (> 3.5 g/day)
- Serum albumin level (decreased)
- Serum cholesterol and triglycerides levels (increased)
- Blood sugar, urea and creatinine level
- HBsAg, VDRL, HIV Elisa
- ANA, Anti ds DNA
- Renal biopsy for confirming the histopathological diagnosis

Complications
- Hypertension
- Hyperlipedemia
- Chronic renal failure
- Renal vein thrombosis
- Thyroid function abnormalities
- Systemic infection

Treatment
- Treatment of hypertension
- Diuretics
- Treatment of the cause
- Corticosteroids for idiopathic glomerulonephritis
- Treatment of renal failure

ACUTE RENAL FAILURE

Definition
Sudden and usually reversible loss of renal function which develops over a period of days to weeks.

Causes of Acute Renal Failure
Pre-renal: Causes which result in decreased renal blood flow and renal damage.
Local causes: Renal artery occlusion - decreased perfusion causes acute tubular necrosis
Systemic causes: Heart failure, severe blood loss or fluid loss

Intrinsic Renal Disease
- Acute tubular necrosis due to toxins or sepsis
- Primary or secondary glomerular disease
- Interstitial renal disease

Post Renal
- Calculus renal disease
  Urogenital tumors

Clinical Features
- History of blood volume loss like severe vomiting, diarrhea, blood loss, burns, etc.
- Hypotension
- Decreased urine output
- Evidence of sepsis and septic shock
- History of nephrotoxic drug intake like NSAIDS, aminoglycosides and sulpha drugs.

Complications
- Hyperkalemia
- Metabolic acidosis
- Pulmonary edema
- Circulatory overload

Investigations
- Blood counts for evidence of sepsis
- Hb% and packed cell volume
  – To defect blood loss
- Urea, creatinine for evidence and severity of renal failure
- Potassium level and blood pH measurement
- Ultrasound abdomen for evidence of calculus, anatomical lesions of the kidney.

Management
- Replacement of blood volume: IV fluids, blood transfusion.
- Dopamine infusion for maintenance of blood pressure and renal perfusion.
- Treatment of the causes like sepsis, relieving the obstruction and stoppage of nephrotoxic drugs.
- Hemodialysis

CHRONIC RENAL FAILURE

Definition
Irreversible deterioration in renal function developing over a period of years.

Aetiology
- Glomerular disease:
  – Chronic glomerulonephritis
  – IgA nephropathy
- Hypertension
- Interstitial disease
- Renal artery stenosis
- Polycystic kidney disease
- SLE, vasculitis, diabetes mellitus

Clinical Features
- Severe anemia and infection
- Vomiting
- Bleeding tendencies
- Generalised pruritis
- Renal bone disease
- Hypertension
- Pedal edema
- Peripheral neuropathy
- Myopathy

Investigations
- Hb% is decreased
- Blood urea and creatinine is increased
- Blood pH is decreased
- Hyperkalemia
- Serum calcium is decreased and phosphorous is increased

For the Causes of Renal Failure
- Estimation of blood sugar for evidence of diabetic nephropathy

- Ultrasound abdomen for polycystic kidney, chronic glomerulonephritis (smooth shrunken - kidneys), renal artery disease (unilateral shrunken kidney), chronic pyelonephritis (irregular scarred kidney)
- Blood tests for SLE, vasculitis
- Renal biopsy for parenchymal disease

Treatment

- Control of hypertension
- Removal of obstruction to the urine flow
- Treatment of urinary tract infection
- Avoidance of nephrotoxic drugs
- Treatment of hypertension and anemia
- Administration of calcium and vit. D_3
- Treatment of hyperkalemia with potassium binding resins.
- Hemodialysis and renal transplantation

Urinary Tract Infection (UTI)

- Multiplication of organisms in the urinary tract results in urinary tract infection.
- UTI is more common in females when compared to males.
- UTI is associated with high concentration of organisms/ml of urine.
- 1,00,000 organisms/ml of urine is called significant bacteriuria.

Common Organisms Causing UTI

Escherichia coli - commonest organism causing 75% of UTI

Other organisms:
- Proteus
- Pseudomonas
- *Staphylococcus epidermidis*
- Klebsiella
- Fungal - candidiasis

Predisposing Factors for UTI

Uncomplicated UTI
- Normal urogenital system
- Normal renal function
- Normal renal defence mechanisms

Complicated UTI: (with underlying systemic/urogenital defect)

- Systemic disease predisposing to UTI, e.g. diabetes mellitus
- Urinary tract abnormalities
  - Calculus disease, obstruction to the urinary tract
  - Vesicoureteric reflux, neurological dysfunction, urinary catheterization, scarred kidney

Different Types of UTI

Upper urinary tract infection: Pyelitis, pyelonephritis
Lower urinary tract infection: Urethritis, cystitis

Pathogenesis of UTI

- Colonisation of bacteria in the urinary epithelium leads onto urethritis and cystitis.
- Shorter urethra and sexual intercourse predispose female patients to develop recurrent UTI.
- Obstruction to the urinary tract, neurogenic bladder, catheterisation of urinary bladder predispose to bacterial colonisation of the bladder.
- Gynaecological and pelvic floor abnormalities result in the colonisation and multiplication of organisms in the urinary tract.

Clinical Features

General Features: Frequency of urination, pain and burning while passing urine.

Urethritis: Frequency and burning while passing urine.

Cystitis: Suprapubic pain and tenderness

Features

Haematuria, passing cloudy foul smelling urine may be present.

Pyelonephritis: High degree of fever, chills and rigors, renal angle tenderness.

Complicated UTI

Urinary tract infections occurring in patients with diabetes mellitus, immunosuppression, urinary obstruction, catheterization of the urinary bladder.

Investigations

- *Urine* shows large number of neutrophils.

- Total WBC count increased
- *Urine culture and sensitivity* Shows >1,00,000 organisms/ml
- *Blood culture and sensitivity* for septicemia
- Ultrasound abdomen for anatomical abnormalities of the genitourinary tract.
- Gynecological evaluation
- Intravenous pyelography and cystoscopy for structural and functional abnormalities of the urinary tract.

Management

General measures
- Excessive fluid intake
- Complete and regular emptying of the bladder
- Emptying bladder before and after sexual intercourse in females .

Specific measures
- Antibiotics depending on the urine culture sensitivity.
  T. Ciprofloxacin 500 1-0-1 for 5 to 7 days
  Or
  Cotrimoxazole/aminoglycosides
- IV antibiotics may be required in patients with upper urinary tract infections.
- Prolonged course of antibiotics is required in patients with complicated UTI.
- Removal of the predisposing cause for UTI.

Asymptomatic Bacteriuria

Presence of more than 1,00,000 organisms/ml of urine without symptoms. If urinary tract abnormalities are present investigation and treatment is required.

WATER, ELECTROLYTE AND ACID BASE DISORDERS

Water Metabolism

Normal Total Water Content of the Human Body
- *In adult males:* 60% of total body weight
- *In adult females:* 50% of total body weight

Water is Distributed in the Body in Two Compartments
- *Intracellular:* 70% of total water content of the body
- *Extracellular:* 30% of total water content of the body

Distribution of Extracellular Water
Water in the interstitial space: around 75%
Water in the intravascular plasma water: around 25%

Maintenance of Water Balance

Intake of water
- *Source of entry:* Gastrointestinal tract
- *Stimulus for water intake:* Thirst
- *Receptors for thirst:* Osmoreceptors in the anterior hypothalamus.

Excretion of water
- *Sources of excretion:* Gastrointestinal tract- Skin, kidney
- *Predominant regulatory factor in water excretion:* Arginine vasopressin (AVP-Antidiuretic Hormone-ADH)

Serum Osmolality
- *Osmolality:* Solute concentration of fluid is called osmolality.
- *Normal serum osmolality:* 270 to 290 mOsmol/kg
- Normal serum osmolality is decided predominantly by water and sodium balance in the body.

Electrolytes
- *Serum sodium:* Normal concentration of serum sodium 135–145 mEq/L
- Sodium is predominantly an extracellular ion.
- *Intake of sodium:* Through the dietary salt intake
- Increase in the sodium intake raises the volume of extracellular fluid.

Excretion of Sodium
- Depends on the extracellular sodium concentration
- Sodium excretion is determined by glomerular filtration rate, absorption of the excreted sodium by the renal tubules.

Aldosterone is a sodium retaining hormone and plays significant role in maintaining serum sodium level.

Serum Potassium

- Normal serum potassium concentration: 3.5 to 5 mEq/L.
- Potassium is predominantly an intracellular ion.
- Potassium balance is important for neuromuscular function
- Regular diet contains significant amount of potassium entering into the gastrointestinal tract.
- Kidney is the main source of potassium excretion.
- Aldosterone and increased potassium level determine serum potassium level.

Acid Base Maintenances

Normal acid base balance depends on the amount of acids/alkali produced or excreted by the homeostatic mechanisms.

Predominant regulatory mechanisms of acid base balance

- Kidney
- Lungs
- Chemical butters

In the extracellular and intracellular fluid

Acidosis: Increase in the hydrogen ion concentration (H^+) is called acidosis.

Alkalosis: Decrease in the hydrogen ion concentration in the blood.

pH: -log 10 of H+ (hydrogen ion concentration)

Anion Gap

- Anion gap represents measurement of negatively charged ions (anions) which are not routinely measured in clinical practice.
- Usual anions which are not measured: Sulphate, lactate, ketones, phosphates and anionic proteins.

Formula for Measurement of Anion Gap

- Anion gap: Plasma sodium concentration - (plasma chloride - plasma bicarbonate)
  Serum Na^+ - (Serum chloride + Serum HCO_3^-)
- Normal value of anion gap = 10–14 mmol/L
- *Acidosis with increased aniongap:* Occurs in

conditions where addition of acid/decrease in the excretion of acid from the body.

For example
- Renal failure
- Diabetic ketoacidosis
- Salicylate and methanol poisoning
- Lactic acidosis

Acidosis with Normal Anion Gap

Occurs in conditions with predominant bicarbonate loss
E.g. renal tubular acidosis, diarrhea
Normal arterial pH: 7.35 to 7.45

Metabolic Acidosis

Characterised by decrease in the plasma bicarbonate and increase in hydrogen ion concentration.

Metabolic Alkalosis

Characterised by decrease in the blood hydrogen ion concentration, increase in the bicarbonate level and increase in the arterial CO_2 concentration as a respiratory compensation.

Respiratory Acidosis

Characterised by increase in the arterial carbon dioxide level (pulmonary defect) and increase in the hydrogen ion (H^+) concentration.

Respiratory Alkalosis

Characterised by decrease in the arterial carbon dioxide concentration and determine the hydrogen ion concentration.

HYPERKALEMIA

Hyperkalemia is defined as level of serum potassium above 5.5 meq/l.

Causes

Pseudo hyperkalemia
- Hemolysis due to abnormal blood sampling
- Tissue damage during blood sampling

True hyperkalemia
- Metabolic acidosis
- Excessive potassium intake

- Blood loss into the body cavities
- Acute and chronic renal failure
- Drug therapy with ACE inhibitors, beta blockers
- Potassium sparing diuretics

Clinical Features
- Features of coexisting disease
- ECG shows tall T waves and arrhythmias
- Cardiac arrhythmias and cardiac arrest when potassium level is > 7 meq/L

Treatment
- Avoidance of potassium intake
- Emergency measures
  - IV Sodium bicarbonate, IV calcium
  - Gluconate/IV dextrose with insulin
  - Hemodialysis
- Chronic hyperkalemia: Administration of potassium exchange resins.

HYPOKALAEMIA
- Hypokalaemia indicates decreased level of potassium in the serum.
- Normal level of serum potassium 3.5 to 5.5 meq/L

Important Causes of Hypokalaemia
- Diarrhea and vomiting
- Decreased intake of potassium
- Diuretic therapy
- Renal tubular disease
- Primary and secondary hyperaldosteronism
- Cushing's syndrome
- Metabolic alkalosis

Features
- Fatiguability
- Muscular weakness
- Paralytic ileus
- Ventricular arrhythmias
- Cardiac asystole
- Potentiation of digitalis toxicity

Management
- Oral potassium supplementation in the form of syrup KCl, fruit juice and tender coconut water.
- IV potassium supplementation

- Correction of fluid, sodium and magnesium defect
- Treatment of the cause.

HYPERNATREMIA
Hypernatremia occurs either due to decrease in intake of water or excess water excretion.

Causes
- Decrease intake of water: Comatose persons, psychogenic
- Increased water loss:
  - Febrile states
  - Hyperthyroidism
  - Diabetes mellitus
  - Diabetes insipidus
  - Hypercalcemia
  - Hypokalemia

Clinical Features
- Excessive thirst
- Dizziness, confusion and coma
- Decrease urine output
- Tachycardia and hypotension
- Signs of dehydration

Treatment
- Replacement of hypotonic fluid
- Treatment of the cause

HYPONATREMIA
Decrease in the serum sodium concentration (normal serum sodium 132–144 meq/l).

Causes
1. Vomiting, diarrhea, burns and pancreatitis
2. SIADH, psychogenic water drinking
3. Nephrotic syndrome, CCF, liver failure.

Clinical Features
- Depends on the cause of hyponatremia and level of serum sodium.
- Anorexia, nausea and vomiting
- Fatiguability, absent tendon reflexes
- Seizures and coma

Management
1. Slow replacement of sodium with isotonic/hypertonic sodium.

2. Avoidance of excess of water intake
3. Treatment of the cause

METABOLIC ACIDOSIS

Metabolic acidosis is characterized by increase in the hydrogen ion concentration in the blood (decrease in the blood pH) and decrease in the bicarbonate concentration in the blood.

Causes
- Diabetic ketoacidosis
- Renal failure (uremia)
- Lactic acidosis
- Methanol and ethylane glycol poisoning

Clinical Features
- Fatigue
- Decrease cardiac output and blood pressure
- Hyperventilation (Kussmaul breathing)
- Cardiac arrhythmias
- Confusion and drowsiness
- Hyperkalemia
- Features of underlying disease

Management
- IV sodium bicarbonate infusion
- Oral sodium bicarbonate for long term therapy in CRF
- Correction of the cause

Metabolic Alkalosis

Metabolic alkalosis is characterised by increase in the plasmas bicarbonate level.

Causes
- Severe vomiting or continuous gastric aspiration
- Diuretic administration
- Endocranial causes:
  – Primary/secondary aldosteronism
  – Cushing's syndrome

– Adrenal enzyme defects
- Administration of IV/oral bicarbonate

Features
- Features of underlying cause for alkalosis
- In severe alkalosis - mental confusion, drowsiness and carpopedal spasm and tetany (due to decrease of ionised calcium).

Treatment
- Correction of underlying cause
- IV normal saline and potassium administration to correct hypokalemia.

RESPIRATORY ALKALOSIS

Respiratory alkalosis occurs due to conditions associated with hyperventilation of lungs with excessive loss of carbon dioxide.

Causes
- Pain and anxiety
- Fever
- Pneumonia/pulmonary edema
- Salicylate intake
- Septicemia

There is decreased level of $PaCO_2$ in the blood with increase in the blood pH.

RESPIRATORY ACIDOSIS

Respiratory acidosis occurs due to detective alveolar ventilation resulting in retention of carbon dioxide in the blood.

Causes
- Chronic obstructive pulmonary disease.
- Acute severe asthma
- Drug (morphine, pethidine) induced respiratory depletion.
- Cerebro vascular accident
- Respiratory muscle paralysis.

There is increased level of $PaCO_2$ in the blood and decrease in the blood pH.

10 Musculoskeletal and Connective Tissue Disorders

Mode of Onset of Symptoms and Duration of Symptoms

1. Acute onset (duration less than 6 weeks)
   Causes
   • Gouty arthritis
   • Septic arthritis
   • Rheumatic arthritis
2. Gradual onset (duration more than 6 weeks), e.g.
   • Rheumatoid arthritis
   • Osteoarthritis
   • Seronegative arthritis
3. Intermittent attacks of arthritis
   For example Gouty arthritis
4. Migratory attacks of arthritis
   For example Rheumatic fever
   • Gonococcal arthritis
   • Viral arthritis

Palindromic Onset

Features

• Individual joints are affected
• Pain and stiffness persists for a few hours to days occurring in recurrent acute episodes.
• Usually progresses to typical rheumatic arthritis.

Pain

Pain is an important symptom of bone and joint disease

Bony pain: Continuous aching pain disturbing sleep
Joint pain: Sharp pain related to posture or movement associated with stiffness.

Pain is usually well localized except pain originating from the hip joint which may be referred to the knee joint.

Assessment of Joint Pain

Mode of onset

1. Acute onset
   – Septic arthritis
   – Rheumatic fever
   – Gouty arthritis
2. Gradual onset
   – Rheumatoid arthritis
   – Osteoarthritis
3. Episodic and intermittent attacks (Gouty arthritis)
   – Palindromic rheumatism (see above)
4. Fleeting (migratory) type of joint pain:
   – Pain begins in one joint at a time and then involves the other joints.
   – Involvement of the other joints occurs after about 3–5 days.
   For exmple Rheumatic fever, gonococcal arthritis
5. Pain severe disturbing sleep:
   – Septic arthritis
   – Gout
6. Effect of activity:
   – Pain appears after activity and decreases with rest, e.g. degenerative arthritis.

Sites of Somatic reference of different Joint Pains

Joint pains	Site of referred pain
Cervical pain:	Head/over the shoulder
Lumbar spine:	Buttocks/posterior thigh
Shoulder:	Lateral aspect of upper arm
Elbow:	Forearm
Hip:	Outer aspect of thigh or knee or both

Referred pain of cervical and lumbar spine disorders increases on coughing, sneezing and straining at stool due to increase in the Intraspinal pressure.

For example, sciatic pain is due to pressure on nerve roots

Joint Swelling

Joint swelling is a predominant manifestation of inflammatory arthritis.

Swelling may be due to synovitis or accumulation of intra articular fluid.

Swelling can also occur in degenerative arthritis due to bony hypertrophy.

Pattern of Joint Involvement

1. Number of joints involved
   Monoarticular - single joint involved
   Acute onset e.g. gout, pseudogout, infective arthritis, trauma to the joint
   Gradual onset, e.g. Rheumatoid arthritis, ankylosing spondylitis, psoriatic arthritis, tubercular arthritis
   Oligo (pauci) articular: 2 or 3 joints are involved, e.g. reactive arthritis, seronegative arthritis.
   Polyarticular: more than three joints, e.g. rheumatoid arthritis, SLE

2. Symmetrical arthritis, e.g. rheumatoid arthritis

3. Asymmetrical arthritis, e.g. gout, rheumatic fever, seronegative arthritis

4. Site of joint involvement
   Upper extremities: Rheumatoid arthritis
   Lower extremities: Reiter's disease, gout

   Axial skeleton: Osteoarthritis, ankylosing spondylitis

Stiffness of Joints

Inflammatory Arthritis

- Early morning stiffness persisting for more than 30 minutes occurs in inflammatory arthritis.
- Morning stiffness persisting more than 1 hour is characteristic of rheumatoid arthritis

- Stiffness is precipitated by prolonged rest and lasts several hours
- Stiffness improves with activity and anti-inflammatory drugs.

Non-inflammatory Arthritis

- Intermittent stiffness
- Stiffness may increase by activity
- Lasts less than one hour
- Stiffness is accompanied only by pain without other inflammatory symptoms
- Stiffness may be due to pain or deformity

Note: Early morning stiffness of pelvic and shoulder girdle is characteristic feature of polymyalgia rheumatica.

Joint Involvement in Specific Disorders

Proximal interphalangeal joint	:	Rheumatoid arthritis
Distal interphalangeal joint	:	Psoriasis
1st Metatarsophalangeal joint	:	Gout
Girdle joint	:	Rheumatoid arthritis Polymyalgia rheumatica
Axial, sacroiliac joint	:	Ankylosing spondylitis
Appendicular skeleton	:	Rheumatoid arthritis
Vertebral column	:	Degenerative arthritis Ankylosing spondylitis
Weight bearing joints	:	Degenerative arthritis

Deformities

Deformity occurs in both inflammatory and degenerative arthritis.

Alteration in the skull spine	Paget's disease and acromegaly
Hands and legs deformities	Rheumatoid arthritis
Jaccoud's arthritis	Rheumatic fever
Deformity due to Heberden's nodes	Osteoarthritis

Deformity of spine can cause gradual loss of height and spinal curvature

Impairment of Movement

Joint and bone disorders cause impairment of movement, occurs due to the following factors.

Table 10.1 Constitutional and Extra-articular symptoms in relation to rheumatic diseases

Symptoms	Associated Rheumatic Disorders
Fever, sweating	Septic arthritis, rheumatic fever
Skin rash	Psoriatic arthritis, Reiter's disease, SLE, rheumatic fever
Dyspnea and chest pain	Rheumatic fever, rheumatoid arthritis, SLE
(pericardial and pleural disease)	
Eyes:	
Conjunctivitis	Reiter's disease
Dry eye	Sjögren's syndrome
Painful iritis	Ankylosing spondylitis
Blue sclera with multiple fractures	Osteogenesis imperfecta
Disturbance of vision and blindness	Giant cell arteritis
Blindness and deafness	Paget's disease of bone
	Scleroderma
GIT disturbances	Inflammatory bowel disease
(Altered bowel habits)	Malabsorption syndromes
Transient diarrhoea	Reactive arthritis
Recurrent mouth ulcers	Bechet's syndrome
Genitourinary symptoms	
Urethritis	Reiter's disease
Asymptomatic urethral discharge	
Second trimester abortion	APLA syndrome
Female vaginal ulcers	Bechet's syndrome
Neurovascular symptoms	
Entrapment neuropathies	Rheumatoid arthritis
Vascular headache	
Psychosis	
Dementia	SLE
Stroke	
Headache, jaw claudication	Giant cell arteritis
Raynaud's phenomenon	SLE, systemic sclerosis, rheumatoid arthritis
Respiratory symptoms	
Symptoms of bronchial asthma	Churg stratus disease
Chronic nasal, sinus and middle ear discharge	Wegener's granulomatosis

- Joint stiffness
- Joint pain
- Tendon damage
- Muscle weakness
- Neurological deficit

Crackling Sensation of Joint
- Crackling sensation on joint movement is a feature of degenerative arthritis
- Osteoarthritis of knee joint characteristically produces crackling sensation on joint movement

- Crackling sound is due to the badly damaged articular cartilage (due to loose bodies fragment of cartilage)

Note: It is normal to hear minor clicks on joint movement

Locking of Joint

Locking
Jamming of the joint occurs at some point after certain range of movement (pain and sweating may be associated with locking).

Mechanism of locking
Part of menisci or cartilage (loose body within the joint) interferes with the movement at articular surfaces.

Constitutional and Extra-Articular Symptoms in Relation to Rheumatic Diseases (Table 10.1

Association of Age, Sex and Race with Rheumatic Disorders

Rheumatic Disorders Affecting Different Age Groups

Younger age
- Rheumatic fever
- SLE
- Reiter's disease

Middle age
- Rheumatoid arthritis
- Fibromyalgia

Elderly age
- Osteoarthritis
- Polymyalgia rheumatica

Rheumatic Disorders Affecting Different Sexes

Predominantly males
- Ankylosing spondylitis
- Gout

Predominantly females
- Rheumatoid arthritis
- SLE, fibromyalgia

Significance of race in Rheumatic Diseases

Disorders predominantly affecting blacks
- Sacroidosis, SLE

Disorders predominantly affecting whites
- Giant cell arteritis
- Wegener's granulomatosis
- Polymyalgia rheumatica

Drugs and Rheumatic Disease
Certain drugs can induce rheumatic disease as given below:

Name of the drug	:	Disorder produced
Statins	:	Arthralgia, myopathy
Steroids	:	Myopathy, osteoporosis
Hydralazine Penicillamine	:	Drug-induced lupus
Salicylates, alcohol	:	Gout
Diuretics, quinidine	:	Arthralgia, drug-induced lupus

Rheumatoid Arthritis

General Features
- Multisystem disease
- Characterised by symmetrical polyarthritis involving minor and major joints with exacerbations and remissions.
- Results in severe deformities and systemic involvement.

Pathogenesis and Pathology
- Females are more commonly affected.
- Formation of abnormal immunoglobulin resulting in autoantibody response to abnormal immunoglobulins (rheumatoid factor) causing joint destruction.
- Antigen antibody complex formation leads to compliment activation, inflammation, synovial damage and systemic involvement.

Clinical Features
- Age group involved: 2nd to 3rd decade. Female > males.
- Insidious onset
- Joints are swollen, tender with limitation of movements.
- Initially symmetrical involvement of proximal interphalangeal joints with later involvement of wrist, ankle and knee.
- Chronic involvement of joints leads onto muscle wasting and deformities.

- Generalised lymphadenopathy, hepato-spleno-megaly, respiratory, cardiac, skin, eye, and peripheral nervous system involvement can occur.

Systemic Involvement in Rheumatoid Arthritis

Musculoskeletal involvement: Weakness and wasting of muscles with joint deformities.

Eyes: Dry eyes, episcleritis and scleritis.

Cardiovascular: Pericarditis and valvulitis

Respiratory: Pleural effusion and pulmonary fibrosis

Renal: Glomerulonephritis

Neurological: Neuropathies

Hematological: Anemia, leucopenia and thrombo-cytopenia.

Dermatological: Rashes, ulcer and subcutaneous nodules

Investigations

- Increased ESR and C reactive protein
- Normocytic normochromic anemia
- Increased level of gammaglobulins
- Rheumatoid factor is positive (in about 60% of patients)
- Synovial fluid analysis shows evidence of inflammation
- X-ray of the joint reveals erosion of articular cartilage.

Deformities in Rheumatoid Arthritis

- Ulnar deviation of hand
- Proximal interphalangeal joint swelling-spindle shaped deformity
- Swan neck deformity
  - Hyperextension of proximal interphalangeal joint and flexion of terminal interphalangeal joint
  - Boutonniere deformity
  - Flexion of proximal interphalangeal joint and hyperextension of distal inter- phalangeal joint
- Z deformity of thumb

Treatment

- Rest to the joints
- NSAIDS: For 2 to 6 weeks, e.g. aspirin/Indo-methacin

- Correction of anemia
- Physiotherapy to the joints

Disease Modifying Drugs

Methotrexate 7.5 mg/wk to 25 mg/wk can be given alone or in combination with chloroquine or sulphasalazine or leflounamide. Treatment can be continued for 1 to 2 years. Careful monitoring of LFT, RFT and hematological parameters are required for the treatment. Early treatment with disease modifying drugs is beneficial in preventing the joint deformities and destruction.

Corticosteroids

- Severe or exacerbation of joint pain require oral or parenteral prednisolone. Intra articular corticosteroid can also be given. Small maintenance dose of steroid may be required in some patients.

Other Forms of Therapy

- Administration of anti-cytokine agents like infliximab.
- Cyclosporine or cyclophosphamide administration.
- Surgical correction of deformities.
- Occupational therapy and rehabilitation.

Dental Aspects of Rheumatoid Arthritis

- Temporomandibular joint may be involved causing stiffness of joints with difficulty in opening the mouth.
- Dry mouth (xerostomia) may occur due to Sjogren's syndrome with rheumatoid arthritis. Oral hygiene should be maintained in these patients.
- Glossitis can occur due to anemia of rheumatoid arthritis or due to its drug therapy.

GIANT CELL ARTERITIS (Temporal arteritis)

Giant cell arteritis is a form of large vessel vasculitis involves predominantly temporal and ophthalmic arteries.

Clinical Features

Age group involved: Elderly around 60 to 70 years of age. Females: males - 4:1

Headache: Temporal or occipital headache with scalp tenderness.

Jaw pain: Pain on chewing or talking, jaw claudication occurs due to ischemia of the masseters.

Visual disturbance: Sudden onset of decrease of vision and blurring of vision. Occurs due to vasculitis of posterior ciliary artery.

Other features: Fatigue, weight loss, fever, depression, cerebral and brain stem ischemia can occur.

Investigations
* Raised ESR and CRP (C reactive protein).
* Temporal artery biopsy shows evidence of vasculitis

Management
* Prednisolone 1 mg/kg body weight for 6 weeks and then to be slowly tapered and stopped.
* Other immune suppressive drugs like azathioprine and methotrexate can be used.

Dental Aspects
* Jaw pain can occur due to giant cell arteritis.
* Rarely gangrene of the tongue can occur due to temporal arteritis.
* Temporal arteritis should be differentiated from trigeminal neuralgia.

Note: Pain, stiffness, weakness across the shoulder and pelvic muscles can occur along with temporal arteritis. This is called as polymyalgia rheumatica.

Systemic Lupus Erythematosus (SLE)

SLE is the common disorder of connective tissue. Females are more commonly affected than males.

Aetiopathogenesis
* Wide spectrum of auto antibody formation occurs due to B and T cell activation.
* Genetic factors and viral infection may initiate the disease.
* Exacerbation of symptoms can occur due to exposure to sunlight, ultraviolet light, infection and pregnancy.

* Drugs like hydralazine and procainamide can initiate lupus like disease.

Clinical Features
General features: Fever and fatiguability
Dermatological: Butterfly rash over the face (photosensitive).
Mucus membrane: Stomatitis and ulceration
Skeletal: Polyarthritis
Respiratory: Pleuritis/pleural effusion
Cardiovascular: Pericarditis, endocarditis and aortic regurgitation
Renal: Glomerulonephritis
Ophthalmic: Conjunctivitis, retinal damage.
Gastrointestinal: Hepatitis, pancreatitis.
Hematological: Anemia and thrombocytopenia

Investigations
* Vary high ESR but CRP is within normal limits.
* Anemia, normocytic, normochromic anemia and thrombocytopenia
* Autoantibodies: Antinuclear antibodies
* Specific for SLE: Antibody against double stranded (ds) DNA.
* Rheumatoid factor may be positive in 30% of patients.
* Other antibodies: Anti histone, anti Sm, antiphospholipid and antineuronal antibodies.
* VDRL may be false positive

Management
* NSAIDS for joint pain
* Chloroquine for skin involvement and skin rash.

Corticosteroids
* Oral prednisolone (1 mg/kg body weight) for 6 weeks and then taper and stop. If required small dose of prednisolone can be maintained. In severe form of the disease IV prednisolone may be required.
* Other form of immune suppression like azathioprine/cyclophosphamide for severe disease not responding to steroids.

Dental aspects of SLE

Following oral lesions can occur in SLE patients
- Erythematous oral lesions
- White patches over the oral mucosa
- Slit- like ulcers over the gingival margins

- Chloroquine therapy can cause lichenoid oral lesions
- Oral candidiasis due to steroid therapy
- Bleeding can occur during dental extraction due to thrombocytopenia.

11 Infectious Diseases

EXANTHEMATOUS FEVERS

Exanthema indicates generalized eruption.

Causes of Exanthematous Fevers

Infections
- Rubella
- Rubeola (measles)
- Epstein-Barr virus infections
- HIV infections

Other Causes
- Drug induced
- Toxic shock syndrome

DIPHTHERIA

Aetiological agent: Corynebacterium diptheriae.
Spread by: Droplet infection
Incubation period: 2–4 days
Organs involved: Either by inflammatory reaction to the organism or by the absorbed exotoxin
Common sites of involvement by corynebacterium: Pharyngeal mucosa, palate and oral mucosa.
Rare site of involvement: Conjunctiva, genital tract. Can contaminate wounds and abrasions. Absorbed exotoxin can damage cardiac muscles and nervous system

Clinical Features
- Insidious onset of symptoms
- Fever
- Tachycardia
- Pseudomembrane formation: Creamy yellow/gray firmly attached membranes over the tonsils spreading on to palate or oral mucosa.
- Tender cervical node enlargement giving a bull neck appearance

Occasionally
- Nasal discharge
- Laryngeal form with high pitched cough

Complications
- Local laryngeal obstruction
- Due to exotoxin
  - Cardiac
  - Myocarditis
  - Arrhythmias
  - Cardiac failure
- Neurological
  - Palatal palsy
  - Paralysis of accommodation reflex
  - Polyneuritis

Management
- Isolation of the patient
- Throat swab for identification of organism
- Antitoxin: Immediate injection 4,000 to 1,00,000 units depending on the severity
- Severe anaphylactic reaction can occur

Antibiotics

Amoxycillin 500 mg 8th hrly for 2 weeks or Erythromycin (500 mg qid 2wks).

Prevention

Active immunization of all children

All contacts
- Give erythromycin
- Give booster dose of toxoid

TETANUS

Aetiological Agent

Sporing bacterium: Clostridium tetani (Cl. tetani).

Spores of *Cl. tetani* will remain in the soil for a long time and can germinate in anaerobic conditions. Tetanus infection develops if the necrosed deep wound gets contaminated with soil (contaminated with human/animal excreta).

Clinical Features

- *Cl. tetani* produces an exotoxin tetanospasmin which causes violent muscular spasm.
- Trismus (lock jaw)
  - Occurs due to painless masseter spasm, commonest early sign.
  - Dental abscess, pharyngeal sepsis also can produce lock jaw but usually painful.
- Risus sardonicus
  - Sardonic smile due to contraction of frontalis and muscles of angle of mouth and
  - There will be closed eyes, raised eyebrows, clenched teeth withdrawing back of lips.
- Spinal muscle spasm
- Produces arching of back called opisthotonus.

There can be severe violent muscle spasm persisting for few seconds to minutes. Muscle spasm can be induced by noise or physical stimulation of the patient. Autonomic dysfunction can cause hypertension and cardiac arrhythmias.

Local Tetanus

Muscle spasm and stiffness occurs only around the infected wound.

Death can occur due to asphyxia (due to laryngeal spasm, bronchopneumonia and autonomic neuropathy).

Management

Management of Wound

- Maxillofacial injuries after road traffic accident can develop tetanus.
- Superficial wound or abrasions
  - Local wound care is to be given

- If already immunized against tetanus, no active immunization is required.
  - If immunization status not known, active immunization with tetanus toxoid.
- Puncture wounds, deeper wounds and bites
  - Local care of wound - wound debridement
  - If already immunized - booster dose of toxoid (not required if immunized within 5 years)

In Patients with Immunisation Status not known

Local Wound Care

- Antibiotics (penicillin)
- Human tetanus immunoglobulin 250 (if within 4 hours)
- Human tetanus immunoglobulin (5000 units if seen after 24 hours)

Other Measures

- Care of blood pressure, respiration and hydration
- Treatment of secondary infection

Treatment in General for Tetanus

To be admitted in intensive care unit
- General measures
  - Adequate hydration and nutritional supplementation
- Neutralising the absorbed toxin
  - Human tetanus antitoxin
  - IV injection of 3,000 IU
- To prevent the further production of toxin:
  - Wound care and wound debridement
  - Inj. crystalline penicillin 600 mg IV 6th hrly into 1 week
  - (I.V metronidazole if penicillin or erythromycin allergy)
- Protection of the airway
  - Tracheotomy if required
  - Helps in ventilatory support

Control of Muscle Spasms

- Avoidance of noise
- Avoid unnecessary stimulation of the patient

- IV Diazepam or heavy sedation
- General anesthesia, paralyzing the patient and ventilatory support.

Complete recovery is possible. After complete recovery person requires active immunization.

Dental Aspects

- Consider tetanus in all patients with trismus and temporomandibular pain dysfunction syndrome.
- Phenothiazine toxicity can cause facial dyskinesias but not trismus.

MUMPS

Infective agent: Paramyxovirus
Affects usually children of 5–9 years
Route of spread: Respiratory by droplet infection
Incubation period: 16–18 days and infectivity lasts for 5-7 days

Disease involves parotid glands other exocrine glands, meninges, ovary and testes

Clinical Features

- Fever
- Bodyache
- Tender parotid enlargement usually bilateral/may be unilateral
- Orchitis, oophoritis, pancreatitis and meningo-encephalitis can occur.

Consider mumps in the differential diagnosis of all parotid swellings.

Treatment

- Symptomatic treatment for pain
- Liquid diet
- If orchitis - course of prednisolone

Prevention

MMR vaccine for mumps, measles and rubella

Measles

Infective agent: Paramyxovirus

Route of transmission: Respiratory route by droplets
Incubation period: 14 days

Clinical Features

- Fever, bodyache
- Upper respiratory symptoms

Koplik's Spots

- Present on the buccal mucosa along side the 2nd molar and may be extensive.
- They appear as 1–2 mm bluish white spots with surrounding redness.
- Koplik's spots are pathognomonic of measles

Rash

- Erythematous non pruritic maculopapular rash can appear all over the body .
- Generalised lymphadenopathy, diarrhea and pneumonia can occur.
- As a late sequelae-subacute sclerosing pan-encephalitis can occur in children causing dementia.

Management

- Symptomatic therapy for fever
- Nutritional support
- Antibiotics for secondary infection

Prevention

Vaccination in children involving mumps, measles and rubella.

Rubella

Etiological agent: A Togavirus - RNA virus
Incubation period: 12 to 23 days.
Infective period: A week before and after the development of rash.
Route of spread: Respiratory via droplets

Clinical Features

- Involves upper respiratory tract with local lymphadenopathy (occipital lymphadenopathy characteristic).
- Skin, joint and placenta can also be involved.

- Maculopapular rash over the face and trunk
- Fever

Forcheimer spots: Petechiae occurring on the soft palate-characteristic of rubella.

- Rubella infection in early pregnancy can result in multiple congenital defects like deafness, congenital heart disease and cataract.

Diagnosis

- Specific IgM antibody indicates recent infection
- Specific IgG antibody indicates previous infection

Prevention

To immunize all children between 12–15 months and a second booster in early childhood.

Chicken Pox (Varicella)

Etiological agent: Varicella zoster virus
Route of spread: Respiratory droplet infection
Incubation period: 11 to 21 days

Clinical Features

- Fever
- Bodyache
- Oral ulcers

Rash

More on the trunk and appear as pink macules which progress to vesicles, pustules with crusting.

Itchy rashes can become secondarily infected with bacterial (streptococcal/staphylococcal) infection.

Occasionally aseptic meningitis, encephalitis, cerebellar ataxia can occur as complications.

Diagnosis

Vesicular fluid can be aspirated and PCR and tissue culture will confirm the diagnosis of viral infection.
Complications
- Meningitis
- Meningoencephalitis

- Cerebellar ataxia
- Secondary bacterial infection
- Herpes zoster

Management

- Symptomatic therapy for pain and fever.
- Administration of acyclovir (400 mg to 800 mg 5 times a day) or famcyclovir 500 mg 3 times a day for 1 week early in the disease and in immune compromised individuals.
- Administration of *varicella zoster* human immune globulin for immune suppressed individuals contacting chicken pox.

HERPES ZOSTER (VARICELLA ZOSTER)

Herpes zoster occurs due to reactivation of varicella zoster virus in the dorsal root ganglion of sensory nerves.

Commonly occurs in elderly/ young age with immune deficiency.

Common Site of Involvement

- Thoracic nerves
- Ophthalmic division of trigeminal nerve
- Causes corneal ulceration
- Ramsay-Hunt syndrome: Herpeszoster of geniculate ganglion.

Features

- Fever, bodyache
- Burning pain in the distribution of nerves
- Rash appears becoming vesicles, pustules with crusting
- Immune compromised can develop multiple involvement of nerves with severe disease and encephalomyelitis.

Complications

Acute
- Encephalomyelitis
- Secondary bacterial infection of the vesicles

Chronic
- Post herpetic neuralgia (persistence of pain for 1–6 months following healing of rash)

Management
- Tab acyclovir 800 mg 1-1-1-1-1 for 5–7 days
- IV Acyclovir 10 mg/kg 8th hrly (in immune suppressed) 7–10 days.

For Post Herpetic Pain
- Amytryptaline 25 mg–50 mg/day
- Gabapentin 300 mg /day

RAMSAY-HUNT SYNDROME

This occurs due to involvement of geniculate ganglion by the herpes zoster virus.

Features
- Rash in the external auditory canal
- Lower motor neuron facial palsy
- Ipsilateral loss of taste and buccal ulceration

Infectious Mononucleosis

Causative organism: Epstein-Barr virus. Organisms multiply in the mouth, pharynx and urogenital tract.

Route of spread: By saliva-droplet spread (kissing by adolescent persons)

Clinical Features
- Fever
- Non specific skin rash
- Pharyngitis
- Posterior cervical lymphadenopathy
- Hepatosplenomegaly
- Hepatitis

Complications
- Pharyngitis and edema of pharynx
- Thrombocytopenia and hemolytic anemia
- Myocarditis
- Glomerulonephritis
- Polyneuritis, transverse myelitis and meningo encephalitis
- Chronic fatigue syndrome

Lab Investigations
- *Peripheral smear:* Presence of atypical lymphocytes
- Monospot-slide test for rapid detection of antibodies
- Positive Paul Bunnel test for detecting heterophil antibody
- Specific Epstein-Barr virus serology

Management
- Symptomatic for pain and fever
- Antibiotics for secondary streptococcal infection, e.g. erythromycin (avoid amoxicillin as it may precipitate maculopapular rashes)
- If pharyngeal edema: T - prednisolone 30 mg into 5 days.

Dental Aspects
- Infectious mononucleosis can cause exudates in the fauces.
- Can cause petechiae at the junction of hard and soft palate.
- Epstein-Barr virus can cause mucosal and gingival ulceration and sialadenitis

HERPES SIMPLEX

Aetiological Agent
- Type I herpes simplex virus: Involves head and neck causing mucocutaneous lesions
- Type II herpes simplex virus: Causes anogenital infection

  Herpes simplex virus can cause keratitis, vulvovaginitis, cervicitis, balanitis and encephalitis.

HERPES LABIALIS (COLD SORE)

It occurs due to reactivation of herpes simplex virus.
  Hyperaesthesia occurs in the lip margin with vesiculation, pustulation and crusting.

Herpes Labialis can be Precipitated by
- High fever
- Menstruation
- Ultra-violet light

Complications of Herpes Simplex Infection
- Fatal infection in the newborn

- May cause severe infection in immune compromised
- Corneal dendrite ulcer
- Encephalitis

Diagnosis
- Virus demonstration by polymerase chain reaction from vesicular fluid
- CSF polymerase chain reaction for the virus
- Serology for confirming primary infection

Management
- T. Acyclovir 200 mg 1-1-1-1-1 or T. Famcyclovir 250 mg 1-1-1 for 7 days.
- In immune suppressed individuals - IV. Acyclovir is indicated

Oral Manifestations of Herpes Simplex Infections

Pharyngitis and Gingivostomatitis
- Common in young adults and children and due to primary infection.
- Fever, myalgia, pain in the oral cavity with enlargement of neck lymph node are the usual symptoms.
- Ulcerations and exudation over the palate, tonsils and oral mucosa can occur.

Herpes Labialis
- Occurs due to reactivation of herpes simplex virus.
- Ulcerations of the vermillion border of lip, oral cavity and external facial skin occurs.
- Herpes labialis can occur after dental extraction.
- Immune compromised patients can develop deeper skin and oral mucosal infection due to Herpes simplex infection.

ENTERIC FEVER (TYPHOID AND PARATYPHOID FEVER)

Aetiological agents
- Typhoid fever: Caused by *Salmonella typhi* (gram negative bacilli)
- Paratyphoid fever: Caused by *Salmonella paratyphi* (Gram negative bacilli)

Mode of spread: Faeco-oral route

Incubation period: 10–14 days
Pathology: Localize mainly in the lymphoid tissues (Payer's patches) of small intestine.

Clinical Features

Typhoid fever

Ist week
- Fever with chills and bodyache
- Step ladder fever (temperature raising daily)
- Relative bradycardia
- Headache, bodyache

End of Ist week
- Rose spots: Red spots over the trunk
- Abdominal distention and tenderness
- Splenomegaly around 7th to 10th day
- Occasionally cough and diarrhea

End of 2nd week and 3rd week
Complications
- Perforation of intestine
- GIT bleeding
- Delirium, coma

Occasionally hepatitis, glomerulonephritis can occur. In 5% of patients baacilli can remain in the gall bladder and can act as carriers.

Paratyphoid Fever
Shorter and milder than typhoid fever. They can cause enteritis. Intestinal complication are less common.

Complications of Enteric (typhoid) Fever
- Gastrointestinal
  - Ileal hemorrhage
  - Ileal perforation
- Septicemia
  - Cholecystitis
  - Pneumonia
  - Myocarditis
  - Arthritis
  - Osteomyelitis
  - Meningitis

Investigations
Ist week
- WBC count is reduced

- Blood and bone marrow culture sensitivity for typhoid and paratyphoid bacilli .

2nd week
- Widal test with raising titer (antibodies against both O and H antigens)
- Urine and stool culture and sensitivity for typhoid and paratyphoid bacilli.

Treatment
- Injection Ciprofloxacin 200 mg IV 1-0-1 × 14 days

  or
- Injection Ceftriaxone 2 grs into 14 days
  Chloramphenicol can also be used if the bacilli are sensitive to the drug. Chronic carriers should be treated with ciprofloxacin into 4 weeks.

MALARIA

Aetiological agents
- *Plasmodium vivax*
- *Plasmodium ovale*
- *Plasmodium malariae*
- *Plasmodium falciparum*

Transmitting agent: Bite of female anopheline mosquitos

Main pathological changes: Hemolysis of infected red cells.

Plasmodium falciparum causes adherence of infected red cells to capillary endothelium of visceral organs causing visceral damage.

Clinical Features of Malaria
In general
- Fever with chills and rigors
- Initial stage of cold, followed by hot stage and then profuse sweating with decrease of temperature
- Anemia
- Splenomegaly

Plasmodium vivax and plasmodium ovale
- Fever with chills and rigors
- Fever occurs every 48 hours in cycles (benign tertian)
- Hepatosplenomegaly
- Anemia

Plasmodium falciparum infection
- Dangerous form of malaria
- Fever, headache, vomiting, cough and diarrhea
- Fever may not follow any particular pattern
- Severe hemolysis, anemia and tender hepato-splenomegaly, renal failure can occur.
- Cerebral malaria causes confusion, coma neurological deficit and death.

PLASMODIUM MALARIAE

Fever occurs on every 3rd day (quartan) and can cause glomerulonephritis and nephritic syndrome.

Complications of Falciparum Malaria
- Cerebral malaria
- Acute renal failure
- Hypoglycemia
- Acute pulmonary edema
- Shock
- Severe anemia
- Secondary bacterial infection
- Hyperpyrexia

Diagnosis
- Thick and thin smear examined for malarial parasite.
- Quantitative Bufly coat technique for malarial parasite.
- Dipstick tests for *Plasmodium falciparum* antigen

Management
- Acute attack of *Plasmodium vivax, plasmodium ovale* and plasmodium malarial infection
  - Tab. chloroquine (250 mg × 4) stat and after 6 hours (250 mg salt × 2) and
  - 250 mg of chloroquine two times/day into 2 days.
- To prevent relapse (Radical cure)
  - T. Primaquine 15 mg to 30 mg into 2 weeks in patients with *plasmodium vivax* and *plasmodium ovale* infection.

Plasmodium Falciparum Infection

Milder form
- T.Quinine 600 mg 1-1-1, 7 to 10 days plus

- Single dose - Sulfadoxime 1.5 g + pyrimethamine 75 mg
- Doxycycline 100 mg/day into 7 days

Complicated Falciparum Malaria
- IV Quinine in dextrosc (10 mg/kg body weight 3 times/ day) 7 to 10 days/metloquine 25m/Kg.
- IV Artemesinin (1.2 to 2.4 mg/ kg/ day 5 to 7 days
- IV fluids and maintenance of electrolytes and hydration
- Exchange transfusion
- Treatment of complications

AMOEBIASIS

Aetiological agent: Entamoeba histolytica

Mode of transmission: Contaminated water and food.

Disease caused: Intestinal amoebiasis (amoebic dysentery)

Extraintestinal amoebiasis: For example hepatic amoebiasis

Intestinal Amoebiasis

Incubation period: 2 weeks to many years

Clinical Features
- Abdominal pain
- Dysentery-passing blood and mucus 2 to 3 times/ day
- Diarrohea alternating with constipation
- Stool with offensive smell
- Tenderness over the caecum and sigmoid colon

Pathology: Flask shaped ulcer involving the caecum and colonic mucosa

Investigation: Stool examination for RBCs and trophozoites.

Sigmoidoscopy: Shows ulcer and scraping should be looked for trophozoites of *Entamoeba histolytica.* Antibodies to *E. Histolytica* usually positive in hepatic amoebiasis

Management
- T. Metranidazole 800 mg 1-1-1 × to 7 days
- T. Diloxanide furoate 500 mg 1-1-1 × 10 days

CHOLERA

Aetiological agent: Vibrio cholerae (two biotypes-classical and El Tor)

Mode of spread: Drinking of contaminated water/ consumption of contaminated food (vomitus/stool of cholera patients).

Clinical Features
- Can occur in epidemics
- Sudden onset of severe diarrhea
- Vomiting may also occur
- No evidence of pain abdomen

Characteristics of Cholera

Diarrhea

Typical rice water stool containing clear fluid with mucus.

Severe diarrhea causes severe dehydration, hypotension, shock, oliguria and death. Occasionally diarrhea may be mild.

CHOLERA SICCA

Typical gastrointestinal symptoms are absent.

Large amount of fluid is lost into the dilated intestinal coils. Severe dehydration and death can occur.

Complications of Cholera
- Fluid and electrolyte imbalance
- Acute tubular necrosis and renal failure

Diagnosis
- Stool examination: Dark field microscopy for evidence of motile vibrio cholerae
- Stool culture and sensitivity

Management
- Immediate replacement of water and electrolytes
- Oral rehydration solution
- Calculation of stool volume and urine volume and replacement of fluid accordingly
- Cap. Tetracycline 250 mg 1-1-1-1into 3–5 days

Prevention
- Strict personal hygiene

- Avoid drinking contaminated water
- *Cholera vaccine:* Parenteral/oral vaccine can be used for protection.

SYPHILIS

Aetiological agent: Treponema pallidum (spirochaete)

Mode of Transmission
- Sexual route
- Rarely - Transfusion related
- Transplacental

Classification
- Congenital syphilis
  - Clinical and latent
  - Stigmata of congenital syphilis
- Acquired syphilis
  Stages
  - Early syphilis
    - Primary syphilis
    - Secondary syphilis
    - Early Latent syphilis
  - Late syphilis
- Latent syphilis
- Tertiary
  - Benign tertiary syphilis
  - Cardiovascular syphilis
  - Neurosyphilis

Acquired Syphilis

Primary Syphilis
Incubation period: 9–90 days

Lesions
- Primary chancre
  - Develops at genital area
  - Red macule develops into papule and becomes an indurated ulcer
  - Associated with inguinal lymphadenopathy
  - Chancre and lymphadenopathy are painless.
  - Chancre can develop over any area - like vagina and cervix
  - Chancre heals even without treatment within 2–6 weeks

Secondary Syphilis
- Develops after 6–8 weeks of primary chancre.
- Dissemination of infection causes multi system disease

Features
- Fever
- Maculopapular rash
- Generalised lymphadenopathy
- Mucosal patches over the mouth, pharynx and genitalia
- Hepatitis, nephritis, meningitis and/or cranial nerve palsies can occur

  Above features may resolve without treatment and then the disease enters into the latent phase.

Latent Syphilis

Person will have positive serological tests for syphilis but no clinical or CSF evidence of nervous system involvement.

Early Latent Syphilis
This phase of syphilis occurs within 2 years of primary infection.

Late Latent Syphilis
This phase of syphilis occurs after 2 years of primary infection.

Late Syphilis
Occurs many years after primary infection.

TERTIARY SYPHILIS

Benign Tertiary Syphilis
Occurs 3–10 years of primary infection
Characteristic lesion: Gumma
Gumma: A chronic granuloma, can invade any structure in the body.
- Gumma can involve the tongue and can cause leukoplakia which may be premalignant.
- Gumma may ulcerate and healing of gumma occurs with scar formation.

CARDIOVASCULAR SYPHILIS

- Occurs after 15 to 20 years after initial infection.
- Syphilis causes aortitis, aortic regurgitation and aortic aneurysm.

Neurosyphilis

Syphilis causes meningo vascular syphilis and parenchymal syphilis like Tabes dorsalis and general paralysis of insane.

Congenital syphilis

Syphilis in the pregnant patient may result in infection of the fetus.

It can result in mental handicap, deafness and blindness in children.

Teeth Abnormalities in Congenital Syphilis

Hutchinson's Teeth

Upper central incisors are peg shaped, widely placed and become centrally notched.

Mulberry Molars

Sixth year molars with multiple poorly developed cusps/deficient enamel.

Other Features of Congenital Syphilis

High arched palate, maxillary hypoplasia, saddle nose, choroiditis, corneal scars and frontal bossing.

Oral Manifestations of Syphilis

Primary Syphilis

Charecteric lesion: Chancre
Features: Large pain less ulcer with induration with unilateral lymphadenopathy.
Sites involved: Tonsils, lips and tongue

Secondary Syphilis

Mucus patches over the palate and oral mucosa. Maculopapular lesions can occur with central ulcerations.

Tertiary Syphilis

Gumma occurs over the palate and tongue.

Congenital Syphilis

Features
- Hutchison's incisors (upper molars) are notched and widely spaced.
- Mulberry molars (cusps of molars are not well developed)
- Fissures at the corner of the mouth and glossitis
- Gumma of the jaw, tongue and palate

Investigations

Non specific tests
- Rapid plasma reagin test (RPR)
- Venereal disease research laboratory test (VDRL)

Treponema specific antibody tests
- *Treponema pallidum* haemagglutination assay (TRHA)
- Fluorescent treponemal antibody absorbed test
- Treponema antigen based immunoassay IgM and IgG.

Management of Syphilis

Table 11.1 lists stages of syphilis alongside drugs of choice for its management.

Table 11.1 Management of syphilis

Stage of syphilis	Drug of choice
Primary Secondary Early latent	Benzathine penicillin intra muscular 2.4 million units (Single dose)
Late latent Cardiovascular	Lumbar puncture - to be done Normal CSF- Benzathine penicillin 2.4 million units IM/Wk into 3 weeks
Benign tertiary	CSF - abnormal treat as neurosyphilis
Neurosyphilis (Symptomatic and asymptomatic)	Procaine penicillin 2.4 million units/day intramuscular + oral Probenecid 500m QID into 10-14 days
Patient allergic to penicillin - tetracycline can be used (Dose :Tetracycline 500 mg 6th hrly x 14 days)	

ACQUIRED IMMUNE DEFICIENCY SYNDROME (AIDS)

Aetiological Agent

Single stranded RNA retro virus. It contains an enzyme called reverse transcriptase. It incorporates into host cell DNA. Virus is called human immune deficiency virus (HIV) type I and type II.

Abnormalities caused by acquired Immune Deficiency Syndrome

- Defective cell mediated immunity
- Susceptibility to increasing number of infections
- Development of rare variety of tumors

Immunological Abnormalities caused by HIV

- Severe defect in the cell mediated immunity
- There will be lymphocytopenia and reduced CD4 lymphocytes (T helper cells)

Chief routes of transmission of Human Immune Deficiency Virus

- Sexual transmission
- Predominantly homosexuals
- Occasionally heterosexual transmission
- Can also be transmitted by blood and blood product transfusion and prick with infected needles and instruments

Major risk groups involved in the Developments of AIDS

- Male homosexuals/bisexuals
- Intravenous drug abusers and needle sharing
- Organ sharing recipients
- Hemophiliacs

Effects of HIV Infection

- Persons who are infected with human immunodeficiency virus develop AIDS.
- Person develops immunodeficiency and all the body system may be affected.
- Persons with AIDS are prone to develop infection with *Pneumocystis carnii*, tuberculosis, fungal and other viral infections.
- There may be manifestations like thrombocytopenic purpura, Kaposi's sarcoma and development of lymphoma.

- African AIDS causes severe diarrhea and wasting syndrome (slim disease).

Clinical features of HIV Infection

Primary infection

Person may be asymptomatic. Primary infection occurs within 2×4 weeks after exposure.

Clinical Manifestations of Primary Infection

- Fever
- Erythematous rash
- Fatigue
- Pharyngitis
- Cervical lymphadenopathy
- Headache, joint pain, myalgia
- Mucosal ulceration

Rarely: Meningoencephalitis, myelitis, polyneuritis, and opportunistic infections.

Symptomatic recovery occurs within 2–10 weeks. Appearance of specific antibody in the serum-sero conversion takes place within 3–12 weeks (usually 8 weeks).

Asymptomatic Infection

- No clinical evidence of disease
- Remains for a variable period of time

Other Features

- Persistant generalized lymphadenopathy: Enlarged lymph nodes- 2 or more groups (>1 cm) for more than 3 months in extra inguinal sites.
- Virus replicates within the lymphoid tissue

Mild Symptomatic Disease

Manifestations

- Fever
- Oral/vaginal candidiasis
- Diarrhea
- Oral hairy leucoplakia
- Weight loss
- Thrombocytopenia, herpes zoster

Acquired immunodeficiency syndrome is characterised by the development of opportunistic infections and neoplasms. There will be associated decrease in the CD_4 count.

Opportunistic Infections and Neoplasms associated with AIDS

Dermatological
- Mucocutaneous candidiasis
- Staphylococcal infection
- Herpes simplex infection
- Herpes zoster infection
- Atypical mycobacterial infection

Respiratory
- Pulmonary tuberculosis
- Atypical mycobacterial infection
- Fungal
  – Aspergillosis
  – Histoplasmosis
  – *Pneumocystis carnii* pneumonia
- Gram negative bacterial infection

Gastrointestinal Tract
- Giardiasis
- Isospora belli infection
- Cryptosporidiosis
- Gram negative bacterial infection

Central Nervous System
- Tuberculosis
- Cryptococcus
- Toxoplasmosis

Disseminated Infection
- Cryptococcus infection
- *Mycobacterium avium intracellulare* infection
- Histoplasma infection

Neoplasms associated with HIV Infection
- Squamous cell carcinoma of mouth, anus and rectum
- Lymphoma
  – Primary cerebral
  – Non Hodgkin's lymphoma
- Kaposi's sarcoma

Miscellaneous Conditions
- Thrombocytopenic purpura
- Encephalopathy
- Seborrheic dermatitis

Oral Manifestations of HIV Infection

Common lesions
- Aphthous ulcers
- Herpes simplex infection
- Oral candidiasis
- Oral hairy leukoplakia
- Herpes zoster
- Syphilitic lesions
- Periodontitis
- Cervical lymphadenopathy
- Mycobacterial infection

Rare Manifestations
- Kaposi's sarcoma
- Lymphoma

Drug induced Mucosal Ulceration
- Due to antiretroviral drugs
- Due to cotrimoxazole (for pneumocystis infection)

HAIRY LEUKOPLAKIA
- Raised white areas of thickening on the lateral border of the tongue.
- Supposed to be caused by Epstein-Barr virus
- It is a premalignant condition
- It may develop into squamous cell carcinoma

KAPOSI'S SARCOMA
- Endothelial cell tumor
- Usually found in oral or perioral mucosa
- Red or purple macule or a nodule on the palate
- Kaposi's sarcoma is characteristic of AIDS

ANGULAR STOMATITIS
Characterised by inflammation of angle of mouth.

Causes
- Candidial infection
- Iron and B complex deficiency

Lab Diagnosis of HIV Infection
- Standard screening test for HIV infection: ELISA Test.
- HIV ELISA detects infection with both HIV-1 and HIV-2.

- HIV ELISA is interpreted as either positive or negative or as indeterminate.
- Most common confirmatory test used for HIV infection is western blot

Protocol for Lab Diagnosis of HIV Infection
- If HIV ELISA is negative Rpt the ELISA if clinically indicated within 3 to 6 months.
- If HIV ELISA is negative on two occasions it is indicative of no HIV infection.
- If HIV ELISA is positive or indeterminate: Confirm with HIV-1 Wester blot.
- If HIV-1 western blot is positive - confirms HIV-1 infection.
- If HIV-1 westernblot is indeterminate suggest repeat westernblot at 1 month and also test for HIV-2 ELISA.

Other tests used in the diagnosis of HIV infection.

HIV - 1: p^{24} antigen capture assay.

HIV - RNA assay

HIV - DNA PCR assay

p^{24} antigen capture assay is positive even before the development of antibodies against HIV infection.

CD_4 T Lymphocyte Court
Human immune deficiency virus specifically affects T helper lymphocyte cells causing immune deficiency. Estimation of T helper lymphocytes (CD_4T cell count) gives an indication of degree of severity of HIV infection.

Significance of CD_4T cell count in a patient of HIV Infection
- CD_4 T cell count less than 350 cells/cmm - indication for starting anti retroviral drugs.
- CD_4 count less than 200 cells/cmm - increases the risk of infection with pneumocystis and indication for cotrimoxazole prophylaxis.
- CD_4 count less than 50 cells/cmm - risk of infection with *Mycobacterium avium intracellularae* and cytomegalo virus.
- Repeat CD_4 count every 3-6 months is indicated while following up a patient of HIV infection.
- Expected increase of CD_4 count is 100-150 cells/

cmm every month after starting antiretroviral therapy.

HIV RNA Load
- HIV RNA load more than 50000 copies/cmm of blood is an indication for antiretroviral therapy.
- HIV RNA load is to be repeated every 3 months after initiation of treatment with antiretroviral drugs.

Baseline investigations in all patients with HIV Infection
- HBsAg
- Mantoux test
- Toxoplasma antibody
- Anti hepatitis C antibody
- VDRL and TPHA
- Anti hepatitis A antibody
- Chest X-ray
- CD4 count
- CMV serology
- HIV RNA load

Dental Treatment
- Risk of transmission with needle stick injury of HIV infected patient is low (Carriers have low titer of virus)
- Risk of infection with hepatitis B is more (26%) compared to HIV virus after needle stick injury.

Drugs used in the treatment of HIV Infection

Anti Retroviral Drugs

Nucleoside reverse transcriptase inhibitors (NRTS)
- Zalcitabine
- Didanosine
- Zidovudine
- Lamivudine
- Stavudine

Non nucleoside reverse transcriptase inhibitors (NNRTS)
- Nevirapine
- Efavirenz

Protease inhibitors
- Indinavir
- Saquinavir
- Retonavir
- Nelfinavir

Oral Side Effects of Antiretroviral Drugs

- Mouth and esophageal ulcers, e.g. zalcitabine
- Drug induced Steven-Johnson syndrome with mouth ulcers.

Treatment of HIV Infection

Indications
- All patients with CD4 counts < 350 cells/ cmm
- All patients with higher viral RNA load (HIV RNA > 50,000 cells/cmm)
- Acute HIV syndrome
- Symptomatic HIV disease
- Post exposure prophylaxis against contact with HIV infection.

Usual HAART (highly active antiretro viral therapy) regimes used

- 2 Nucleoside analogues + 1non nucleosidal antiretroviral
  For example Zudovidine + Lamivudine + Nevirapine or
- 2 Nucleoside analogues + 1 Protease inhibitor
  For example, Zudovidine + Lamuvudine + Protease inhibitor (indinavir)
  During treatment monitoring of drug side effects, CD 4 counts, viral RNA load is required. Change of drug regime is required, depending on the patient's response and drug side effects. Therapy to be continued for life long.

Factors which favours the increase risk for HIV transmission after post exposure

- Severely ill patient with advanced HIV disease
- Presence of visible blood on the instrument
- Deeper injuries of the patient
- Contact with instruments which are placed in the vascular system of the patient.

Recommended Post Exposure Prophylaxis

For routine exposure
28 days of treatment with 2 drugs
For example, Zudovidine + Lamividine

For complicated and high risk exposure
28 days of treatment with Zudovidine + Lamividine + 3rd drug like Indinavir

Oral Candidiasis (Oral Thrush or Moniliasis)
- Oral candidiasis is caused by *Candida albicans*. Lesions will have sheets of curdy white patches difficult to remove and leave behind a raw surface after removal.

Common Conditions Associated with Oral Candidiasis
- Immune suppressive and corticosteroid therapy
- Long term antibiotic therapy
- Diabetes mellitus
- Acquired immune deficiency syndrome

Different forms of Oral Candidiasis
- Pseudomembrane formation type
  - Soft creamy colored raised patches.
  - Wiping the lesion leaves behind red area.
  - Involves buccal mucosa and soft palate
  - Gram stain well show long tangled masses of fungal hyphae
  - Treatment: Nystatin lozenzes (500000IU)
- Antibiotic induced stomatitis due to candidiasis
  - Occurs after broad spectrum antibiotics
  - Red oedematous oral mucosa with one or two flecks of thrush.
  - Angular stomatitis is an associated feature
  - Treatment: Topical antifungal application
- Denture induced stomatitis and candidiasis.
  - Erythematous lesions of whole of denture bearing area with thrush.
  - Treatment: leaving dentures out of mouth at night and storing them in hypochlorite solution.
  - Topical antifungal should be used.
- Candidial leukoplakia
  - Firmly adherent white plaques over the tongue either on the dorsum or edges of the tongue.

- Candidiasis and its association with immune deficiency.
  - Candidiasis is associated with conditions like AIDS, Digeorge syndrome (natural immune deficiency) and immune suppression after organ transplantation.
- Chronic mucocutaneous candidiasis
  - May have familial association
  - In severe form of chronic mucocutaneous candidiasis there may be granuloma formation over the skin and oral mucosa with susceptibility to bacterial infection.

  - Occasionally candidiasis may be associated with autoimmune endocrinopathies like hypoparathyroidism Addisson's disease and thymomas.

Treatment of Oral Candidiasis
- Nystatin lozenzes (500000 Units) or Amphotericin lozenzes (10 mg) QID (four times a day) × 1 week.
- Miconazole local application can be done for candidial leukoplakia and for candidial angular stomatitis.

12 Skin Diseases and Infections with Oral Manifestations

INFECTIVE DISEASES WITH ORAL MANIFESTATIONS

HERPES SIMPLEX

Aetiological agent: Herpes simplex virus type I
Type I herpes simplex virus can cause
1. Acute gingival stomatitis
2. Fever
3. Cervical lymphadenopathy

Primary Herpetic Gingivostomatitis

- Resolves within 10 days
- Lesions involve gingiva, palate, tongue and oral mucosa.
- Lesions are associated with greenish-gray slough with halitosis.
- Requires antipyretics, analgesics and good oral hygiene and chlorhexidine mouth wash.
  Acyclovir is essential to control infection in immune compromised patients.
  Recurrent infection with herpes simplex virus can affect mucocutaneous junction of lips called cold sore (Herpes labialis).

Treatment
Acyclovir ointment - locally or oral acyclovir

VARICELLA ZOSTER

Table 12.1 gives oral manifestations of different infectious diseases. Reactivation of varicella zoster virus can affect maxillary or mandibular division of trigeminal nerve and can cause facial pain, oral ulceration and vesicles unilaterally over the tongue (see infectious diseases).

ORAL MANIFESTATIONS OF DIFFERENT SKIN DISEASES

LICHEN PLANUS

Common skin disease frequently involving the oral cavity.

Skin Lesions
- Small purplish or violaeous itchy papules affecting the flexor aspects of the wrist.

Oral Lesions of Lichen Planus
- Usually bilateral affecting the posterior aspect of buccal mucosa.
- Can involve the tongue and gingiva
- They can be papular or whitish plaques

Oral lesions of lichen planus can mimic lesions produced by pemphigus. Symptomatic oral lesions require local steroids and severe form may require intralesional and systemic steroids.

Steven-Johnson Syndrome (Figs 12.1a to c)

Steven-Johnson syndrome is characterised by the development of blisters with purpuric macules.

Causes
- *Infections:* Mycoplasma, coxsakie and herpes simplex infections
- *Drug induced:* Sulfa drugs, penicillins, barbiturates and NSAIDs

Features
- Fever, painful skin and mucosal ulcers, eye lesions
- Gastro intestinal and pulmonary involvement

Table 12.1 Oral manifestations of different infectious diseases

Diseases	Oral manifestations
AIDS	Candidiasis, hairy leukoplakia, Kaposi's sarcoma, cervical lymphadenopathy
Chickenpox	Oral ulcers
Diphtheria	Exudates/membrane over the palate, palatal palsy
Herpes simplex	Oral ulceration, ulcers can involve palate, gingiva, lips.
Herpes zoster	Oral ulceration in zoster of maxillary and mandibular division of the trigeminal nerve. Vesicles and ulcers on the palate and pinna of the ear in Ramsay-Hunt syndrome.
Infectious mononucleosis	Exudates over the tonsils, petechiae over the palate, oral ulceration
Measles	Koplik's spots, pharyngitis
Mumps	Papillitis at salivary duct orifices, Sialdenitis
Rubella	Pharyngitis

Management

- Stoppage of drugs causing the lesions.
- Ocular care
- Supportive therapy with hydration and nutritional supplementation
- Corticosteroids and IV immunoglobulin

PEMPHIGUS

- Dermatological disorder characterised by widespread formation of vesicles, blisters and ulceration.
- Age group affected: Middle aged women

Pathology

- Deposition of antibodies along the intercellular junctions leading on to destruction of epithelium.

Clinical

- Vesicles or bullae formation in the oral mucosa and skin.
- Extensive skin damage leading onto fluid and electrolyte loss and secondary infection.

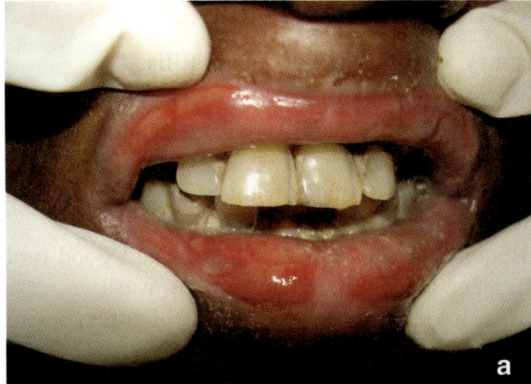

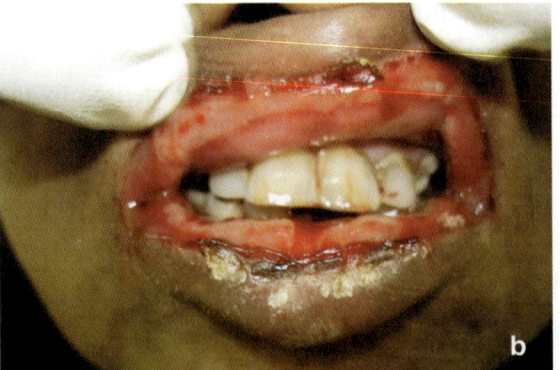

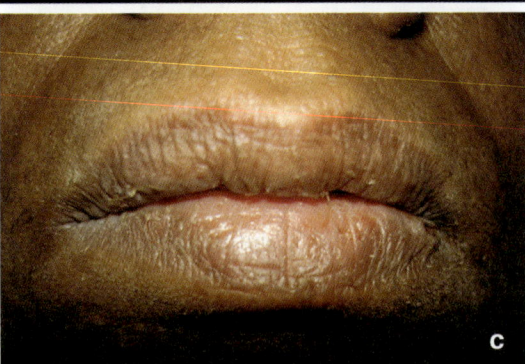

Fig. 12.1a to c Drug induced Steven-Johnson syndrome

Mucus Membrane Pemphigoid

- Presence of intact bullae/vesicles along the oral mucosa.

Investigations

- Smear from vesicles shows detached epithelial (Tzanck) cells.
- Biopsy from the lesion: demonstration of antibody deposition by immunoflorescent technique.

Management

- Local application of steroids (beclomethasone) for oral lesions
- Combination of 100–150 mg/day of azathioprine with 40–80 mg of prednisolone.
- Methotrexate or cyclophosphamide can be used instead of azathioprine.

ERYTHEMA NODOSUM

Features

- Fever, bodyache and joint pain

Lesions

- Usually involves the lower limb
- Painful palpable bluish red nodules
- May resolve slowly leaving white scars

Causes

- Drug induced: Sulphonamides and cotrimoxazole

Infections

- Tuberculosis, leprosy, brucellosis, streptococcal infection, fungal infection

Pathology

- Vasculitic type of reaction to subcutaneous fat and dermis.

Treatment

- NSAIDS
- Short course of corticosteroids
- Treatment of underlying cause

BEHCET'S SYNDROME

- Multisystem disease charecterised by vasculitis, classically associated with clinical triad of uveitis, oral and genital ulcers.
- Behcet's syndrome is supposed to be an antigen mediated disease and features are due to circulating immune complexes.

Clinical Features

- *Oral ulcerations:* Recurrent aphthous ulcers. Minor or major or herpitiform lesions. Ulcers are usually deep and multiple.
- Recurrent genital ulcers
- *Eye involvement:* Uveitis, vasculitis of retina and optic atrophic
- *Dermatological:* Pustular lesions and erythema nodosum
- *Musculoskeletal:* Arthralgia
- *Renal:* Haematuria and proteinuria
- *Neuropsychiatric:* Brain stem signs, depression etc.

Investigations

- Raised ESR and immunoglobulin levels.
- Pathergy: Development of pustules (within 48 hrs) after skin pricking.

Management

- *Oral lesions:* Topical steroid application
- *Systemic involvement:* Colchicine, thalidomide, immune suppressive drugs.

13 Medical Emergencies in Dental Practice

Vasovagal Attack (Common faint)

Fainting and Approach to a Patient of Sudden Fainting (collapse) During Dental Procedure
- Fainting is the most common cause of sudden loss of consciousness.
- Patient can faint before or during dental treatment.

Predisposing Factors for Fainting during Dental Treatment
- Anxiety
- Pain due to procedure /injection
- Fasting state
- High febrile states
- Fatigue

Symptoms and Signs of Fainting
- Fatigue, nausea and dizzy feeling
- Pallor
- Skin becomes cold and moist
- Initially pulse becomes slow and weak, later it becomes rapid and full.
- Loss of consciousness

Mechanism of Vasovagal Attack (Common faint)
Psychological factors like pain, site of blood, injection needle can cause reflex stimulation of autonomic nervous system and cause peripheral vasodilation, bradycardia and fainting.

Common Fainting should be differentiated from
- Seizure
- Hypoglycemia
- Acute myocardial infarction
- Stroke
- Adrenal insufficiency
- Drug reaction

- Complete heart black and bradycardia

Clinical Aspects of Fainting
- It is preferable to give injections with the patient in lying down position before procedures.
- If the diagnosis is not very clear for the loss of consciousness:
  - Make the patient laid flat, patients with common faint will have instantaneous recovery.
  - If the recovery is not immediate check the patient's pulse. If the pulse is not felt person may be having cardiac arrest, take necessary measures.
- It the patient's pulse is rapid and full give oral glucose.
- If the patient is unconscious give IV glucose (50%-100 ml). Patients with hypoglycemia will immediately recover (especially in a diabetic).
- If after administration of glucose improvement does not occur:
  - Maintain the airway and administer oxygen
  - IV hydrocortisone may be required in suspected adrenal insufficiency
  - Call for urgent medical help

Respiratory Emergencies

Respiratory emergencies may be due to anesthetics, respiratory failure or respiratory obstruction.

Respiratory Failure
- Usually due to anesthetics or hypoxia induced.
- Person will have stoppage of breathing, person

becomes cyanosed, pulse may become irregular and then cardiac arrest may occur.

Management
- Stop the administration of anesthetic/sedation
- Clear the airway and administer oxygen inhalation
- Keep the patient in flat position
- Start cardio pulmonary respiratory resuscitation. (if there is cardiorespiratory arrest)
- Call for medical assistance.

If there is Respiratory Obstruction either due to Foreign Body or Laryngospasm

Perform
- Airway suction
- Removal of foreign body if it is in the pharynx.
- If obstruction below the pharynx, do tracheostomy
- Do urgent chest X-ray to locate the foreign body and remove the foreign body with the medical help.

Acute Chest Pain

Acute severe chest pain is usually caused by angina or myocardial infarction.
- Patient will complain of severe retrosternal chest pain.
- Nausea, vomiting, dyspnea and sweating may occur.
- Pulse may be weak/irregular

Management
- Reassurance
- Sublingual glyceryl trinitrate 0.5 mg sublingual
- O_2 inhalation if the person is breathless
- Call for medical help

An Attack of Asthma

Precipitating Causes
- Anxiety
- Local anesthetic
- NSAID administration

Features
Previous history of dyspnea with wheeze

- Patient is severely breathless
- Accessory muscles of respiration acting
- Presence of rhonchi on respiratory auscultation.

Management
- Reassurance
- Immediate salbutamol nebulisation
- If there is no relief within in 5–10 minutes- administer injection terbutaline 0.5 mg subcutaneously.
- Injection hydrocortisone 200 mg IV may be required, if there is no relief with salbutamol
- Give 100% oxygen inhalation
- Call for medical help

Drug Reactions and Interactions

Main drug reactions and interactions include
- Reactions with local anesthetics
- Overdose of intravenous barbiturates
- Hypotension resulting from interactions with IV barbiturates and antihypertensive drugs
- Hypertension from interaction of pethidine with monoamine oxidase inhibitors

Local Anaesthetic Reactions
Following reactions can occur after administration of local anesthetics
- Fainting
- Intravascular injection of local anesthetic
- Local anesthetic allergy
- Temporary facial palsy or diplopia (due to local anesthetic injections in dental practice).
- Cardiovascular reactions

Intravascular injection of local anesthetic rarely occurs can cause agitation, confusion, drowsiness, convulsions or loss of consciousness. Local anesthetic reactions usually recover within half an hour.

Temporary Facial Palsy after Local Anaesthetic Administration

After local anesthetic injection for dental extraction local anesthetic track downwards towards the facial nerve or orbital contents causing facial palsy. But facial palsy disappears after the effect of the anesthetic.

Cardiovascular Reactions after Local Anaesthetic Administration

- Local anesthetics can occasionally cause cardiovascular reactions.

Management of Cardiac Arrest

- Call medical assistance or ambulance service
- Keep the patient flat
- Do cardiopulmonary resuscitation

Cardiopulmonary Resuscitation (CPR)

- Two firm blows with the closed fist to the mid sternum (occasionally this may restart the heart in normal rhythm).
- Clearing the airway: Tilt the head backwards with chin lifted. Remove the denture and foreign body if any.
- Start artificial ventilation (mouth to mouth breathing) airway with face mask/endotracheal intubations-2 breathing/every 15 chest compressions.

Schematic Approach for Administering Basic Life Support (Fig. 13.1)

1. Ascertain whether the person is alive by shaking and shouting at the patient.
2. Opening the airway by tilting the head, lifting the chin and thrusting the jaw
3. Observe whether there is effort of breathing
   - Look for movement of chest
   - Auscultate for breath sounds
   - If breathing administer 2 effective breaths.
4. Check for circulation-carotid pulse for 10 seconds only
   - If circulation present continue breathing while monitoring circulation every minute.
   - No circulation - Start CPR
     - Chest compressions 100/minute
     - Administer 2 breaths for every 15 compressions

Technique of CPR

Place the hand of one side over the lower sternum and keep the heel of the other palm over the dorsum of the lower hand.

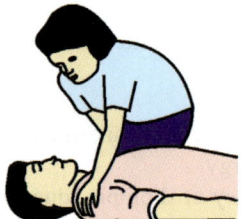

Check for responsiveness

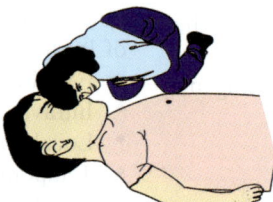

Check for breathing

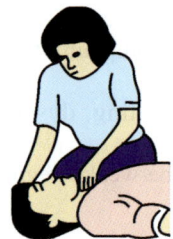

Check for signs of circulation

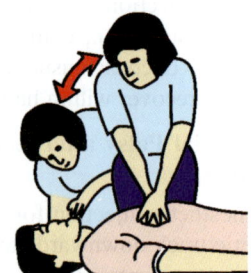

Start cardiopulmonary resuscitation

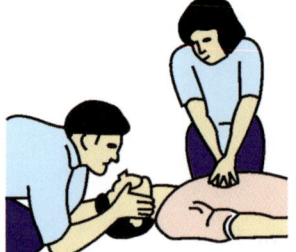

Mouth to mouth ventilation

Fig. 13.1 Schematic approach for administering basic life support

- Apply sufficient pressure to depress the sternum around 2 inches with abrupt relaxation.
- Depress the sternum approximately 100 times/minute.
- Administer 100 ml IV sodium bicarbonate (8.4%) at a rate of 10 ml/minute.
- Defibrillation and advanced cardiac support may be required.
- Record pulse, blood pressure and respiratory rate.
- It the patient does not resuscitate within 15 minutes, less chance to recover.

Other Medical Emergencies

SHOCK

Clinical term used to describe a state where in oxygen delivery fails to meet the metabolic requirement of the body despite a normal oxygen content of the arterial blood.

Invariably shock is synonymous with hypotension and is state of circulatory failure.

Classification

Hypovolemic Shock

Due to severe reduction in the circulating blood volume
Massive internal or external bleeding, severe dehydration, severe burns.

Septic shock
Systemic infection causing endothelial dysfunction, vasodilatation, microvascular occlusion, tissue and organ damage.

Anaphylactic
Allergen induced causing severe vasodilatation.

Cardiogenic
Acute myocardial infarction, myocarditis

Neurogenic
Severe form of brain or spinal injury causing disruption of neurogenic vasomotor control.

Obstructive
Obstruction to blood flow causing decreased cardiac output.
For example, cardiac tamponade, massive pulmonary embolism, tension pneumothorax

Clinical Features
- Cold clammy extremities and skin
- Drowsiness and irritability
- Tachycardia
- Hypotension (systolic BP less than 100 mmHg)
- Urine output is less than 30 ml/hr
- Rapid shallow breathing
- Central venous pressure - usually decreased
- Multiple organ dysfunction

Management
- All forms of shock require early diagnosis and treatment.
- Monitoring central venous pressure, pulse volume and hematocrit helps in the diagnosis and treatment of shock.
- Administer specific therapy depending on the cause.
- Delay in the management results in tissue hypoxia and irreversible organ damage.

Acute Respiratory Distress Syndrome (ARDS)

Acute, diffuse inflammatory response of the lung either to direct or indirect insult (outside the lung) is called ARDS.

KEY POINTS 13.1

- Cold clammy extremities, low volume pulse and evidence of decreased cardiac output consider cardiogenic, hypovolemic and obstructive shock.

- Warm extremities, high volume pulse and evidence of high cardiac output consider septic, anaphylactic and neurogenic shock.

- JVP is reduced in anaphylactic and hypovolemic shock. JVP is elevated in cardiac failure and obstructive shock.

Causes

Due to direct injury to the lungs
- Pneumonia
- Lung contusion
- Aspiration of gastric contents
- Near drowning
- Toxic gas inhalation

Due to indirect injury to the lungs
- Severe sepsis
- Fat embolism
- Multiple trauma
- Severe burns
- Pancreatitis
- Barbiturates and heroin
- Major blood transfusion reaction

Criteria for diagnosis
- Evidence of hypoxia
- Pulmonary capillary wedge pressure not elevated/ no evidence of elevated left atrial pressure.
- Bilateral alveolar opacities in the lung.
- Impaired lung compliance

Clinical features
- Features suggestive of predisposing condition
- Breathlessness
- Bilateral crepitations in the lung
- Evidence of other organ failure (kidney, bowel, liver, nervous system, etc.) and coagulation failure.

Management
- Treatment of underlying conditions like sepsis, trauma and burns
- Adequate nutritional support
- Treatment of secondary infection
- Prevention of complications like thrombolism and gastrointestinal bleed.

- Glucocorticoids, supplementation of oxygen and ventilatory support

Organophosphorous Poisoning

Organophosphorous compounds are used as insecticides.

Mechanism of Action of Organophosphorous Compounds

Inhibit acetyl choline esterase enzyme leading onto accumulation of acetylcholine at the neuromuscular junction.

Features of Acute Consumption of Organophosphorous Compounds
- Vomiting, diarrhea
- Loss of memory
- Sweating
- Drowsiness
- Pin point pupil
- Respiratory paralysis
- Hypersalivation
- Coma
- Dyspnoea

Diagnosis is made by history (consumption of poison) and measuring blood - ACE (acetyl choline esterase) level which will be very low.

Treatment
- Gastric lavage
- Cleaning the skin (poison can be absorbed through the skin).
- Inj. atropine till the person is fully atropinised and to be continued.
- Specific antidote: Inj. Oxime, 1g: QID for 48–72 hrs
- Artificial ventilation
- Anticonvulsants for seizures.

14 Preoperative Assessment for General Anaesthesia

Enquire about the Following Disorders in all Patients who are Undergoing General Anaesthesia
- Cardiovascular disorders and hypertension
- Diabetes mellitus
- Respiratory disorders
- Neuromuscular disorders
- Smoking and alcoholism
- Drug allergies and present medications
- Previous anaesthetic complication
- Pregnancy
- Any evidence for airway obstruction
- Cough, dyspnea, palpitation, chest pain, pedal edema, about arrhythmias causing palpitation.

Following Disorders require Evaluation before General Anaesthesia

- Cardiovascular and respiratory disorders.
- Endocrine disorders
- Hepatic dysfunction and jaundice
- Convulsive disorders and fainting
- Renal disorders
- Anaemia and bleeding disorders
- Gastro intestinal disorders

In all patients who are undergoing general anesthesia, possible airway obstruction, possible injury to the airway and intubation difficulty should be considered.

Investigations before Anaesthesia

- Hb% and peripheral smear
- Urine routine
- Chest X-ray
- Renal function tests
- ECG
- Liver function tests

- Sickling test
- Electrolytes
- Blood sugar

Indications for Local Anaesthesia
- Minor form of surgery
- Contraindication for general anaesthesia
- No immediate general anaesthesia available

Indications for General Anaesthesia
- Allergy to local anaesthetics
- Severe acute infection
- Major surgical procedures

Contraindication for General Anaesthesia
- Significant cardiac disease
- Severe form of respiratory disease
- Infection in the floor of the mouth

Precautions before General Anaesthesia
- Patient's identifications
  - Name
  - Reason for anesthesia
  - Operation site

- Emptying the urinary bladder.
- Keeping the stomach empty 4 hrs before administering anaesthesia.
- Psychological preparation of the patient: Patient should be given enough confidence and reassurance and discussion regarding surgical procedures.
- Premedication is used usually 30 to 40 minutes before surgery.
- Artificial dentures to be removed before general anesthesia.

Different types of Premedications used
- *Narcotic analgesia* (pethidine, morphine): Causes sedation. But can cause nausea, vomiting and respiratory depression.
- *Benzodiazepines:* Have anxiolytic action, e.g.: diazepam and lorazepam.
- *Atropine derivatives,* e.g. atropine and hys-cenine have antiemetic and parasympatholytic action. Atropine derivatives should be given carefully in elderly, patients with cardiac arrhythmias and in glaucoma patients.

Denture Removal
- Fragile, loose teeth may be damaged during administration of general anesthesia.
- Artificial dentures should be removed before general anesthesia.

Local Anaesthesia

Different Local Anaesthetics used
- Lignocaine 2% plain gives brief anesthesia
- Lignocaine 2% + adrenaline 1 in 80,000 - effective analgesia for more than 90 minutes.
- Pilocarpine 4% plain: Gives brief analgesia
- Pilocarpine 3% + felypressin 0.03 IU/ml

Drugs for IV Anaesthesia
- Ketamine
- Thiopentone

Drugs for IV Sedation
- Diazepam - up to 20 mg
- Midazolam - 0.07 mg/kg

General Anaesthetics used
- Halothane
- Nitrous oxide
- Enflurane

Postoperative care after General Anaesthesia
- Closely watch the patient till he is fully recovered from anesthesia/conscious recovers.
- Keep the patient semiprone and clear airway should be maintained.
- If necessary postoperative analgesia and antibiotics to be given.
- Patients can develop drowsiness, headache after general anesthesia. Sore throat may develop due to intubation.

- Postoperative atelectasis (collapse of part of the lung) can develop. Patient should be given chest physiotherapy, breathing exercises and encourage to cough.

Postoperative Fever may Develop Due to
- Pulmonary infection
- Hematoma formation
- Wound infection

Postoperative hemorrhage is usually due to local cause and care should be taken to prevent significant bleeding.

Postoperative Collapse of the Patient
Patient can develop hypotension, loss of consciousness, pallor, sweating and tachycardia postoperatively. These may be due to,
- Pulmonary embolism
- Cardiac arrest (may be due to cardiac arrhythmias)
- Massive hemorrhage
- Adrenal insufficiency

Postoperative Complications

Immediate complications
- Nausea and vomiting
- Post operative pain
- Delayed recovery of consciousness
- Cardiorespiratory complications

Delayed Complications
- Wound infection
- Jaundice
- Respiratory and cardiac problems

Immediate Complications

Nausea and vomiting
- Usually due to the effect of the anesthetic agent.
- Metoclopramide or prochlorperazine may be effective

Postoperative pain
- Appears after the effect of anesthesia has disappeared.
- Requires potent analgesics, e.g. Injection Pethidine

Delayed Recovery of Consciousness

Due to

- Overdose of anaesthetic agents
- Hyperglycemia
- Cardiac complications
- Cerebrovascular accident

Delayed Complications

- Post operative pneumonia should be recognized early and to be treated.
- Myocardial infarction can occur especially in patients with IHD.

Jaundice

- Postoperative jaundice may be due to
  - Hepatotoxic drugs and hepatotoxic anesthetics
  - Viral hepatitis
  - Aggravation of preexisting liver disease
  - Ischemic hepatic damage due to circulatory failure
  - Transfusion reaction
  - Resolution of massive hematoma
- Wound infection
  - Requires proper dressing of the wound and antibiotics.

15 Antibiotics and Chemotherapeutic Agents

Different categories of Antibiotics and Chemotherapeutic Agents

1. Amino glycosides
2. β lactams
3. Folate antagonists
4. Glycopeptides
5. Macrolides and lincosamides
6. Nitroimidazoles
7. Quinalones
8. Tetracyclines and chloramphenicol
9. Carbapenems

For example: Gentamycin 3–5 mg/kg/day
               Amikacin 15 mg/kg/day
               Netilmycin 6 mg/kg/day
               Tobramycin 5 mg/kg/day

Side Effects

- Renal toxicity and renal failure (usually reversible)
- Blockage of neuromuscular junction with rapid IV administration
- Ototoxicity (toxic damage to 8th nerve - not reversible)

Uses

- Gram negative infections
- They have got synergism with β lactams.

Beta - Lactams (Key points 15.2)

Adverse Reactions

- Allergic reactions - anaphylaxis
- Diarrhoea
- Leucopenia, thrombocytopenia
- Interstitial nephritis
- Rarely seizures and encephalopathy

Different types of β-Lactams

1. **Naturally occurring**
   For example benzyl penicillin/phenoxymethyle penicillin
   Dose: Benzyl penicillin 1.2 to 2.4 g QID
   Effective against gram positive organisms and anaerobes

2. **Penicillinase resistant penicillins**
   For example flucloxacillin 500 mg QID
   Acts against *staphylococcus aureus.*

3. **Aminopenicillins**
   For example ampicillin 500 mg QID
   Amoxycillin 500 mg 8th hrly
   Effective against gram positive organisms and enterobacteriacae

4. **Carboxy and ureido penicillins**
   For example Ticarcillin & peperacillin
   Effective against pseudomonas
5. **β-lactamase Inhibitors**
   For example, clavulanic acid
   Adding clavulanic acid to penicillin increases its spectrum of activity

Monobactams

For example Aztreonam 1 to 2 g 12th hrly
Effective against gram negative organisms
No action against gram positive organisms

Cephalosporins

First Generation Cephalosporins

For example, Cephalexin 250 mg QID /Cephazolin
Effective against gram positive organisms

2nd Generation Cephalosporines

For example Cefuroxime 500 mg bd oral or 750 mg IV 8th hrly
Effective against both gram positive and gram negative infections

Third Generation Cephalosporins

For example Ceftriaxone 1 to 2 gr 8th hrly
For example Ceftazidime: 1gr 8th hrly IV
Effective against gram negative bacilli and pseudomonas

Fourth Generation Cephalosporins

For example Cefipime, cefpirome
Broad spectrum against both gram positive and gram negative organisms

Side Effects
- Allergic reactions
- Nephrotoxicity
- Pseudomembranous enterocolitis

Folate Antagonists

For example Cotrimoxazole (trimethoprim and Sulphaamethoxazole)
Dose: 80/400 or 160/800 mg twice daily

Uses
- Active against gram negative infection and some gram positive infections
- For Pneumocystis infection in HIV patients

Side Effects
- Skin and mucus membrane reactions including Stevens-Johnson syndrome
- Bone marrow dysplasia
- Hemolytic in G-6P D deficient patients

Glycopeptides

For example, Vancomycin 500 mg or 1g BD IV,Teicoplanin 200 mg–400 mg/day IV.

Uses
- Effective against methicillin resistant *Staphylococcus aureas* (MRSA)
- Some action against Enterococci and coagulase negative staphylococci.

Side Effects

Vancomycin
- Rapid IV infusion can cause histamine release leading onto anaphylaxis and Redman syndrome
- Combination with aminoglycosides can cause nephrotoxicity

Teicoplanin

Rarely can cause allergic reactions

Macrolides and Lincosamides

For example Erythromycin 250 mg–500 mg QID
Azithromycin 500 mg / day (very long half life)

Lincosamides

For example Lincomycin 300/600 mg 8th hrly
Clindamycin-300/600 mg 8th hrly

Uses
- Active against gram positive organisms
- Useful in patients with penicillin allergy
- Active against mycoplasma, chlamydia and rickettsial infection

Side effects of Macrolides and Lincosamides
- GIT side effects - vomiting
- Erythromycin estolate causes:
  – Cholestatic jaundice

– Can cause prolonged QT interval and ventricular tachycardia
- Clindamycin can cause pseudomembranous enterocolitis.

Nitrimidazoles

For example Metronidazole 400 mg 8th hrly/ Tinidazole 500 mg Bid.

Uses

- Anaerobic infection (bacteroides, clostridium species)
- Giardiasis
- Amoebiasis
- Trichomonas infection

Side Effects

- Metallic taste in the mouth
- If taken along with alcohol will produce antabuse effect.

Quinalones

For example, norfloxacin 400 mg bid, ciprofloxacin 500 mg bid, ofloxacin 400 mg bid, levofloxacin 500 mg od

Uses

- Very active against gram negative and atypical organisms
- Minimal activity against gram positive and anaerobic organisms

Side Effects

- Skin reactions
- Dizziness, tremors and convulsive disorders
- Quinalone and theophylline administration together can cause insomnia and seizures
- Can interfere with cartilage growth in children

Carbapenems

For example, Imepenem/meropenem: 500 mg 1g 12th or 8th hrly.

Broadest spectrum of β-lactams

Active against anaerobic and gram positive and negative organisms
- Expensive drug

Other Antimicrobials which are used Occasionally

Linezolid

- Belongs to oxazolidinones
- Active against gram positive organisms including methicillin resistant staphylococcus (MRSA).

Fusidic Acid

- Useful against gram positive bacterial infections

Nitrofurantoin

- Useful against gram positive and gram negative organisms
- Very good urinary tract antibiotic
- Safe in pregnancy and children
- Can cause pulmonary infiltrates with eosinophilia

Tetracyclines

For example, Doxycycline 100 mg bd

Uses

- Active against mycoplasma, chlamydia, rickettsiae, and spirochetes.
- Useful in patients with hyponatremia due to SIADH (Syndrome of inappropriate ADH secretion)

Side Effects

- Causes nausea and diarrhea
- Contraindicated in renal failure (except Doxycycline)
- Causes discoloration of teeth in children

Chloramphenicol

Dose: 500 mg QID
Uses
- Typhoid Fever
- Against *H. Influenzae*, *Strep. pneumonia*, nisseria, rickettsiae, chlamydiae and mycoplasma and anaerobes.

Side Effects
- Idiosyncratic – Aplastic anemia (not dose related)

- Bone marrow suppression (dose dependent and reversible)
- Gray baby syndrome-cyanosis and circulatory collapse in children

Drugs Used in the Treatment of Fungal Infections

Amphotericin B: A polyene antifungal agent

Uses
- Active against aspergillosis, crypttococcosis and candidiasis
- In neutropenia with fever with suspected fungal infection
- Amphotericin B lozenges are available for mucosal fungal infection

Side Effects
- May produce anaphylaxis
- Insoluble particles can produce embolisation during therapy
- Nephrotoxicity

Flucytosine
- Active against candida and cryptococcus
- Flucytosine should be combined with another anti fungal agent
- Can produce reversible pancytopenia

Azole group of Antifungal Agents

For example   Miconazole
                       Clotrimazole
                       Ketoconazole
                       Flucanazole
                       Itraconazole

Ketoconazole
- Oral antifungal agent
- Active against Candida and Aspergillus's species
- Produces hepatotoxicity

Flucanazole
- Active against candida infection
- Easily administrable with good safety profile

Itraconazole
- Oral antifungal drug
- Active against Aspergillus species

TOPICAL ANTIFUNGAL AGENTS
(For mucocutaneous fungal infection)

Nystatin
- Can be used as only topical agent
- Very useful against mucosal candidiasis
- If absorbed produces severe nephrotoxicity

Griseofulvin
- For extraneous fungal infection like Tinea corporis, Tinea pedis and Tinea capitis
- Oral administration for 4–8 weeks or more than that is required
- Dose: 500 mg to 1000 mg / day

Terbinafine
- Useful in nail and cutaneous fungal infection
- Can be given once daily
- Causes hepatotoxicity

Antiviral Drugs

Commonly used Antiviral Drugs

Acyclovir

Available Preparations
Oral/Intravenous or topical application

Uses
- Infection with
  - Varicella
  - Herpes simplex
  - Herpes zoster
- Oral tabs: 400 mg 5 times/day
- Side effect: Hypersensitivity, gastrointestinal and neurotoxicity

Famcyclovir

- Available preparations: Oral 250 mg to 750 mg 5–7 days.

Valcyclovir

Uses
- Herpes zoster

- Genital herpes simplex
- Valcyclovir 1g 1-1-1. 5-7 days

Side Effects of Valcyclovir
Thrombotic thrombocytopemic purpura. Hemolytic uremic syndrome.

Ribavirin

- Preparations available: oral/IV

Uses
- Chronic hepatitis B & C
- Respiratory syncytial virus infection

Side Effect
- Hemolytic anemia
- Hypersensitivity reaction

Gancyclovir

Preparations
- Oral / intravenous
- Dose: 5 mg/kg 14–21 days

Uses
- For Cytomegalovirus infection

Side Effect
- Cytopenias

Lamivudine

Preparations
- Oral

Uses
- HIV infection
- Chronic hepatitis B infection

Side Effect
- Toxicity against bone marrow
- Dose: 100–150 mg/day

Amantadine

Preparations
- Oral tablets

Uses
- Against influenza A infection
- Prophylaxis against influenza

Side Effects
- CNS side effects

Table 15.1 gives oral manifestations which may occur due to drug therapy.

Table 15.1 Oral manifestations that may occur due to drug therapy

Manifestations	Drugs responsible
Oral candidiasis	Corticosteroids, broad spectrum antibiotics, immune suppressive drugs
Teeth discoloration	Oral iron, tetracyclines, chlorhexidine, fluorides
Erythema multiforme (Stevens-Johnson syndrome)	Penicillin, phenytoin, phenobarbitone, sulfonamide, carbamezapine, busulphan
Angio edema	Aspirin, penicillin
Gingival hyperplasia	Calcium channel blockers, phenytoin, cyclosporin, phenobarbitone, contraceptive pills, primidone
Pigmentation of oral cavity	Heavy metals, ACTH, anticonvulsants, busulphan, chloroquine
Salivary gland enlargement	Insulin, antithyroid drugs, iodides, isoprenaline, phenothiazines, phenylbutazone, sulfonamides
Hypersalivation	Anticholinesterases, phenobarbitone, ethionamide, haloperidol, iodides, ketamine
Drugs causing dry mouth	Amphetamine, adriamycin, atropine, antiparkinsonian drugs, anti-histaminics, benzhexol, clonidine, tricyclics
Drugs causing disturbed taste	Biguanides, clofibrate, anti thyroid drugs, griseofulfin, metronidazole, gold salts
Cervical lymphadenopathy	Phenytoin, primidone
Involuntary facial movements	L- Dopa, methyl dopa, metoclopramide, tricyclics, carbamezapine

Interferons

- Cytokines with broad spectrum antiviral drug
- Interferon preparations are available as injections
- Useful in chronic hepatitis B and chronic hepatitis C infection
- Can cause influenza like illness and cytopenias. Table 15.2 lists contraindications to some of the drugs used in dentistry.

Table 15.2 Contraindications for certain drugs which may be used in dentistry

Drugs	Contraindications
Aspirin	Aspirin allergy, bronchial asthma, bleeding disorders, children with fever, renal and liver disease
Atropine	Elderly, urinary retention, prostatic hypertrophy, hyperthyroidism, glaucoma
Adrenaline	Hypertension, hyperthyroidism, IHD, pheochromocytoma
Amoxycillin/Ampicillin	Penicillin allergy, infectious mononucleosis
Carbamezapine	Liver disease, bone marrow suppression
Cephalosporins	Penicillin allergy, allergy to cephalosporins
Codeine	Hypothyroidism, liver disease, elderly
Corticosteroids	Hypertension, peptic ulcer, tuberculosis
Co-Trimoxazole	Liver disease, G-6PD deficiency, renal disease, pregnancy, porphyria
Dextropropoxyphene	Respiratory disease, liver disease, pregnancy
Diazepam	COPD, hypothyroidism, neuromuscular disease, porphyria, severe liver disease, cerebrovascular accident, children and elderly
Erythromycin Estolate	Liver disease, cardiac arrhythmias
Ketoconazole	Liver and renal disease
Metronidazole	Renal disease, blood dyscrasias, pregnancy
Opiates	COPD, head injury, hypothyroidism, liver disease, pregnancy, prostatic enlargement, urinary retention, bronchial asthma
Paracetamol	Liver disease, renal disease
Penicillin	Allergy, renal disease
Pentazocine	Liver disease, kidney disease, head injury pregnancy
Pethidine	Hypothyroidism, COPD
Rifampicin	Liver disease
Sulphonamides	G-6PD deficiency, porphyria, pregnancy renal disease, allergy
Tetracyclines	Children below 12 years, pregnancy, renal disease
Thiopentone	Cardiovascular disease, hypothyroidism, liver disease, myasthenia gravis, porphyria, barbiturate sensitivity
Tranexamic acid	Thromboembolic disease, haematuria
Tricyclics	Elderly, liver disease, cardiovascular disease, epilepsy

16 Normal Laboratory Data

URINE ANALYSIS

- Volume: 750–1200 ml/day
- Specific gravity: 1.002–1.025
- Titrable acidity: 20–40 mEq/d
- Amylase: 100–600/day
- Protein: less than 150 mg/day
- Potassium: 25–100 mEq/24hrs
- Sodium: 100–260 mEq/24hrs

CELLULAR COMPONENTS

Urinary Sediment
Normal cellular constituents
- Epithelial cells: 3–5/HPF
- RBC's: 3–5/HPF
- WBC's: 5/HPF

Urinary Casts
- Casts are formed when the tubular glycoprotein Tomm-Horsfall protein is precipitated in the tubular lumen.
- Cells, cellular debris, crystals get into the precipitated Tomm-Horsfall protein (cast matrix) to form different types of casts.

Hyaline Casts
- Formed of only Tomm-Horsfall protein.
- Does not contain any cellular material.
- Fever, dehydration, exercise can cause small increase in the hyaline casts.
- Broad, long hyaline casts suggest underlying renal disease.

Broad Casts
Represent tubules of hypertrophied nephrons/ large collecting ducts indicate advanced renal disease.

Granular Casts
Formed due to aggregation of tubular cell debris. Large numbers of coarsely granular casts are found in patients with acute tubular necrosis.

Waxy Casts
May represent terminal phase of degeneration of granular casts suggest advanced renal disease.

Fatty Casts/Lipiduria
Usually present in patients with nephrotic syndrome/ in patients with fat embolism.

RBC Casts
Suggest glomerular source of bleeding.

WBC Casts
Usually suggests acute/chronic pyelonephritis.

Bacterial Casts
Seen in acute pyelonephritis

Bacteriuria
Significant bacteriuria is indicated by the presence of more than 100000(105) organisms/ml of midstream sample of urine.

STOOL ANALYSIS

- Protein content - nil
- Stool nitrogen <1.7 g/day
- Fat < 6 gm/day (measured on a 3 days stool collection on a diet containing at least 50 gm of fat).

NORMAL CEREBRO SPINAL FLUID ANALYSIS

- CSF pressure: 50–180 mm of water
- Total protein: 20–50 mg /dl

- Chloride: 116–122 mEq /L
- Glucose: 40–70 mg/dl
- Cells: Up to 5 cells/mm^3 (all mononuclear cells).

TUMOR MARKERS (Table 16.1)

HEMATOLOGICAL INDICES

Hemoglobin concentration
- Males: 13–18 gm/dl
- Females: 12–16 gm/dl

Haematocrit (PCV)
- Males: 0.42–0.52 (42–52%)
- Females: 0.37–0.48 (37–48%)

RBC counts
- In males 4.8 × 106 cells/micro L
- In females 5.4 × 106 cells/micro L

Reticulocyte count : < 2%

Erythrocyte sedimentation rate (ESR)
- Males: 0–15 mm/hr
- Females: 0–20 mm/hr

Mean corpuscular hemoglobin (MCH): 28.33 PG/cell

Mean corpuscular hemoglobin concentration (MCHC): 32–36 gm/dl
Life span of RBC's -120 days
Total WBC count 4 to 11 ×10/mm3

Differential count
- Neutrophils: 40–75%

- Eosinophils: 0–7%
- Basophils: 0–2%
- Lymphocytes: 20–45%
- Monocytes: 4–10%

Platelet count: 1.3 lakh - 4 lakh/mm^3
Bleeding time (Ivy): 2–8 minutes
Prothrombin time: 10.5–14.5 seconds
Vitamin B$_{12}$ level: 170–1600 ng/L
Serum Folate: 3–16 ng/ml
Serum Iron: 50–150 micrograms/dl
Total Iron-binding capacity: 250–370 micrograms/dl
Ferritin: 150-400 ng/ml

CHEMICAL CONSTITUENTS OF BLOOD

- Albumin: 3.5–5.5 g/dl
- Alkaline phosphatase: 40–125 U/L
- Amylase: 60–180 U/L
- AST and ALT: 0–35 U/L
- Bicarbonate: 23–28 mmol/lit
- Total Bilirubin: 0.3–1.0 mg/dl
  – Direct: 0.1–0.3 mg/dl
  – Indirect: 0.2–0.7 mg/dl
- Calcium: 9–10.5 mg/dl
- Calcium ionized: 4.5–5.6 mg/dl
- Chloride: 98–106 mEq/L
- Copper: 70–140 micrograms/dl
- Magnesium: 1.8–3 mg/dl
- Osmolality: 282–295 mOsmol/kg
- Potassium: 3.5–5.0 mEq/L
- Sodium: 136–145 mEq/L
- Uric acid: 2.5–8 mg/dl
- Urea: 10–20 mg/dl
- Creatinine less than 1.5 mg/dl
- Cholesterol: Total cholesterol<200 mg/dl
  – LDL< 130 mg/dl
  – HDL>60 mg/dl
- Triglycerides<160 mg/dl
- Glucose
  – Fasting (plasma): 70–110 mg/dl (plasma)
  – Postprandial (2 hrs after food): 140mg/dl (plasma)
- Impaired glucose tolerance
  – Fasting:110–125 mg/dl
  – Postprandial: 140–199 mg/dl

Table 16.1 Tumor markers

Tumors	Markers
Breast carcinoma	CA 15-3
Colonic carcinoma	Carcinoembryonic antigen
Hepato cellular carcinoma	Alpha-feto protein
Medullary carcinoma of thyroid	Calcitonin
Ovarian malignancy	CA-125
Carcinoma prostate	Prostate specific antigen Acid phosphatase
Multiple myeloma	Bence-Jones protein
Testicular malignancy	HCG (Human chorionic gonadotrophin)
Chorio carcinoma	
Pancreatic carcinoma	CA 19-9

- Diabetes mellitus
  - Fasting sugar equal to or more than 126 mg/dl
  - Post prandial sugar: Equal to or more than 200 mg/dl

HORMONE LEVELS

Thyroid hormones
- TSH: 0.4–5 microunits/ml
- T_4: 5–12 microgram/dl
- T_3: 70–190 ng/dl

Adrenal hormones
- Cortisol 8 am: 5–25 micrograms/dl
- Cortisol 4 pm: 3–12 micrograms/dl

ACTH upto 20 mu/L

Parathyroid hormones: 0.4–0.9 ng/ml

Insulin: Fasting serum levels 6–26 micro units/ml

Growth hormone: Usually less than 2 mu/L (varies with stress).

Prolactin: 2–15 ng/ml

Gonadotrophins and Gonadal Steroids

Estradiol
- Men < 50 pg/ml
- Women 20–60 pg/ml (higher level at ovulation)

Testosterone
- Males: 3–10 ng/ml
- Females: < 1 ng/ml

Progesterone
- Males<2 ng/ml
- Females (Luteal phase): 2–20 ng/ml

FSH and LH levels (Table 16.2)

Table 16.2 FSH and LH levels		
	FSH	*LH*
Adult women	1.4–9.6 mIU/ml	0.8–26 mIU/ml
At ovulation	2.3–21 mIU/ml	25–27 mIU/ml
Post menopausal	34–96 mIU/ml	40–104 mIU/ml
Men	0.9–15 mIU/ml	1.3–13 mIU/ml

Index